Target Organ Toxicology Series

Endocrine Toxicology

Second Edition

Target Organ Toxicology Series

Target Organ Toxicology Series

Endocrine Toxicology

Second Edition

Editors

John A. Thomas, Ph.D.
Vice President for Academic Services
Professor of Pharmacology
Department of Academic Services
University of Texas
Health Science Center at San Antonio
San Antonio, Texas

Howard D. Colby, Ph.D.
Professor
Department of Pharmacology and Toxicology
Philadelphia College of Pharmacy and Science
Philadelphia, Pennsylvania

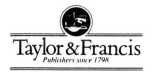

Taylor & Francis
Publishers since 1798

USA	Publishing Office	Taylor & Francis 1101 Vermont Avenue, N.W., Suite 200 Washington, DC 20005-2531 Tel: (202) 289-2174 Fax: (202) 289-3665
	Distribution Center	Taylor & Francis 1900 Frost Road, Suite 101 Bristol, PA 19007-1598 Tel: (215) 785-5800 Fax: (215) 785-5515
UK		Taylor & Francis Ltd. 1 Gunpowder Square London EC4A 3DE Tel: +44 171 583 0490 Fax: +44 171 583 0581

The material contained in this volume was submitted as previously unpublished material, except in the instances in which credit has been given to the source from which some of the illustrative material was derived.

Great care has been taken to maintain the accuracy of the information contained in the volume. However, neither Taylor & Francis Publishers nor the editors can be held responsible for errors or for any consequences arising from the use of the information contained herein.

Materials appearing in this book prepared by individuals as part of their official duties as U.S. Government employees are not covered by the below-mentioned copyright.

ENDOCTRINE TOXICOLOGY: Second Edition

1 2 3 4 5 6 7 8 9 0   B R B R   9 8 7

A CIP catalog record for this book is available from the British Library.

♾ The paper in this publication meets the requirements of the ANSI Standard Z39-48-1984 (Permanence of Paper).

Library of Contgress Cataloging-in-Publication Data

Endocrine toxicology / John A. Thomas & Howard D. Colby, editors.—
    2nd ed.
        p. cm. — (Target organ toxicology series)
        Includes bibliographical references and index.

    1. Endocrine toxicology.   I. Thomas, J. A. (John A.), 1933–
II. Colby, Howard D.   III. Series.
        [DNLM: 1. Endocrine Diseases—chemically induced.   2. Endocrine
Glands—drug effects.   WK 100 E527 1966]
RC649 E523 1996
616.4—dc20
DNLM/DLC
for Library of Congress   95-39059

ISBN 1-56032-613-1

Contents

Contributing Authors

Nasir Bashirelahi, Ph. D. *Professor of Biochemistry, Department of Oral and Craniofacial Biological Sciences, University of Maryland Dental School, 666 West Baltimore Street, Baltimore, Maryland 21201*

Wayne P. Bocchinfuso, BSc. Ph.D. *Postdoctoral Fellow, Laboratory of Reproductive and Developmental Toxicology, National Institute of Environmental Health Sciences, 111 Alexander Drive, Research Triangle Park, North Carolina 27709-2233*

Charles C. Capen, D.V.M., Ph.D. *Professor and Chairperson, Department of Veterinary Biosciences, Professor, Internal Medicine, College of Medicine, Ohio State University, 1925 Coffey Road, Columbus, Ohio 43210-1093*

Bandana Chatterjee, Ph.D. *Professor, Department of Cellular and Structural Biology, University of Texas Health Sciences Center at San Antonio, 7703 Floyd Curl Drive, San Antonio, Texas 78284-7762*

Howard D. Colby, Ph.D. *Professor, Department of Pharmacology and Toxicology, Philadelphia College of Pharmacy and Science, 600 South 43rd Street, Philadelphia, Pennsylvania 19104*

John M. Connors, Ph.D. *Associate Professor, Department of Physiology, West Virginia University Robert C. Byrd Health Sciences Center, Morgantown, West Virginia 26506-9229*

Timothy P. Coogan, Ph.D. *Senior Scientist, Drug Safety Evaluation, Robert Wood Johnson Pharmaceutical Research Institute, Welsh and McKean Roads, Spring House, Pennsylvania 19477*

Sylvia W. Curtis, M.A. *Biologist, Laboratory of Reproductive and Developmental Toxicology, National Institute of Environmental Health Sciences, 111 Alexander Drive, Research Triangle Park, North Carolina 27709-2233*

Vicki L. Davis, Ph.D. *Senior Staff Fellow, Environmental Toxicology Program, National Institute of Environmental Health Sciences, 111 Alexander Drive, Research Triangle Park, North Carolina 27709-2233*

Lawrence J. Fischer, Ph.D. *Professor, Institute for Environmental Toxicology, Michigan State University, C-231 Holden Hall, East Lansing, Michigan 48824*

Yajue Huang, Ph.D. *Professor, Department of Pharmacology and Toxicology, Philadelphia College of Pharmacy and Science, 600 South 43rd Street, Philadelphia, Pennsylvania 19104*

Quinshi Jiang, Ph.D. *Professor, Department of Pharmacology and Toxicology, Philadelphia College of Pharmacy and Science, 600 South 43rd Street, Philadelphia, Pennsylvania 19104*

Myeong H. Jung, Ph.D. *Instructor, Department of Cellular and Structural Biology, University of Texas Health Sciences Center at San Antonio, 7703 Floyd Curl Drive, San Antonio, Texas 78284-7762*

B. Koffman, Ph.D. *Professor, Department of Biochemistry, University of Maryland Dental School, 666 West Baltimore Street, Baltimore, Maryland 21201*

Kenneth S. Korach, Ph.D. *Chief, Receptor Biology Section, Laboratory of Reproductive and Developmental Toxicology, National Institute of Environmental Health Sciences, 111 Alexander Drive, Research Triangle Park, North Carolina 27709-2233*

Sabine Rehm, D.V.M. *Veterinary Pathologist, Department of Toxicology, Smithkline Beecham Pharmaceuticals, 709 Swedeland Road, King of Prussia, Pennsylvania 19406*

Arun K. Roy, Ph.D. *Professor, Department of Cellular and Structural Biology, University of Texas Health Sciences Center at San Antonio, 7703 Floyd Curl Drive, San Antonio, Texas 78284-7762*

Zsuzsa Sandor, M.D. *Research Fellow, Department of Pathology and Laboratory Medical Services, University of California at Irvine, Veterans Affairs Medical Center, 5901 East 7th Street, Long Beach, California 90822*

Lowell E. Sever, Ph.D. *Program Manager, Battelle Seattle Research Center, 4000 North East 41st Street, Seattle, Washington 98105*

James T. Stevens, Ph.D. *Head of Short-Term/Long-Term Toxicology, Department of Toxicology, Ciba Crop Protection Division, Ciba-Geigy Limited, Werk Stein, WST-452.1.08, CH-4332 Stein, Switzerland*

Robert J. Sydiskis, Ph.D. *Associate Professor, Department of Oral and Craniofacial Biological Sciences, University of Maryland at Baltimore, 666 West Baltimore Street, Baltimore, Maryland 21201*

Sandor Szabo, M.D., Ph.D. *Professor of Pathology and Pharmacology, University of California, Irvine, and Chief, Pathology and Laboratory Medical Services, Veterans Affairs Medical Center, 5901 East 7th Street, Long Beach, California 90822*

John A. Thomas, Ph.D. *Vice President for Academic Services and Professor of Pharmacology, Department of Academic Services, University of Texas Health Sciences Center, San Antonio, Texas 78284-7722*

Robert L. Vellanoweth, Ph.D. *Assistant Professor, Department of Chemistry and Biochemistry, California State University at Los Angeles, 5151 State University Drive, Los Angeles, California 90032*

Jeffrey M. Voight, Ph.D. *Associate Professor, Department of Pharmacology and Toxicology, Philadelphia College of Pharmacy and Science, 600 South 43rd Street, Philadelphia, Pennsylvania 19104*

Michael P. Waalkes, Ph.D. *Chief, Inorganic Carcinogenesis Section, National Cancer Institute, Frederick, Maryland 21702-1201*

Jerrold M. Ward, D.V.M., Ph.D. *Chief, Veterinary and Tumor Pathology Section, Office of Laboratory Animal Sciences, National Cancer Institute, Frederick, Maryland 21702-1201*

Preface

The *Target Organ Toxicology Series* contains a range of topics from the molecular events surrounding hormone action(s) to the epidemiologic studies involving the effects of environmental and occupational chemicals on reproductive organs. Endocrine systems perturbed by chemicals include the adrenal cortex, the thyroid and parathyroid, the gonads and the endocrine pancreas. A number of chapters describe the general characteristics of the steriod receptor as well as specific molecular and genetic characteristics of the estrogen receptor(s) and the androgen receptor(s). Chemicals and drugs that mimic hormonal action upon female or male sex steroid biochemical events can provoke changes in the reproductive systems. Likewise, chemical-induced changes in thyroid biosynthesis and interruption of calcium metabolism can disturb hormonal function. This monograph describes some of the underlying toxic mechanisms involving pancreatic ß cells and metal-induced changes in male sex assessory glands. Chemicals can not only suppress cellular activity of endocrine cells, but under certain hormonal conditions produce cellular hyperplasia.

John A. Thomas
Howard D. Colby

Introduction

The second edition of *Endocrine Toxicology* might be considered complimentary to the first edition. A decade has elapsed since one of the target organ toxicity symposia pertaining to endocrine toxicology was held at West Virginia University Medical Center. Some of the topics covered in the earlier symposium are again revisited and updated.

Ten years ago, the terms *endocrine disruptors, xenoestrogens,* or *environmental estrogens* had not been coined, yet the student of endocrinology understood their implications. Perhaps the most rapid advances that have generally occurred in the field of endocrine toxicology have been in the elucidation of the molecular characteristics of the steroid receptor(s).

It has been interesting to reflect on what has occurred the past ten years based on the 1985 reviews of the first edition of *Endocrine Toxicology*. Such reviews provide not only a historical reference point but also reveal some of the advances that have occurred in the field of chemical perturbation of the endocrine system. The first edition is "devoted to fairly specific toxic agents (cadmium, lead and chlordecone)" (cited in *Adverse Drug Reactions*, 1985). The *Quarterly Review of Biology*, 1985 stated, ". . . An excellent series dealing with the effects of chemicals on peripheral target organs and on their controlling the endocrine organs . . . this first edition is strongly recommended, and it is hoped that the series will grow from strength to strength." From a review in the *Lancet* (1985), "over 80% of this book is devoted to the effects of xenobiotics on the reproductive system." "It succeeds as a study of pathophysiological mechanisms; it does not seek to catalogue toxic agents . . . ." From *Veterinary & Human Toxicology* (1985), the first edition "will serve as a reinforcement to investigators in a variety of fields (such as physiology, biochemistry, pharmacology and toxicology) who seek to understand the delicate relationship between hormones and the chemical environment in which the endocrine system must function." In a review in *Toxicology* (1985), it was stated that the first edition "will prove indispensable for all those interested in reproductive toxicology." Finally, the *Journal of Toxicology & Environmental Health's* (1985) review of *Endocrine Toxicology* described its contents as "oriented towards the cellular/biochemical level . . . with a generous amount of (reasonable) speculation on mechanisms."

This interesting composite of these 10-year-old reviews in prestigious journals reinforces the importance of endocrine toxicology and seeks to better understand how chemicals and drugs can affect hormonal events. The second edition will prove as valuable as the first edition of *Endocrine Toxicology*.

John A. Thomas
Howard D. Colby

Endocrine Toxicology, 2nd ed.,
Edited by J. A. Thomas and H. D. Colby
Copyright © 1997 Taylor & Francis

1

Chemically-Induced Injury of the Parathyroid Gland: Pathophysiology and Mechanistic Considerations

Charles C. Capen

Department of Veterinary Biosciences, The Ohio State University, Columbus, Ohio 43210-1093

NORMAL DEVELOPMENT, STRUCTURE, AND FUNCTION OF PARATHYROID GLAND

Functional Cytology

Parathyroid glands are composed of a single cell type concerned with the biosynthesis of one hormone (Fig. 1). Chief cells have a normal secretory cycle, with the majority being in the inactive stage under steady-state conditions. In response to a low calcium ion signal, chief cells enter the active phase with synthesis and packaging of a "batch" of hormone. After secretion of parathyroid hormone (PTH), the chief cell involutes back to the resting (inactive) phase. In response to long-term stimulation, chief cells undergo a sequence of morphologic changes culminating in the formation of water-clear cells. Conversely, long-term suppression by elevated blood calcium ion results in parathyroids with predominantly inactive and atrophic chief cells. Mitochondrion-rich oxyphil cells form in parathyroids of humans and certain animal species with advancing age. Synthetic and secretory organelles are largely crowded out by the proliferation of mitochondria in the cytoplasm, suggesting that oxyphil cells are not actively involved in the biosynthesis of PTH.

Chief cells that are interpreted to be inactive (resting or involuted) predominate in the parathyroid glands under normal conditions. Inactive chief cells are cuboidal and have uncomplicated interdigitations between contiguous cells (24). The relatively electron-transparent cytoplasm contains poorly developed organelles and infrequent secretory granules. The cytoplasm often has either numerous lipid bodies and lipofuscin granules or aggregations of glycogen particles. Chief cells in the active stage occur less frequently in the parathyroid glands of most species. The cytoplasm of active chief cells has an increased electron density due to the

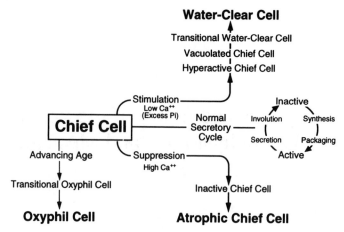

FIG 1. Functional cytology of parathyroid gland under normal and pathologic conditions.

close proximity of organelles and secretory granules, increased density of the cytoplasmic matrix, and loss of glycogen particles and lipid bodies.

The second cell type in the parathyroid glands of certain animal species and human beings is the oxyphil cell (Fig. 1). They are absent in parathyroids of the rat, chicken, and many species of lower animals. Oxyphil cells are observed either singly or in small groups interspersed between chief cells. They are larger than chief cells, and their abundant cytoplasmic area is filled with numerous large, often bizarre-shaped mitochondria. Glycogen particles and free ribosomes are interspersed between the mitochondria. Granular endoplasmic reticulum, Golgi apparatuses, and secretory granules are poorly developed in oxyphil cells of normal parathyroid glands, suggesting that oxyphil cells do not have an active function in the biosynthesis of PTH. Oxyphil cells have been shown histochemically to have a higher oxidative and hydrolytic enzyme activity than chief cells, associated with the marked increase in mitochondria.

Cells are observed with cytoplasmic characteristics intermediate between those of chief and oxyphil cells. These transitional oxyphil cells have numerous mitochondria, but other organelles are present, including rough endoplasmic reticulum, Golgi apparatuses, and secretory granules. The significance of oxyphil cells in the pathophysiology of parathyroid glands has not been elucidated completely. They are not altered in response to short-term hypocalcemia or hypercalcemia in animals, but both oxyphil cells and transitional forms may be increased in response to long-term stimulation of human parathyroid glands. Therefore, oxyphil cells do not appear to be degenerate chief cells, as had previously been suggested, but rather are derived from chief cells as the result of aging or some other metabolic derangement.

Biosynthesis of Parathyroid Hormone by Chief Cells

Parathyroid chief cells in humans and many animal species store relatively small amounts of preformed hormone; instead they respond quickly to variations in need for hormone by changing the rate of synthesis. Like many peptide hormones, PTH is first synthesized as a larger biosynthetic precursor molecule that undergoes post-translational processing in chief cells. Pre-proparathyroid hormone (pre-proPTH) is the initial translation product synthesized on ribosomes of the rough endoplasmic reticulum in chief cells. It is composed of 115 amino acids and contains a hydrophobic signal or leader sequence of 25 amino acid residues that facilitates the penetration and subsequent vectorial discharge of the nascent peptide into the cisternal space of the rough endoplasmic reticulum (80). Pre-proPTH is rapidly converted (within 1 minute or less of its synthesis) to proparathyroid hormone (proPTH) by the proteolytic cleavage of 25 amino acids from the NH_2-terminal end of the molecule (57). The intermediate precursor, proPTH, is composed of 90 amino acids and moves within membranous channels of the rough endoplasmic reticulum to the Golgi apparatus (Fig. 2). Enzymes

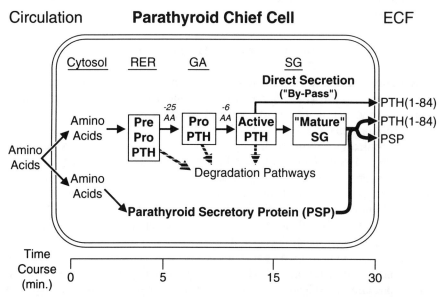

FIG 2. Biosynthesis of parathyroid hormone (PTH) and parathyroid secretory protein-I (PSP) chromogranin A PSP-I by chief cells. Preproparathyroid hormone (preproPTH) is the initial translation product from ribosomes of the rough endoplasmic reticulum, which is rapidly converted to proparathyroid hormone (ProPTH). Active PTH either is stored in the cytosol as mature secretory granules (SG) or may be secreted directly from chief cells ("By-pass"). Chief cells also synthesize another protein designated parathyroid secretory protein-I (PSP) which is incorporated into secretory granules along with active PTH. PSP is released in parallel with PTH by a low calcium ion concentration in extracellular fluids.

within membranes of the Golgi apparatus cleave a hexapeptide from the NH_2-terminal (biologically active) end of the molecule forming active PTH. Active PTH is packaged into membrane-limited, macromolecular aggregates in the Golgi apparatus for subsequent storage in chief cells. Under certain conditions of increased demand (ie, low calcium ion concentration in extracellular fluid compartment), PTH may be released directly from chief cells without being packaged into secretion granules by a process termed "bypass secretion."

Although the principal form of active PTH secreted from chief cells is a straight chain peptide of 84 amino acids (molecular weight 9500 d), the molecule is rapidly cleaved into amino- (N-) and carboxy- (C-) terminal fragments in the peripheral circulation and especially in the liver. The purpose of this fragmentation is uncertain since the biologically active N-terminal fragment is no more active than the entire PTH(1–84) molecule. The plasma half-life of the N-terminal fragment is considerably shorter than that of the biologically inactive C-terminal fragment of PTH. The C-terminal and other portions of the PTH molecule are degraded primarily in the kidney and tend to accumulate with chronic renal disease. The immunoheterogeneity caused by the multiple circulating fragments of PTH created significant problems in the development and application of highly specific radioimmunoassays to diagnostic problems in human patients and experimental animals (54).

Control of Parathyroid Hormone Secretion

Secretory cells in the parathyroid gland store small amounts of preformed hormone but are capable of responding to minor fluctuations in calcium concentration by rapidly altering the rate of hormonal secretion and more slowly by altering the rate of hormonal synthesis (135). In contrast to most endocrine organs under complex controls involving both long and short feedback loops, the parathyroids have a unique feedback controlled by the concentration of calcium (and to a lesser extent magnesium) ion in serum. If the blood calcium is elevated by the intravenous infusion of calcium, there is a rapid and pronounced reduction in circulating levels of immunoreactive parathyroid hormone (iPTH). Conversely, if the blood calcium is lowered by ethylenediaminetetraacetic acid (EDTA), there is a brisk and substantial increase in iPTH levels.

The concentration of blood phosphorus has no direct regulatory influence on the synthesis and secretion of PTH; however, several disease conditions with hyperphosphatemia in both animals and man are associated clinically with secondary hyperparathyroidism. An elevated blood phosphorus level may lead indirectly to parathyroid stimulation by virtue of its ability to lower blood calcium. If the blood phosphorus is significantly elevated by an infusion of phosphate and calcium administered simultaneously in amounts to prevent the accompanying reduction of blood calcium, plasma iPTH levels remain within the normal range. Magnesium ion has an effect on parathyroid secretion rate similar to that of calcium, but its effect is not equipotent to that of calcium (98).

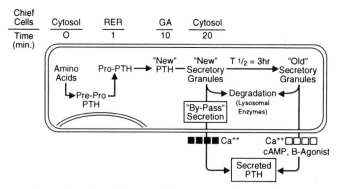

FIG 3. Bypass secretion of parathyroid hormone in response to increased demand signaled by decreased blood calcium ion concentration. Recently synthesized and processed active PTH (1–84) may be released directly and not enter the storage pool of mature ("old") secretory granules in the cytoplasm of chief cells. PTH from the storage pool can be mobilized by cyclic adenosine monophosphate (cAMP) and ß (B)–agonists (such as epinephrine, norepinephrine, and isoproterenol) as well as by lowered blood calcium ion, whereas secretion from the pool of recently synthesized PTH can be stimulated only by a decreased calcium ion concentration. RER, rough endoplasmic reticulum; GA, Golgi apparatus; Redrawn from Cohn and MacGregor, *Endocrine Review* 2:1–20, 1981.

Calcium ion controls the rate not only of biosynthesis and secretion of PTH but also of other metabolic and intracellular degradative processes within chief cells. An increase of calcium ions in extracellular fluids rapidly inhibits the uptake of amino acids by chief cells, synthesis of proPTH and conversion to PTH, and secretion of stored PTH. A shift in the percentage of flow of proPTH from the degradative pathway to the secretory route represents a key adaptive response of the parathyroid gland to a low calcium diet. During periods of long-term calcium restriction, the enhanced synthesis and secretion of PTH would be accomplished by an increased capacity of the entire pathway in individual hypertrophied chief cells and through hyperplasia of active chief cells.

In response to increased demand, recently synthesized and processed active PTH may be released directly after passing through the Golgi complex, most likely in small vesicles. It thus bypasses the storage pool of mature secretory granules in the cytoplasm of chief cells. Bypass secretion of PTH can be stimulated only by a low circulating concentration of calcium ion, whereas β-agonists, as well as low calcium, can mobilize PTH stored in secretory granules (Fig. 3).

Parathyroid chief cells have several adaptive responses to hypocalcemia, which otherwise would be life-threatening. The first is bypass secretion of PTH in response to a low calcium ion signal. The second is to increase the efficiency of conversion of inactive proPTH into active PTH and its subsequent release from chief cells. This process under normal conditions is quite inefficient and therefore provides a point of regulation in response to increased demand for hormone. Longer-term adaptive responses to hypocalcemia are the result of hypertrophy and hyperplasia of parathyroid chief cells.

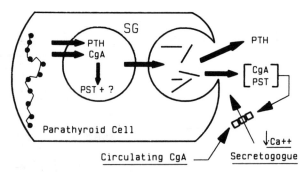

FIG 4. Autocrine/paracrine action of chromogranin A (CgA)–derived peptides. PTH and CgA are co-released from chief cells in response to a low calcium ion signal. Pancreastatin (PST) is a 49 amino acid peptide derived from CgA that exerts local negative feedback on chief cells and decreases PTH secretion from chief cells. From Cohn *et al.*, 1993.

Chief cells synthesize and secrete another major protein, parathyroid secretory protein (I) (PSP) or chromogranin A. This protein has a higher molecular weight (70 kD) than PTH and is composed of 430–448 amino acids; it is stored and secreted with PTH. A similar molecule has been found in secretory granules of a wide variety of peptide hormone–secreting cells and in neurotransmitter secretory vesicles. An internal region of the PSP or chromogranin A molecule is identical in sequence to pancreastatin, a C-terminal amidated peptide that inhibits glucose-stimulated insulin secretion. This 49-amino-acid, proteolytic cleavage product (amino acids number 240–280) of PSP has recently been reported to inhibit low calcium–stimulated secretion of PTH and chromogranin A from parathyroid cells. These findings suggest that chromogranin A–derived peptides may act locally in an autocrine manner to inhibit the secretion of active hormone by endocrine cells, such as those of the parathyroid gland (11,34,50) (Fig. 4).

Biologic Actions of Parathyroid Hormone

PTH is the principal hormone involved in the minute-to-minute fine regulation of blood calcium in mammals. It exerts its biologic actions directly by influencing the function of target cells primarily in bone and kidney and indirectly in the intestine by maintaining plasma calcium at a level sufficient to ensure the optimal functioning of a wide variety of body cells. The action of PTH on bone is to mobilize calcium from skeletal reserves into extracellular fluids (120). The increase in blood calcium results from an interaction of PTH with osteoblasts and osteoclasts in bone and from increased tubular reabsorption of calcium in the kidney (66,145).

Target Cells in Bone

Osteoclasts appear to be primarily responsible for the catabolic action of PTH on bone by increasing bone resorption (30,31,121,161). PTH has been known for some

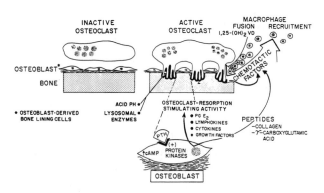

FIG 5. Paracrine control of bone resorption. Specific receptors for parathyroid hormone are present on osteoblasts but not osteoclasts.

time to stimulate an increased activity of preformed osteoclasts. This is interesting in light of recent findings that have failed to demonstrate specific receptors for PTH on osteoclasts, although receptors were present on osteoblasts (117,139). Isolated osteoclasts do not respond to PTH without the concurrent presence of osteoblasts (99).

The mechanisms by which binding of PTH to osteoblasts results in stimulation of osteoblastic secretory products capable of stimulating osteoclastic bone resorption are not known. However, they may include direct effects on the osteoblast and stimulation of osteoclastic secretory products capable of stimulating osteoblastic bone resorption (Fig. 5) (154). If the increase in PTH is sustained, the size of the active osteoclast pool in bone is increased by activation of osteoprogenitor cells in the endosteal bone-cell envelope.

The initial binding of PTH to osteoblasts lining bone surfaces appears to cause the cells to contract, thereby exposing the underlying mineral to osteoclasts (125) (Fig. 5). The change in shape of osteoblasts associated with PTH may be critical to mediation of osteoclastic bone resorption stimulated by the hormone. Osteoblastic contraction is associated with microfilament disaggregation (161). The alteration in osteoblast shape exposes osteoid-covered bone matrix to osteoclasts; however, osteoclasts attach preferentially to mineralized bone matrix.

Osteoblasts also may elaborate unidentified paracrine chemical mediators of osteoclastic bone resorption. None of the known bone-resorbing factors (eg, PTH, prostaglandin E_2 [PGE_2], lymphokines, growth factors) have been shown to stimulate osteoclasts directly, without the presence of osteoblasts (40). The only substance that was found to stimulate bone resorption by isolated chicken osteoclasts in one investigation was murine splenic-conditioned medium (40). Bone resorption by isolated osteoclasts is inhibited by calcitonin and PGE_2, which induce cyclic adenosine monophosphate (cAMP) production in osteoclasts.

PTH stimulation of osteoblasts results in induction of bone resorption due to osteoclast activation and increased osteoclast numbers. The plasma membrane of osteoclasts in intimate contact with the resorbing surfaces is modified to form a series of membranous projections ("brush" or "ruffled" border). The brush border of activated osteoclasts is isolated from the extracellular fluids by adjacent transitional ("sealing") zones, thereby localizing the lysosomal enzymes and acidic environment to the immediate area undergoing dissolution. PTH and other bone-resorbing agents increase proteolytic, lysosomal, and acid-producing enzymes in osteoclasts, including acid phosphatase, β-glucuronidase, and carbonic anhydrase (161). Carbonic anhydrase is localized to the brush border and induces acidification of the brush border area.

Binding of PTH to specific receptors on bone cells results in the activation of adenylate cyclase in the plasma membrane (Fig. 5). Adenylate cyclase catalyzes the conversion of adenosine triphosphate (ATP) to cAMP in target cells. The accumulation of cAMP in target cells functions as an intracellular messenger of PTH action in osteoblasts. PTH also induces an increase in cytoplasmic calcium and stimulates phosphatidyl inositol turnover in osteoblasts (Fig. 5); however, it has not been determined which intracellular messenger is required for induction of bone resorption by PTH stimulation of osteoblasts (44,49,65). The increase in cytosolic calcium is partially dependent on cAMP accumulation. Calcium concentration in the osteoblast may also be increased by the activation of protein kinase C, resulting in the production of inositol triphosphate and subsequent release of calcium from the endoplasmic reticulum (164).

Target Cells in Kidney

PTH has a rapid (within 5–10 minutes) and direct effect on renal tubular function leading to decreased reabsorption of phosphate and phosphaturia (78). The site of PTH on blocking tubular reabsorption of phosphate has been localized by micropuncture methods to the proximal tubule of the nephron. Parathyroidectomy decreases renal phosphate excretion. PTH binds to a receptor on the basolateral aspect of renal epithelial cells. The hormone stimulates adenylate cyclase, increasing intracellular cAMP and thereby activating protein kinases that phosphorylate proteins that make the luminal membrane less permeable to phosphorus. PTH also increases the transport of calcium across the basolateral renal cell membrane and increases intracellular calcium, which inhibits the formation of cAMP, thus decreasing the phosphaturic effects of PTH (12,78). PTH is capable of stimulating inositol triphosphate and diacylglycerol production in renal tubular cells (67) (Fig. 6). Therefore, regulation of phosphate transport by PTH may be mediated by two transmembrane-signaling systems, one that activates adenylate cyclase and another that activates protein kinase C and increases intracellular calcium (35).

Although the effects of PTH on the tubular reabsorption of phosphate have been considered to be of major importance, evidence has accumulated indicating

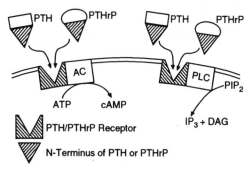

FIG 6. Parathyroid hormone (PTH) and parathyroid hormone-related protein (PTHrP) have a high degree of homology in the primary or tertiary structures of the N-terminal regions. This permits binding and activation of PTH receptors resulting in the stimulation of adenylate cyclase (AC) and phospholipase C (PLC) in target cells in bone and kidney with the formation of cAMP and conversion of phosphatidylinositol diphosphate (PIP_2) to inositol triphosphate (IP_3) and diacylglycerol (DAG). (reprinted by permission from Rosol, T.J., and Capen, C.C. Mechanism of cancer-induced hypercalcemia. *Lab. Invest.* 67:680–702, 1992).

that the ability of PTH to enhance the reabsorption of calcium plays a considerable role in the maintenance of calcium homeostasis. This effect of PTH on tubular reabsorption of calcium appears to be due to a direct action on the distal convoluted tubule (145). The biochemical mechanism by which PTH enhances calcium reabsorption is unknown, but it is coupled to increases in intracellular cAMP (58). There are two calcium-active transport systems in the basolateral membrane of renal cells, a high-affinity calcium adenosine triphosphatase (ATP-ase) and a Na^+/Ca^{++} exchanger.

The other important effect of PTH on the kidney involves the regulation of the conversion of 25-hydroxycholecalciferol to 1,25-dihydroxycholecalciferol and other metabolites of vitamin D. PTH has been shown to promote the absorption of calcium from the gastrointestinal tract in animals under a variety of experimental conditions (112). This effect is not as rapid as the action on the kidney and is not observed in vitamin D–deficient animals. The increase in intestinal calcium transport appears to be an indirect effect of PTH on absorptive cells, namely by acting on mitochondria in renal tubular epithelial cells to stimulate synthesis of the biologically active metabolite of vitamin D (40). The effects of PTH on the metabolism of 25-hydroxycholecalciferol appear to be mediated by cAMP and not dependent on calcium ion concentration (64). The active metabolites of vitamin D make bone cells more sensitive to the direct effects of PTH ("permissive effect"), as well as greatly enhancing the gastrointestinal absorption of calcium and thereby amplifying the effect of PTH on plasma calcium concentration.

In addition, vitamin D metabolites exert negative feedback control on parathyroid chief cells at the level of transcription to decrease mRNA for pre-proPTH (Fig. 7). As blood levels of 1,25-dihydroxycholecalciferol are increased and PTH acts to increase intestinal calcium absorption, the animal requires less PTH synthesis and release from the parathyroid gland to maintain calcium homeostasis.

The kidney is also a major organ for the degradation of PTH. Biologically active PTH from the peritubular capillaries is degraded by specific proteases on the surface of renal tubular cells. In addition, both biologically active (NH_2—1–34)

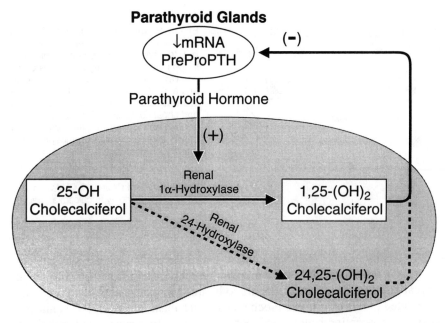

FIG 7. Circulating levels of 1,25-dihydroxycholecalciferol exert negative feedback control on parathyroid chief cells at the level of transcription to decrease mRNA for preproPTH and the syntheses of parathyroid hormone. Conversely, parathyroid hormone is one major controlling factor for the renal α–hydroxylase that synthesizes 1,25-(OH)$_2$-cholecalciferol from 25-OH-cholecalcif-

and inactive (34–84 COOH) fragments are degraded intracellularly by lysosomal enzymes within renal tubular cells (67).

The PTH receptor has recently been cloned and sequenced from cDNA isolated from kidney cells (74). It belongs to a class of receptors that has seven transmembrane domains and is linked to a specific G protein in the target cells. The expressed receptor binds PTH and PTH-related protein (PTHrP) with equal affinity, resulting in the activation of adenylate cyclase and phospholipase C (see Fig. 6). The PTH–PTHrP receptor has a striking degree of sequence homology (approximately 56%) with the calcitonin receptor but lacks similarity with other G protein–linked receptors other than secretin (88). The receptors for these calcium-regulating hormones appear to belong to a new family of G protein–linked receptors with seven transmembrane-spanning domains that activate adenylate cyclase and phospholipase C (Fig. 8).

AGE-RELATED CHANGES IN PARATHYROID STRUCTURE AND FUNCTION

Serum immunoreactive PTH (iPTH) (as well as immunoreactive calcitonin [iCT]) has been reported to be different in young compared with aged Fischer 344 (F344) rats; however, the serum calcium concentration does not change with

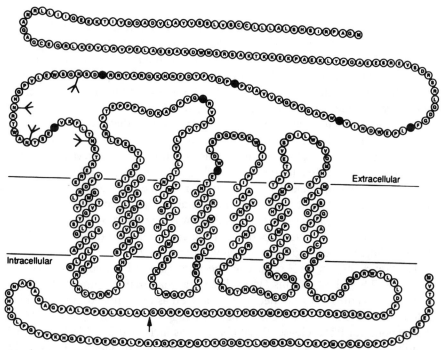

FIG 8. PTH-PTHrP receptor (NH$_2$ terminus at top) cloned and sequenced from cDNA isolated from kidney cells. (Y) Potential N-glycosylation sites; (•) Cysteine residues conserved in the calcitonin receptor. From Jüppner, H., Abou-Samra, A.B., Freeham, M., *et al*. A G protein-linked receptor for parathyroid hormone and parathyroid hormone-related peptide. *Science 254*: 1024–1026, 1991.

age (162). This suggests that the regulation of iPTH (and iCT) secretion may be affected by the process of aging. Parathyroid glands from F344 rats of different ages (young, 2–3 months; adult, 12–13 months; and old, 24–27 months) have been removed and incubated in vitro with media containing either low (1.0 mM) or high (2.5 mM) calcium for 3 hours. iPTH secretion per pair of glands was significantly higher in older rats regardless of the medium concentration of calcium. The decrease in iPTH secretion in response to high (2.5 mM) calcium was smaller in old rats compared with the response of glands from young rats.

The decreased responsiveness of chief cells to calcium may be due to age-related changes in the regulation of the secretory pathway. This could include age-related changes in the effect of calcium on release of stored PTH, intracellular degradation of PTH, or modification of adenylate cyclase activity as observed in other tissues that utilize calcium as an intermediary signal (17). Therefore, the sensitivity of parathyroid chief cells to calcium appears not to be fixed, but rather may change during development and aging and in response to certain disease processes.

The increased secretion of iPTH with advancing age in rats could be due to several factors, including (1) an increased number of parathyroid secretory cells with age and (2) an altered regulation of chief cells in response to calcium ion associated with the process of aging (162). For example, a decreased sensitivity of chief cells to negative feedback by calcium ion could result in the higher blood levels of iPTH noted in aged F344 rats. Wada *et al.* (155) reported that the early age-related rise in plasma PTH in F344 rats was a consequence of neither low plasma calcium nor renal insufficiency. Age-related changes in the responsiveness of chief cells to circulating levels of other factors that modulate iPTH secretion, particularly 1,25-dihydroxycholecalciferol and α- and β-adrenergic catecholamines, also could contribute to the variations in blood levels of iPTH in rats of different ages. In addition, target cell responsiveness to PTH also decreases with advancing age in rats. PTH does not increase the renal production of 1,25-dihydroxyvitamin D in adult (13-month-old) male F344 rats compared with young (2-month-old) rats, in which its production was increased 61% (4). Older rats have a decreased calcemic response and decreased renal production of 1,25-dihydroxycholecalciferol compared with young rats (4,75).

The "set point" for PTH release has been investigated in male F344 rats at 3, 6, 12, 18, 24, and 28 months (153). The basal maximally stimulated and suppressed levels of iPTH were determined, as well as the concentration of ionized calcium sufficient to produce half-maximal suppression of the plasma iPTH— the set point for PTH release. Basal iPTH levels increased 2.3-fold from 3 to 28 months of age, whereas basal blood ionized calcium remained unchanged. The set point for PTH release increased steadily from 1.19 ± 0.09 mM at 3 months to 1.37 ± 0.13 mM at 24 months; basal serum iPTH levels correlated significantly with the set point. Neither maximally stimulated nor suppressed iPTH levels had any significant change with advancing age. These results suggest that the age-related increase in basal iPTH in the rat was related in part to the increased set point for PTH release from parathyroid chief cells (153).

Studies in male Sprague–Dawley rats revealed that basal iPTH (NH_2-terminal assay) was 68% higher in aged (24–26-month-old) compared with adult (6-month-old) rats. The initial (5–10 minutes) secretory response to acute constant hypocalcemic stimulus (0.32 mM decrease in ionized Ca^{++} for 2 hours by ethylenediaminetetraacetic acid [EDTA]) was reduced in aged compared with adult rats (1.9-fold decrease vs. 3.1-fold increase), suggesting reduced PTH stores. However, higher sustained iPTH levels (30 minutes to 2 hours) were maintained in aged rats, indicating increased synthesis and secretion. The EDTA infusion rate necessary to maintain a constant hypocalcemia was lower in aged rats, suggesting a possible skeletal resistance to PTH. Slow EDTA and calcium infusions were used to determine iPTH secretion at plasma CA^{++} levels from 0.7 to 1.5 mM. In aged rats, iPTH levels were higher at all Ca^{++} concentrations, but the set point for iPTH release by Ca^{++} was the same as in adult rats. Therefore, the elevated iPTH secretion in aged Sprague–Dawley rats was not caused by a change in the set point for iPTH release; however, it did result in decreased PTH stores in the gland (51).

Lee *et al.* (86) reported an increase in urinary phosphorus excretion in old (28–29-month-old) F344 rats compared with younger (12–15-month-old) adult rats fed equal amounts of dietary phosphorus. The increase in renal phosphorus excretion in old F344 rats was PTH-independent because the phosphaturia was not reversed by thyroparathyroidectomy and the renal cortical generation of cAMP in response to PTH was not different between the two age groups of rats. However, in response to PTH there was a clear decrease in phosphorus uptake by renal brush border membrane vesicles prepared from old (28–29-month-old) rats compared with those from younger (12–15-month-old) rats. Alkaline phosphatase activity in the renal cortical vesicles was not different between the two age groups of rats.

Kiebzak and Sacktor (77) demonstrated a significant age-related phosphaturia (ie, elevated urinary phosphorus excretion and fractional excretion) in Wistar-derived male rats fed a normal (0.5%) phosphorus diet. Studies compared young, rapidly growing (2–3 month-old), young adult (6-month-old), and mature adult (12-month-old) rats, as well as those approaching senescence (18-month-old) and the senescent (24-month-old). Plasma phosphorus decreased significantly and progressively with advancing age. There was an age-related decrease in the transport of phosphorus by renal brush border membrane vesicles, but the Na^+ gradient–dependent uptake of glucose and proline was unaffected, demonstrating the specificity of the phosphorus transport decrement. An elevation in serum PTH did not appear to be related to the renal phosphorus conservation since urinary cAMP was not elevated in the intact senescent rat and phosphorus excretion was not normalized in the senescent rats 3 days after parathyroidectomy. Both the senescent and young adult Wistar rats adapted to a low (0.1%) phosphorus diet by a marked (>100%) increase in phosphorus intake by renal brush border membrane vesicles compared with those prepared from rats fed a normal phosphorus diet. Therefore, the kidney of senescent Wistar rats retained the ability to respond appropriately to a low intake of dietary phosphorus.

DEVELOPMENTAL DISTURBANCES

Parathyroid Cyst

Embryologically, the parathyroid glands are of entodermal origin, derived from the pharyngeal pouches in close association with the primordium of the thymus (Fig. 9). Mice and rats have a single pair of parathyroids (37). Parathyroid (Kürsteiner's) cysts develop from persistence and dilatation of remnants of the duct that connects the parathyroid (anterior portion) and thymic (caudal portion) primordia during embryonic development. The cyst fluid has been reported to contain higher levels of iPTH (1–84 intact molecule and 39–84 COOH fragments) than serum (10). The lining cells stain for PTH by immunohistochemistry. Similar cysts may be present in the anterior mediastinum when remnants of the embryonic duct are displaced with the caudal migration of the thymus.

Small cysts are occasionally observed in mice within the parenchyma of the parathyroids or in their immediate vicinity. Parathyroid cysts usually are lined by

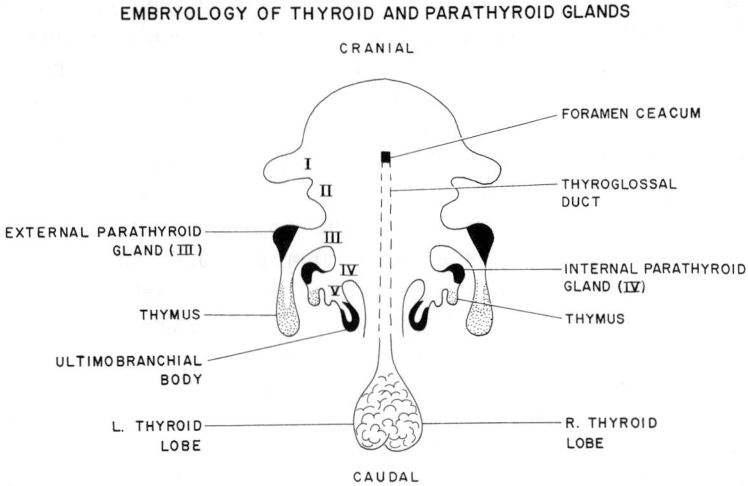

EMBRYOLOGY OF THYROID AND PARATHYROID GLANDS

FIG 9. Embryology of parathyroid glands and relationship to primordia of thyroid gland and ultimobranchial body.

a cuboidal-to-columnar (often partially ciliated) epithelium and contain a densely eosinophilic proteinic material. The cyst contents may be uniformly dense or contain crystalloid or spherical structures. The lining epithelial cells have an electron-dense cytoplasm and numerous microvilli projecting into the lumen of the cyst; their synthetic and secretory organelles are poorly developed.

Parathyroid cysts are distinct from midline cysts, which are derived from remnants of the thyroglossal duct. The latter are lined by multilayered thyroidogenic epithelium that often has colloid-containing follicles. They are usually located near the midline from the base of the tongue caudally into the mediastinum.

Ectopic Thymic Tissue in Parathyroid Gland

A frequently encountered change in the mouse parathyroid gland is ectopic (aberrant) thymic tissue incorporated into the gland or present in the immediate vicinity. Smith and Clifford (140) reported a 21% or greater incidence of ectopic thymus in parathyroids of fetal, young, and adult mice. Pour *et al.* (118) reported finding thymic tissue in the parathyroid regularly in BALB/c mice and with a 1% frequency in OFI mice. The ectopic thymic tissue varied considerably in size but often exerted pressure on the adjacent parathyroid gland. A fine fibrous connective tissue capsule often partially surrounded the ectopic thymic tissue and separated it from the adjacent parathyroid gland. Since the parathyroid and thymus arise embryologically from similar pharyngeal pouch primordia, it is not surprising that an admixture of these two tissues may occur due to incomplete division.

Ectopic Parathyroid Tissue in Thymus

Parathyroid tissue ectopically situated in the thymus is occasionally detected microscopically in the mouse. Most often a small aggregation of normal-appearing chief cells is located peripherally in the thymus in the surface connective tissue or septa extending into the thymus (52). Small capillary branches penetrate the thin surrounding layer of connective tissue and extend between the cords of chief cells. The infrequent finding of parathyroid tissue near or within the thymus appears to be related to incomplete separation of these two tissues, which arise from similar embryologic primordia.

XENOBIOTIC-INDUCED TOXIC INJURY OF PARATHYROIDS

Ozone

Inhalation of a single dose of ozone (0.75 ppm) for 4–8 hours has been reported to produce light and electron microscopic changes in parathyroid glands (8). Subsequent studies have utilized longer (48-hour) exposure to ozone to define the pathogenesis of the parathyroid lesions (6,9). Initially (1–5 days postozone exposure), many chief cells undergo compensatory hypertrophy and hyperplasia with areas of capillary endothelial cell proliferation, interstitial edema, degeneration of vascular endothelium, formation of platelet thrombi, leukocyte infiltration of the walls of larger vessels in the gland, and disruption of basement membranes. Chief cells had prominent Golgi complexes and endoplasmic reticula, aggregations of free ribosomes, and swelling of mitochondria (7).

Inactive chief cells with few secretory granules predominated in the parathyroids in the more chronic stages of ozone exposure. There was evidence of parathyroid atrophy 12–20 days postozone exposure with mononuclear cell infiltration and necrosis of chief cells. The reduced cytoplasmic area contained vacuolated endoplasmic reticulum, a small Golgi apparatus, and numerous lysosomal bodies. Plasma membranes of adjacent chief cells were disrupted resulting in coalescence of the cytoplasmic area. Fibroblasts with associated collagen bundles were prominent in the interstitium, and the basal lamina of the numerous capillaries often was duplicated.

The parathyroid lesions in ozone-exposed animals were similar to isoimmune parathyroiditis in other species (89). Antibody against parathyroid tissue was localized near the periphery of chief cells by indirect immunofluorescence, especially 14 days following ozone injury (9).

Aluminum

Evidence for a direct effect of aluminum on the parathyroids was suggested from studies of patients with chronic renal failure treated by hemodialysis with aluminum-containing fluids or orally administered drugs containing aluminum. These patients often had normal or minimal elevations of iPTH, little histologic evidence of osteitis fibrosa in bone, and a depressed parathyroid response to acute hypocalcemia (15). Studies by Morrissey *et al.* (105) have reported that an increase in aluminum concentration in vitro over a range of 0.5–2.0 mM in a low calcium medium (0.5 mM) progressively inhibited the secretion of PTH. At 2.0 mM aluminum, PTH secretion was inhibited by 68%, while high-medium calcium (2.0 mM) without aluminum maximally inhibited PTH secretion only 39%. The inhibition of PTH secretion by aluminum does not appear to be due to an irreversible toxic effect since normal secretion was restored when parathyroid cells were returned to a 0.5-mM-calcium medium without aluminum. The incorporation of [^{3}H]-leucine into total cell protein, parathyroid secretory protein, proparathyroid hormone (proPTH), or PTH was not affected by aluminum; however, the secretion of radiolabeled protein by dispersed parathyroid cells was inhibited by aluminum (105).

The molecular mechanism by which aluminum inhibits PTH secretion appears to be similar to that of calcium ion by reducing diglyceride levels in chief cells (104). Aluminum appears to decrease diglyceride synthesis, which is reflected in a corresponding decrease in synthesis of phosphatidylcholine and possibly triglyceride. However, phosphatidylinositol synthesis is not affected by aluminum.

Toxicity of Excess Vitamin D and Metabolites

Experimental Hypervitaminosis D

Ultrastructural changes in secretory activity of parathyroid glands in response to persistent hypercalcemia have been investigated in cows given 30 x 10^6 units of vitamin D$_2$ (irradiated ergosterol) daily for intervals of 3–30 days (26). The parathyroid glands had ultrastructural alterations suggesting suppression of PTH synthesis and secretion (27). Hypercalcemia did not appear to affect the entire population of chief cells uniformly. After 3–7 days of vitamin D, the blood calcium was increased to 12.3 mg/100 mL, and parathyroid glands contained inactive chief cells, as well as occasional atrophic and active chief cells.

The most striking initial alteration in response to vitamin D–induced hypercalcemia was an accumulation of numerous secretory granules within some chief cells. These cells appeared to have entered a phase of active hormonal synthesis prior to or during the development of hypercalcemia. Subsequently, they returned to the inactive phase, but the products of synthesis accumulated as increased numbers of granules. Secretory granules were present throughout the cytoplasm but often in large aggregates near the plasma membrane.

The changes in the parathyroid glands in response to hypercalcemia of longer duration (10–30 days) were similar but became progressively more severe. Inactive chief cells predominated in the parathyroid glands, but atrophic cells became more numerous. Atrophic chief cells were more electron-dense and smaller than inactive chief cells. The nucleus was irregularly shrunken, and the cytoplasmic matrix was dense and contained lipofuscin and lipid bodies, ribosomes, a small Golgi apparatus, and often many secretory granules. The intercellular spaces between adjacent atrophic chief cells were widened. Cells with characteristics intermediate between inactive and atrophic chief cells were observed, suggesting that the latter are derived from inactive chief cells.

Chronic hypercalcemia appeared to inhibit but not prevent chief cells from actively synthesizing PTH. Occasional chief cells were observed with lamellar aggregations of endoplasmic reticulum and clusters of ribosomes, suggesting active hormonal synthesis in cells with many peripherally situated storage granules. The number of secretory granules in chief cells decreased progressively from the 10th to the 30th day of hypercalcemic suppression. The increased lysosomal bodies (sometimes partially surrounding a secretory granule), together with the presence of partially degraded granules within autophagic vacuoles, suggests a mechanism by which chief cells degrade their secretory product in response to chronic hypercalcemia.

Solanum malacoxylon Intoxication

Livestock grazing on calcinogenic plants develop a progressive debilitating disease with widespread soft tissue mineralization that has been recognized worldwide. Ingestion of *Cestrum diurnum* (day-blooming jessamine) in Florida and and other states in the southern United States and *Trisetum flavescens* in the Bavarian and Austrian Alps produces calcinosis in horses, cattle, and sheep (41,81,158). *Solanum malacoxylon*, found in Argentina and Brazil, produces a disease in cattle (called *enteque seco* or *espichamento*) characterized by hypercalcemia, hyperphosphatemia, and widespread soft tissue mineralization (28,43).

The leaves of these calcinogenic plants contain substances possessing vitamin D–like biologic activity (157). The dried leaves of *S. malacoxylon* have been reported to contain a steroid–glycoside conjugate in which the steroidal component is identical with 1α, 25-dihydroxycholecalciferol (1α, $[OH]_2D_3$) (60,156). This active principle in *S. malacoxylon* stimulates intestinal calcium absorption and enhances calcium-binding protein synthesis (38,119).

Other evidence for the potent vitamin D–like action of *S. malacoxylon* comes from studies on experimental *S. malacoxylon* intoxication of cattle. After ingestion of the dried leaves of *S. malacoxylon*, there is a rapid rise in serum calcium levels accompanied by an increase in inorganic phosphorus. Chronic *S. malacoxylon* intoxication in cattle results in widespread mineralization of the cardiovascular system, lung, kidney, and other organs (42). Experimental intoxication of cattle with pharmacologic levels of the parent vitamin D compound results in similar lesions and changes in levels of serum electrolytes (26).

After feeding *S. malacoxylon* to cattle, parathyroid chief cells initially accumulated secretory granules and later underwent involution and atrophy (36). There was an accumulation of mature secretory granules near the plasma membrane of chief cells after feeding leaves (0.4 g/kg) of *S. malacoxylon* for only 1 day. The plasma membranes were straight and had occasional uncomplicated interdigitations with adjacent chief cells.

Chief cells of cattle fed *S. malacoxylon* leaves for 6 days (0.067 g/kg/day) and 32 days (0.029 g/kg/day) appeared to be predominately inactive. The cytoplasmic area was diminished and the nucleus was more irregular. Secretory granules were reduced compared with animals fed *S. malacoxylon* for 1 day, but there were increased numbers of lysosomal and lipofuscin bodies. The intercellular spaces between adjacent inactive chief cells were widened and traversed by numerous interdigitating cytoplasmic processes (36).

L-Asparaginase

Tettenborn *et al.* (149) and Chisari *et al.* (33) reported that rabbits administered L-asparaginase develop severe hypocalcemia and tetany characterized by muscle tremors, opisthotonos, carpopedal spasms, paralysis, and coma. This drug was of interest in cancer chemotherapy because of the beneficial effects of guinea pig serum against lymphosarcoma in mice.

Parathyroid chief cells appeared to be selectively destroyed by L-asparaginase (168). Chief cells were predominately inactive and degranulated, with large autophagic vacuoles present in the cytoplasm of degenerating cells. Cytoplasmic organelles concerned with synthesis and packaging of secretory products were poorly developed in chief cells. The rabbits developed hyperphosphatemia, hypomagnesemia, hyperkalemia, and azotemia in addition to the acute hypocalcemia. Rabbits with clinical hypocalcemic tetany did not recover spontaneously; however, administration of parathyroid extract prior to or during treatment with L-asparaginase decreased the incidence of hypocalcemic tetany.

The development of hypocalcemia and tetany has not been observed in other experimental animals administered L-asparaginase (113). However, this response may not be limited to the rabbit, since some human patients receiving the drug also have developed hypocalcemia (73). The L-asparaginase–induced hypoparathyroidism in rabbits is a valuable model to investigate drug–endocrine cell interactions, somewhat analogous to the selective destruction of pancreatic β cells by alloxan with production of experimental diabetes mellitus.

Fluoride

Drinking water containing large doses of fluoride (200 ppm) has been reported to cause parathyroid hyperplasia in sheep (48). Chief cells were primarily in the active stage of the secretory cycle after 1-month exposure. The endoplasmic reticulum was aggregated into lamellar arrays and the Golgi apparatus was well developed in chief cells. iPTH levels in the blood were elevated 5-fold after 1 week and remained elevated over the experimental period of a month. Faccini (47) interpreted these changes suggesting stimulation of chief cells by fluoride as a response to an increased PTH demand resulting from decreased mobilization of calcium from fluoroapatite-containing bone. Apatite crystals in fluorotic bone are known to be of larger size than in normal bone and appear to be more stable and less reactive in surface exchange reactions.

Secondary hyperparathyroidism has been reported in patients with skeletal fluorosis (148). The parathyroid glands have morphologic evidence of hyperactivity and the patients have elevated circulating levels of iPTH. Ream and Principato (123) reported increased glycogen accumulation in hyperactive chief cells of rats following the ingestion of large doses (150 ppm) of fluoride in drinking water.

IMMUNE-MEDIATED INJURY OF PARATHYROIDS

Isoimmune hypoparathyroidism has been induced experimentally by repeated injections of parathyroid emulsions with Freund's adjuvant for 4 months (89). The parathyroids had lymphocytic infiltration, atrophy and disorganization in the pattern of arrangement of chief cells, and progressive fibrosis. Mitochondria in chief cells were irregularly swollen, and cristae were disrupted, giving a vacuolated appearance. The granular endoplasmic reticulum was poorly developed and secretory granules were reduced in number.

Hypoparathyroidism results when subnormal amounts of PTH are secreted by pathologic parathyroids or the hormone secreted is unable to interact normally with target cells (20). Hypoparathyroidism often is associated with a diffuse lymphocytic parathyroiditis resulting in extensive degeneration of chief cells and replacement by fibrous connective tissue. In the early stages of lymphocytic parathyroiditis, there is infiltration of the gland with lymphocytes and plasma cells with nodular regenerative hyperplasia of the remaining chief cells. The lymphocytic parathyroiditis appears to develop by an immune-mediated mechanism, since a similar destruction of secretory parenchyma and lymphocytic infiltration has been produced experimentally by repeated injections of parathyroid tissue immulsions. Bone resorption is decreased because of a lack of PTH, and blood calcium levels diminish progressively.

PARATHYROID CHANGES ASSOCIATED WITH METABOLIC DISORDERS

Renal Hyperparathyroidism

Secondary hyperparathyroidism as a complication of chronic renal failure is a metabolic state characterized by an excessive, but not autonomous, rate of PTH secretion (23). The secretion of hormone by the hyperplastic parathyroid gland usually remains responsive to fluctuations in blood calcium. The primary etiologic mechanism in this disorder is long-standing progressive renal disease resulting in severely impaired function. When the renal disease progresses to the point at which there is significant reduction in glomerular filtration rate, phosphorus is retained and progressive hyperphosphatemia develops (Fig. 10). Although the concentration of blood phosphorus has no direct regulatory influence on the synthesis and secretion of PTH, when elevated, it contributes to parathyroid stimulation by virtue of its ability to lower blood calcium levels.

Parathyroid stimulation associated with chronic renal disease can be attributed directly to the hypocalcemia. An impaired intestinal absorption of calcium due to an acquired defect in vitamin D metabolism plays an important role in the development of hypocalcemia associated with renal insufficiency. Chronic renal disease interferes with the production of 1,25-dihydroxycholecalciferol by the kidney, thereby diminishing intestinal calcium transport. All parathyroids are considerably enlarged as a result initially of hypertrophy of chief cells and subsequently of hyperplasia as compensatory mechanisms to increase hormonal synthesis and secretion in response to the hypocalcemic stimulus.

Chronic renal insufficiency in animals occurs frequently as a result of several acquired, induced, or congenital kidney lesions (22). All four parathyroid glands undergo marked chief cell hyperplasia and the bones have varying degrees of generalized osteitis fibrosa. Ultrastructurally, chief cells in the parathyroid glands of dogs with chronic renal disease are primarily in the actively synthesizing stage. Chronically stimulated chief cells have extensive lamellar aggregations of endoplasmic reticulum, numerous ribosomes, large mitochondria, and prominent

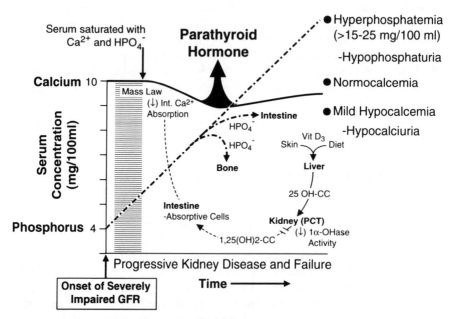

FIG. 10. Alterations in serum calcium and phosphorus during the pathogenesis of secondary hyperparathyroidism associated with progressive renal disease and failure.

Golgi apparatuses with many prosecretory granules. The numbers of mature storage granules are less than in chief cells from normal dogs, and they are situated in the peripheral parts of the cell. Plasma membranes of adjacent cells are frequently interdigitated.

Nutritional Hyperparathyroidism

The increased secretion of PTH in this disorder is a compensatory mechanism directed against a disturbance in mineral homeostasis induced by nutritional imbalances (Fig. 11) (19). The disease occurs in many animal species, including dogs, cats, monkeys, and laboratory rodents, among others, fed improper diets. Dietary mineral imbalances of etiologic importance in the pathogenesis are a low content of calcium, excessive phosphorus with normal or low calcium, and inadequate amounts of cholecalciferol (vitamin D_3) in New World nonhuman primates housed indoors without exposure to sunlight. The significant end result is hypocalcemia, which results in parathyroid stimulation (Fig. 11).

A diet low in calcium fails to supply the daily requirement, even though a greater proportion of ingested calcium is absorbed, and hypocalcemia develops. Ingestion of excessive phosphorus results in increased intestinal absorption and elevation in blood phosphorus levels. Hyperphosphatemia does not stimulate the parathyroid gland directly but does so indirectly by lowering blood calcium

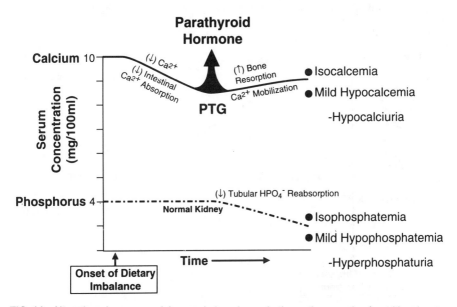

FIG. 11. Alterations in serum calcium and phosphorus in the pathogenesis of nutritional secondary hyperparathyroidism caused by feeding a diet low in calcium or deficient in cholecalciferol but with normal amounts of phosphorus.

levels and suppressing the synthesis of 1,25-$(OH)_2$-cholecalciferol by the kidney. In response to the nutritionally induced hypocalcemia, all parathyroid glands undergo cellular hypertrophy and hyperplasia.

In response to the diet-induced hypocalcemia, chief cells undergo hypertrophy and eventually hyperplasia. The expanded cytoplasmic area is lightly eosinophilic and vacuolated compared with chief cells in control animals. Perivascular spaces are narrow and there are few fat cells in the interstitium. Ultrastructurally, the cytoplasmic area of chief cells is increased, and organelles concerned with protein synthesis and packaging of secretory products are well developed after low-calcium diet for 1 week. An increased number of chief cells have the endoplasmic reticulum aggregated into lamellar arrays and an enlarged Golgi apparatus associated with many prosecretory granules (25).

Hypoparathyroidism

Hypoparathyroidism is a metabolic disorder in which either subnormal amounts of PTH are secreted by pathologic parathyroids or the hormone secreted is unable to interact normally with target cells (20). Hypoparathyroidism is often associated with a diffuse lymphocytic parathyroiditis resulting in extensive degeneration of chief cells and replacement by fibrous connective tissue (Fig. 12). In the early stages of lymphocytic parathyroiditis, there is infiltration of the gland with lymphocytes and plasma cells, with nodular regenerative hyperplasia of the remaining chief cells. The lymphocytic parathyroiditis appears to develop

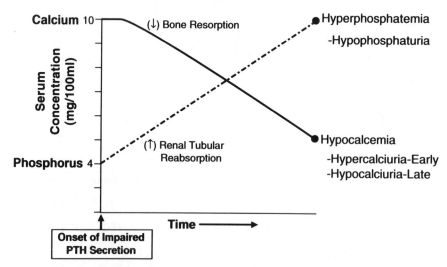

FIG. 12. Alterations in serum calcium and phosphorus in response to an inadequate secretion of parathyroid hormone. There is a progressive increase in serum phosphorus and a marked decline in serum calcium levels that often results in neuromuscular tetany.

by an immune-mediated mechanism, since a similar destruction of secretory parenchyma and lymphocytic infiltration have been produced experimentally by repeated injections of parathyroid tissue immulsions.

The functional disturbances and clinical manifestations of hypoparathyroidism are primarily the result of increased neuromuscular excitability and tetany. Because of the lack of PTH, bone resorption is decreased and blood calcium levels diminish progressively (4–6 mg/100 mL) (Fig. 12). Affected animals are restless, nervous, and ataxic, with weakness and intermittent tremors of individual muscle groups that progress to generalized tetany and convulsive seizures. Concurrently, blood phosphorus levels are substantially elevated owing to increased renal tubular reabsorption.

Primary Hyperparathyroidism

In primary hyperparathyroidism, PTH is produced in excess by a functional tumor in the parathyroid gland. The normal control of PTH secretion by the concentration of blood calcium is lost in primary hyperparathyroidism. Hormone secretion is autonomous, and the parathyroid produces excessive hormone in spite of the increased blood calcium (Fig. 13). PTH acts initially on cells in the renal tubules to promote the excretion of phosphorus and retention of calcium. A prolonged increased secretion of PTH results in accelerated bone resorption and increased renal production of $1,25-(OH)_2$-cholecalciferol. The lesion in the parathyroid gland responsible for the excessive secretion of PTH is usually an adenoma composed of active chief cells (21).

Parathyroid Suppression by Feeding High Calcium Diets

To investigate the mechanisms by which high calcium prepartal diets predispose to the development of profound hypocalcemia at parturition, adult cows were fed a high calcium diet (150 g/day or six times the recommended quantity) with normal phosphorus (25 g/day) content for 50 days prepartum (13). The serum calcium increased after 10 days (11.8 mg/100 mL) and remained elevated above values in controls fed a balanced diet with recommended amounts of calcium (25 g/day) and phosphorus. However, the ability to respond to the hypocalcemic challenge associated with parturition and the initiation of lactation was less in animals fed the high calcium diet, and the decrease in serum calcium at parturition was greater than in controls.

Plasma iPTH did not increase significantly prepartum in animals fed the high calcium diet and decreased from 1240 pg/mL at parturition to 735 pg/mL at 48 hours postpartum (13). Control cows fed the balanced diet with only the recommended amount of calcium had consistently higher iPTH levels prepartum, which increased from 2970 pg/mL at parturition to 7880 pg/mL at 48 hours postpartum. Inactive chief cells predominated in parathyroids of animals fed the high calcium

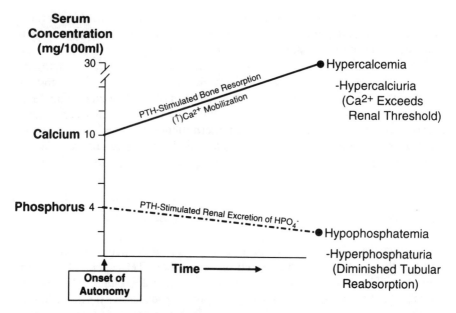

FIG. 13. Alterations in serum calcium and phosphorus in response to an autonomous secretion of parathyroid hormone in primary hyperparathyroidism.

diet. The cytoplasm contained numerous lipid bodies, dispersed individual pro-files of endoplasmic reticulum, small Golgi apparatuses, and occasional lipofuscin granules but infrequent mature secretory granules.

Atrophic chief cells were frequently present in parathyroids of cows fed high calcium diets. They were irregular in outline, had an electron-dense cytoplasm, and were shrunken from adjacent chief cells. Synthetic cytoplasmic organelles were poorly developed and secretory granules were infrequent. Active chief cells with lamellar arrays of endoplasmic reticulum, large Golgi apparatuses, and many secretion granules predominated in parathyroids of control parturient animals (13).

NEOPLASMS OF PARATHYROID GLAND

Chief Cell Adenoma and Carcinoma

Parathyroid adenomas in adult-aged rats vary from microscopic in size to uni-lateral nodules several millimeters in diameter, located in the cervical region by the thyroids or infrequently in the thoracic cavity near the base of the heart. Parathy-roid neoplasms in the precardiac mediastinum are derived from ectopic parathy-roid tissue displaced into the thorax with the expanding thymus during embryonic development. Tumors of parathyroid chief cells do not appear to be a sequela of long-standing secondary hyperparathyroidism of either renal or nutritional origin. The unaffected parathyroid glands may be atrophic if the adenoma is functional, normal if the adenoma is nonfunctional, or enlarged if there is concomitant chief cell hyperplasia.

Adenomas are solitary nodules that are sharply demarcated from adjacent parathyroid parenchyma. Since the adenoma compresses the rim of surrounding parathyroid to varying degrees depending on its size, there may be a partial fibrous capsule either from compression of existing stroma or proliferation of fibrous connective tissue. Adenomas are usually nonfunctional (endocrinologically inactive) in adult-aged rats. Chief cells in nonfunctional adenomas are cuboidal or polyhedral and arranged either in a diffuse sheet, lobules, or acini with or without lumina. Some parathyroid adenomas in the rat become cystic. The cystadenomas contain solid areas of tumor cells and large cystic areas lined by neoplastic chief cells. The cysts contain a densely eosinophilic proteinaceous fluid.

Larger parathyroid adenomas, such as those detected macroscopically, often nearly incorporate the entire affected gland. A narrow rim of compressed parenchyma may be detected at one side of the gland or the affected parathyroid may be completely incorporated by the adenoma. If functionally active, chief cells in this rim often are compressed and atrophic due to pressure and the trophic effects of the persistent hypercalcemia.

Chief cell carcinomas are rarely encountered in laboratory rats. Carcinomas can result in a macroscopically detectable enlargement of one gland. Parathyroid carcinomas are often more fixed in position than chief cell adenomas due to invasion of either the adjacent thyroid lobe or adjacent cervical skeletal muscle. Some of the enlargement may be due to central necrosis and hemorrhage in the carcinoma. The malignant chief cells either form acinar structures, palisade along blood sinusoids, or are arranged in solid sheets subdivided into lobules by a fibrovascular stroma. There is usually complete incorporation of the affected gland and evidence of invasion through the parathyroid capsule. Evidence of vascular invasion and formation of tumor cell emboli are infrequently observed. Malignant chief cells may be more pleomorphic than those in adenomas, but mitotic figures are infrequent.

Factors Influencing the Development of Parathyroid Tumors

Age

There are relatively few chemicals or experimental manipulations reported in the literature that significantly increase the incidence of parathyroid tumors. Long-standing renal failure with intense diffuse hyperplasia does not appear to increase the development of chief cell tumors in rats. In studies conducted by the National Toxicology Program (NTP), the historical incidence of parathyroid adenomas was 0.3% (4 in 1315) in untreated control male F344 rats and 0.15% (2 in 1330) in female F344 rats. Parathyroid adenomas in F344 rats are an example of a neoplasm whose incidence increases dramatically when 2-year studies are compared with life-span data. Solleveld *et al.* (141) reported that the incidence of parathyroid adenomas increased in males from 0.1% at 2 years to 3.1% in lifetime studies. Corresponding data for female F344 rats was 0.1% at 2 years and 0.6% in lifetime studies.

Gonadectomy

Oslapas *et al.* (115) reported an increased incidence of parathyroid adenomas in female (34%) and male (27%) rats of the Long–Evans strain administered 40 µCi sodium ^{131}I and saline at 8 weeks of age. There were no significant changes in serum calcium, phosphorus, and parathyroid hormone compared with controls. Gonadectomy performed at 7 weeks of age decreased the incidence of parathyroid adenomas in irradiated rats (7.4% in gonadectomy vs. 27% in intact controls), but there was little change in incidence of parathyroid adenomas in irradiated females. X-irradiation of the thyroid–parathyroid region also increased the incidence of parathyroid adenomas. When female Sprague–Dawley rats received a single absorbed dose of x-rays at 4 weeks of age, they subsequently developed a 24% incidence of parathyroid adenomas after 14 months (116).

Xenobiotic Chemicals

Parathyroid adenomas have infrequently been encountered following the administration of a variety of chemicals in 2-year bioassay studies in Fischer rats. In a study involving F344 rats and the pesticide rotenone, there appeared to be an increased incidence of parathyroid adenomas in high-dose (75 ppm) males (4 of 44 rats) compared with either low-dose (38 ppm) males, control males (1 of 44 rats), or NTP historical controls (0.3%) (1). It was uncertain whether the increased incidence of this uncommon tumor was a direct effect of rotenone feeding or the increased survival in high-dose males. Chief cell hyperplasia was not present in parathyroids that developed adenomas.

Irradiation and Hypercalcemia Induced by Vitamin D

Wynford-Thomas *et al.* (163) reported that irradiation significantly increased the incidence of parathyroid adenomas in inbred Wistar albino rats and that the incidence could be modified by feeding diets with variable amounts of vitamin D. Neonatal Wistar rats were given either 5 or 10 µCi radioiodine (^{131}I) within 24 hours of birth. In rats 12 months of age and older, parathyroid adenomas were found in 33% of rats administered 5 µCi ^{131}I and in 37% of rats given 10 µCi ^{131}I compared with 0% in nonirradiated controls. The incidence of parathyroid adenomas was highest (55%) in normocalcemic rats fed a low vitamin D diet and lowest (20%) in irradiated rats fed a high vitamin D diet (40,000 IU/kg) that had a significant elevation in plasma calcium.

PARATHYROID HORMONE–RELATED PROTEIN

Relationship to Parathyroid Hormone

The presence of PTH-like activity in tumors associated with humoral hypercalcemia of malignancy (HHM) (127–129) and the similarities of HHM to primary hyperparathyroidism led to the isolation and discovery of PTH-related protein (PTHrP) (91,142). PTHrP was initially purified from human tumors associated with HHM (107,144). Subsequently, the cDNA and gene for PTHrP were isolated, sequenced, and characterized (95,97,147). The PTHrP gene is complicated and contains at least six exons, two 5' untranslated regions each with its own promoter, a pre-prohormone coding region, a main coding region, and two additional 3' regions that have coding and noncoding regions (92,93,146). There is alternate splicing of PTHrP mRNA so that three mature peptides can be formed composed of 139, 141, and 173 amino acid residues (94,150). The PTH gene is simpler and has only three exons (5'-untranslated region, pre-prohormone coding region, and main coding region with a 3' noncoding region) and encodes for a mature protein of 84 amino acids.

The rat, mouse, and chicken cDNA or genes for PTHrP have also been isolated and sequenced (76,92,93,136). There is extensive primary amino acid sequence homology between the species. The first 111 N-terminal amino acids have only two divergent amino acids in the rat, human, and mouse forms of PTHrP. Nonhuman species have only the 139 or 141 amino acid forms of PTHrP and also have a simpler genomic organization with fewer exons.

PTHrP binds to PTH receptors in bone and kidney with similar affinity as PTH (Fig. 6) (29,114). The first 34 N-terminal amino acids of PTHrP contain the PTH-like biologic activity. This is similar to PTH in which the first 34 N-terminal amino acids contain most of the biologic activities. There is 70% sequence homology of the first 13 N-terminal amino acids of PTHrP compared with PTH, but little homology after amino acid 13. The N-terminus is important in the activation of the PTH receptor (120). Sequence homology in this region is important for the ability of PTHrP to stimulate PTH receptors. By comparison, amino acids 20–34 are important for the binding of PTH to its receptor. There is little sequence homology between PTH and PTHrP in this region; however, PTHrP binds to the PTH receptor with this region of its sequence (3). These findings suggest that two different primary amino acid sequences permit high affinity binding to the same receptor.

The PTH–PTHrP receptor has recently been cloned and sequenced from cDNA isolated from opossum kidney cells and rat osteoblasts (2,74). There is 78% homology between the rat and opossum receptors, indicating conservation across mammalian species. The PTH–PTHrP receptor belongs to a newly recognized class of receptors that contains seven transmembrane domains and includes the calcitonin and secretin receptors (87). Therefore, evidence to date indicates that PTHrP binds to PTH receptors in bone and kidney and that distinct PTHrP receptors do not exist in these organs.

Role in Cancer-Associated Hypercalcemia

Cancer-associated hypercalcemia (CAH) is one of the most frequently occurring paraneoplastic syndromes (108,111). CAH is a syndrome consisting of multiple pathogenic mechanisms and a variety of inciting neoplasms (56,143). Certain neoplasms are consistently associated with CAH, and there are sporadic reports of a variety of neoplasms associated with hypercalcemia.

There are two primary mechanisms by which tumors can induce hypercalcemia: (1) release of humoral factors that act systemically to increase osteoclastic bone resorption or increase calcium reabsorption from the kidney or calcium absorption from the intestinal tract; and (2) stimulation of local bone resorption associated with neoplasms metastatic to bone (Fig. 14) (110). Some neoplasms that induce CAH may stimulate hypercalcemia by both mechanisms simultaneously. The complete syndrome of CAH appears not to be induced by a single factor, but rather by the cooperative or synergistic action of multiple factors produced either by neoplastic cells or host cells.

Humoral hypercalcemia of malignancy (HHM) is a form of cancer-associated hypercalcemia that is induced by the secretion of humoral factors that have effects distant to the site of the neoplasms (Fig. 15) (96). Some neoplasms that cause HHM may metastasize to bone, but the primary mechanism of hypercalcemia is due to distant effects of humoral factors and not to localized bone resorption. This form of CAH has been the focus of intense investigation during the past decade. There are multiple humoral factors that have been associated with HHM, including PTH, PTHrP, cytokines, steroids such as 1,25-dihydroxyvitamin D, and prostaglandins (69,109). It is of interest that many of the humoral factors produced by tumor cells that alter calcium metabolism and bone resorption can also be produced by osteogenic cells, such as osteoblasts.

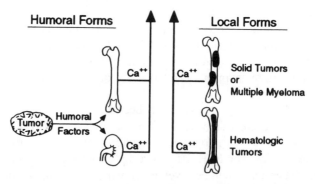

FIG. 14. Humoral and local forms of cancer-associated hypercalcemia increase circulating concentrations of calcium by stimulating osteoclastic bone resorption or increased renal tubular reabsorption of calcium. (Reprinted by permission form Rosol, T. J., and Capen, C. C. Mechanism of cancer-induced hypercalcemia. *Lab. Invest. 67*: 680–702,1992.)

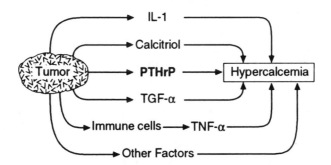

FIG. 15. Humoral factors such as parathyroid hormone-related protein (PTHrP), interleukin-1 (IL-1), tumor necrosis factors (TNF), or transforming growith factors (TGF) produced by tumors induce humoral hypercalcemia of malignancy (HHM) by acting as systemic hormones and stimulating osteoclastic bone resorption or increasing renal tubular reabsorption of calcium. (Reprinted by permission form Rosol, T. J., and Capen, C. C. Mechanism of cancer-induced hypercalcemia. *Lab. Invest. 67*: 680–702, 1992.)

PTHrP plays a central role in the pathogenesis of HHM (128,142). It is produced by most tumors associated with hypercalcemia (16,62,167) and is present in the circulation at increased concentrations in human patients and animals with HHM (63,122,134). The administration of anti-PTHrP antibodies in animal models of HHM has been reported to decrease serum calcium levels and bone resorption (83,84).

Parathyroid Changes in Cancer-Associated Hypercalcemia

HHM is a common clinical syndrome in dogs with several forms of cancer. The two most common malignancies that induce HHM are lymphoma and adenocarcinomas derived from apocrine glands of the anal sac (128). The apocrine adenocarcinoma of the anal sac occurs in the perirectal area of predominantly older female dogs and results in persistent hypercalcemia in 90% of tumor-bearing animals but rarely metastasizes to bone (101,124). Tumor excision results in a return to normocalcemia. Tumor recurrence is associated with a return of hypercalcemia due to secretion of PTHrP by the neoplastic cells (133,134).

Parathyroid glands from dogs with hypercalcemia and apocrine adenocarcinomas were composed of inactive or atrophic chief cells (103). They were arranged in narrow cords with prominent perivascular and interstitial spaces containing collagen fibers. Ultrastructurally, the reduced cytoplasmic area of chief cells, straight cell borders with uncomplicated interdigitations between adjacent cells, and the poorly developed synthetic and secretory organelles suggested that chief cells in dogs with persistent hypercalcemia were either inactive or atrophic.

Lymphoma induces HHM in about 30% of the affected dogs and usually is associated with the T-cell phenotype (159). Hypercalcemia is induced by the secretion of PTHrP and other lymphokines that are capable of stimulating bone resorption (128,134). Ultrastructurally, parathyroid glands in hypercalcemic dogs with lymphosarcoma were predominately composed of inactive chief cells (102). Chief cells interpreted to be inactive had a reduced cytoplasmic area, straight plasma membranes, and increased intracytoplasmic lipid. The Golgi apparatus was small and associated with a few small granules.

In order to further determine the effects of PTHrP on parathyroids, chief cells were examined from four groups of nude mice (NIH:Swiss) with different serum calcium concentrations associated with CAH (55). A tumor line, derived from an adenocarcinoma of the apocrine glands of the anal sac of a hypercalcemic dog and designated CAC-8 (132), was transplanted into mice. The mice were euthanatized when the transplanted adenocarcinoma (CAC-8) induced hypercalcemia (6–8 weeks post-transplantation). CAC-8 in mice and has been reported to produce PTHrP and transforming growth factors α and β (100,133). The mean serum PTH concentration in CAC-8 tumor–bearing hypercalcemic mice decreased and serum 1,25-dihydroxyvitamin D increased compared with control mice (131). In order to evaluate directly the effects of PTHrP on chief cells, mice were infused with synthetic PTHrP(1–40) for 7 days (130). To evaluate the effect of low calcium intake on chief cells, mice were fed a low calcium diet (0.01% calcium, 0.55% phosphorus) for 14 days (126). To exclude water as a possible calcium source, these mice had access to distilled water only. Control mice were fed an identical diet containing 0.85% calcium. Serum calcium concentrations were significantly different for CAC-8 tumor–bearing mice and PTHrP-infused mice as compared with controls. CAC-8 tumor–bearing mice were markedly hypercalcemic (17.0 ± 3.1 mg/dL), and mice infused with PTHrP(1–40) for 7 days developed less severe hypercalcemia (13.6 ±1.5 mg/dL), when compared with the control group (9.3 ± 0.8 mg/dL) or with mice fed a low calcium diet (8.6 ± 0.6 mg/dL).

Chief cells from each mouse were evaluated quantitatively and qualitatively by electron microscopy. CAC-8 tumor–bearing and PTHrP-infused mice had significantly larger mean areas of chief cells (48 ± 18 μm^2 and 45 ± 12 μm^2, respectively) compared with the control mice (40 ± 18 μm^2) and with mice fed a low calcium diet (37 ± 13 μm^2). The majority of chief cells in CAC-8 tumor–bearing mice had decreased tortuosity of plasma membranes and only a few membranous interdigitations between adjacent cells. The plasma membranes of the PTHrP-infused mice were similar to the CAC-8 tumor–bearing group, whereas the control mice had many chief cells with tortuous cell membranes. Mice fed a low calcium diet had more prominent interdigitations of plasma membranes of adjacent chief cells than controls.

Mature secretory granules had diameters ranging from 150 to 200 nm, a narrow submembranous space, and a electron-dense core. Depending on the plane of section through the cell, they were usually concentrated in one area of the cytoplasm, and their numbers varied considerably among chief cells. The greatest number of secretory granules was present in chief cells from control mice (5.2 ±

2.8/cell). PTHrP-infused mice (4.3 ± 2.6/cell), CAC-8 tumor–bearing mice (2.1 ± 1.3/cell), and mice fed a low calcium diet (1.7 ± 1.8/cell) had significantly fewer secretory granules compared with control mice.

Chief cells in mice with hypercalcemia induced by PTHrP developed unique membranous whorls associated. The highest incidence of cytoplasmic membranous whorls was present in severely hypercalcemic CAC-8 tumor–bearing mice, which had a mean of 24 whorls/500 chief cells (range, 1–45 whorls/500 cells). In PTHrP-infused mice, the mean was 8 whorls/500 cells (range, 0–16 whorls/500 cells). Only one whorl was found in chief cells from mice fed a low calcium diet, and whorls were not observed in chief cells from control mice. The cytoplasmic area occupied by membranous whorls ranged from 9 to 39 μm^2 in CAC-8 tumor–bearing mice and from 7 to 14 μm^2 in PTHrP-infused mice.

The formation of membranous whorls appeared to be similar in all affected mice. The unique whorls consisted of membranes, presumably derived from rough endoplasmic reticulum, plus entrapped cytoplasmic organelles. They often contained lipid droplets near the center of the whorl. The formation of membranous whorls appeared to begin with a circular aggregation of membranes from the rough endoplasmic reticulum. Membranes that made up larger whorls did not contain attached ribosomes. The initial stages of membranous whorl formation were observed most often in the PTHrP-infused mice and less frequently in CAC-8 tumor–bearing mice.

One frequently reported ultrastructural change in parathyroid chief cells of mice, with and without hypercalcemia, is the development of unique cytoplasmic membranous whorls under varied conditions such as starvation or after the administration of glucocorticoids, reserpine, or vitamin D (70–72,85). These myelin-like structures do not resemble the lamellar bodies found in human parathyroid chief cells in chronic renal failure or in parathyroid adenomas (45,46,59). In contrast, a parathyroid autograft from a human patient with chronic renal failure was reported to have myelin-like structures in about 5% of the chief cells similar to those described in mice (46). Membranous whorls have also been reported in a parathyroid adenoma from a patient with acute hyperparathyroidism (14).

Membranous whorls in the chief cells of hypercalcemic nude mice do not appear to be the result of enhanced endocytosis of plasma membranes, as has been reported in rats after vitamin D_3 administration (160). Rather, they appear to originate from coiling and condensation of rough endoplasmic reticulum with a gradual loss of ribosomes. Detachment of ribosomes from rough endoplasmic reticulum membranes and subsequent formation of intracellular myelin-like whorls are common ultrastructural changes in injured cells. Fragmentation of intracellular membranes with accumulation of phospholipids and reassembling with cholesterol may be important in the formation of myelin-like membranous whorls. Formation of whorls in chief cells appears to be an indicator of suppressed secretory activity and results from the accumulation of membranous material derived from endoplasmic reticulum. Whorling of cytoplasmic membranes in parathyroid cells of mice appears to be associated with suppression of secretory activity independent of cause, rather than only with elevated serum calcium or PTHrP concentrations (71,72).

Mice infused with PTHrP had similar changes in chief cells compared with CAC-8 tumor–bearing mice with HHM but to a less severe degree. This suggests that a longer duration and greater magnitude of hypercalcemia results in more profound ultrastructural changes in parathyroid chief cells.

Emerging Concepts of PTHrP in Normal Physiology

In contrast to PTH, produced only by the parathyroid gland, PTHrP is produced by many normal tissues. These include stratified squamous epithelium, endocrine glands (adrenal cortex and medulla, fetal and adult parathyroid glands, adenohypophysis, thyroid), skeletal and smooth muscle, kidney, bone, lactating mammary gland, brain, pancreas, ovary, testicle, myometrium, avian oviduct, and placenta (5,68,79,137,151). Present evidence suggests that PTHrP acts as an autocrine or paracrine regulator in these tissues, but its exact function in most normal adult tissues is unknown (Fig. 16) (53). PTHrP can function as an autocrine growth factor in human renal cell carcinoma (18).

PTHrP is produced by the fetal parathyroid glands and placenta and appears to function in an endocrine manner to control the serum calcium concentration and the transport of calcium and magnesium across the placenta (90,138) In contrast to the PTH-like effects of PTHrP associated with the N-terminus of the protein, the midmolecule region is important in stimulating calcium transport by the placenta. Rat and human fetuses have a wide distribution of PTHrP immunoreactivity, suggesting that PTHrP plays a role in cell growth and differentiation (106). PTHrP is

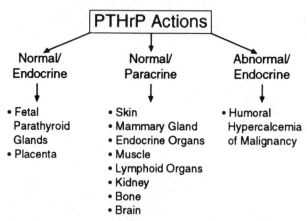

FIG. 16. Sites of parathyroid hormone-related protein (PTHrp) production and action. PTHrp can function either in an endocrine or paracrine manner in normal tissues depending on whether it acts locally or is secreted into the circulation and in an abnormal endocrine manner when it is produced by cancer cells. (Reprinted by permission form Rosol, T. J., and Capen, C. C. Mechanism of cancer-induced hypercalcemia. *Lab. Invest. 67*: 680–702,1992.)

produced by the lactating mammary gland, with expression stimulated by suckling and prolactin (165), and there are high concentrations of PTHrP in milk (152). PTHrP may have a systemic role in the lactating female and neonate since suckling increases urinary cyclic adenosine monophosphate (cAMP) and phosphate excretion in lactating rats (166). However, neutralization of PTHrP by passive immunization did not alter calcium homeostasis in lactating or neonatal mice (82).

The expression of the PTHrP gene in a variety of normal tissues may explain why so many different types of neoplasms can induce HHM. It is surprising that PTHrP can be produced by many normal tissues of the body and not be associated with significant concentrations in the circulation. PTHrP in most normal tissues appears to act locally and is likely to be readily metabolized and degraded by the tissues in which it is produced. For example, immunohistochemical studies have demonstrated that epidermal keratinocytes contain abundant PTHrP (39,61). Total production of PTHrP by the skin and other organs should be much greater than the production of PTH by the parathyroid glands, yet little of the PTHrP produced appears to enter the systemic circulation, since circulating concentrations of PTHrP are very low in normal animals and human beings.

SPECIAL METHODS TO EVALUATE THE STRUCTURE AND FUNCTION OF PARATHYROIDS

Morphologic Evaluation by Light and Electron Microscopy

The parathyroid gland is infrequently injured directly in experimental animals by the acute or chronic administration of xenobiotics. However, parathyroid function may be altered by a wide variety of chemicals that either elevate or lower the blood concentration of calcium, particularly calcium ion. In response to hypocalcemia, chief cells undergo hypertrophy and eventually hyperplasia. On formalin- or Bouin's-fixed tissue sections, the expanded cytoplasmic area is lightly eosinophilic and vacuolated, compared with chief cells in normal animals. Perivascular spaces are narrow in hyperplastic parathyroids, and there are few fat cells in the interstitium. In response to sustained hypercalcemia, the cytoplasmic area of chief cells is decreased and more densely eosinophilic, often with a widening of intercellular and pericapillary spaces. If the hypercalcemia is prolonged, there is an overall reduction of glandular parenchyma, with increased fibrous or adipose connective tissue in the interstitium. Subtle differences between treated and control groups can be best evaluated by morphometric evaluation of parenchyma-to-interstitium ratio, cell and nuclear areas, numbers of mitochondria, and numbers of secretory and prosecretory granules in chief cells (55).

Ultrastructural evaluation of chief cells is a sensitive means of morphologically assessing whether a particular drug or chemical affects the parathyroid gland. Perfusion of the thyroid–parathyroid area with glutaraldehyde-based fixatives followed by postfixation with osmium tetroxide results in the best retention of structural detail in parathyroids of animals. Morphometric studies at the ultrastructural level can be used to quantitate total cytoplasmic area and area occupied by a particular organelle (eg, secretory granules) (55).

In response to an acute lowering of blood calcium, a larger percentage of chief cells ultrastructurally will appear to be actively synthesizing and secreting PTH than under steady-state conditions. This is indicated by a peripheral migration of secretory granules and alignment along the plasma membrane, aggregation of the endoplasmic reticulum into lamellar arrays, and enlargement of the Golgi apparatus associated with many small dense granules in the process of formation. It should be pointed out that chief cells of rats have few mature secretory granules compared with most animal species and human beings. Conversely, chief cells in response to hypercalcemia are predominantly inactive, as evaluated by electron microscopy, with dispersed profiles of endoplasmic reticulum, small Golgi complexes with more few granules, and often accumulations of either glycogen or lipid in the cytoplasm. Atrophic chief cells develop in response to sustained and/or more severe hypercalcemia. Their cytoplasm is more electron-dense and irregularly shrunken, with widened intercellular spaces. Cytoplasmic organelles are poorly developed and may have early degenerative changes suggested by mitochondrial vacuolation with disruption of cristae and distention of endoplasmic reticulum with loss of ribosomes.

Assay Methods for Parathyroid Hormone

PTH in the circulation of animals can be measured by sensitive radioimmunoassays (RIA) or immunoradiometric assays (IRMA). Although the hormone is secreted from chief cells primarily as a straight chain (1–84 amino acids) peptide, molecular fragments (amino- and carboxy-terminals) are formed in the periphery (primarily by Kupffer cells in the liver). The immunoheterogenicity created by the multiple circulating fragments of PTH has caused significant problems in the development of sensitive assays in both human patients and experimental animals. The two-site IRMA method is a frequently used procedure that recognizes both the N- and C-terminal ends of the intact PTH(1–84) molecule. Proper storage and handling of the serum sample are necessary to insure that degradation of intact PTH does not occur prior to analysis. Serum should be separated and frozen immediately, and the sample sent on ice to an appropriate laboratory (32).

Since the N-terminal end of the molecule (the portion that interacts with the receptor in target cells) is highly conserved between man and all mammalian species thus far tested, assays directed against this end of PTH are the most sensitive and accurate in assessing parathyroid function. The N-terminal assay is particularly useful in measuring ongoing or recent functional changes in the parathyroid following exposure to various xenobiotics or physiologic perturbations. However, the assay is cumbersome and slow (6 days) and the commercial availability of reagents for this procedure has recently been restricted. Circulating levels of PTH using N-terminal assays in most animals are near 20 pg/mL (eg, mouse, 19 ± 3 pg/mL; rat, 29 ± 7 pg/mL; dog, 20 ± 5 pg/mL; and cat 17 ± 2 pg/mL), with levels in nonhuman primates being slightly lower.

The measurement of the stable N-terminus of PTH by the two-site IRMA methodology (kit available from the Nichols Institute, San Juan Capistrano, Calif) may be useful for toxicity testing since the assay is rapid and detects a wide range of PTH concentrations without need for sample dilution. The assay can be run on either serum (preferred) or plasma that has been separated and frozen (–70°C in either glass or plastic tubes) as soon as possible after collection. In contrast to some peptide hormones, PTH as quantitated by RIA is relatively stable in serum at ice or refrigerator temperatures, so that it is possible to collect representative specimens from large numbers of experimental rats (as at the end of a chronic study).

PTH assays utilizing antibody generated against the carboxy- (C-) terminal end and midregion of the PTH molecule usually give less consistent results in animals than in human patients. The amino acid sequence of the C-terminal portion of PTH is less well conserved than the N-terminal region between animal species and man, thereby rendering the antibody less specific and the assay less sensitive. It is important to emphasize that the C-terminal fragment in the circulation is biologically inactive and has a longer plasma half-life than the N-terminal end of the PTH molecule. Since the kidney is the organ primarily concerned with the degradation and excretion of the C-terminal and midregion fragments, they tend to accumulate in the serum of animals with renal disease or toxic injury to the kidney. C-terminal assays for PTH in species in which a specific antibody is available tend to give a more integrated evaluation of parathyroid function over time due to the slower turnover rate of this portion of the molecule in the circulation.

REFERENCES

1. Abdo KM, Eustis SL, Haseman J, Huff JE, Peters A, Persing R. Toxicity and carcinogenicity of rotenone given in the feed to F344/N rats and B6C3F1 mice for up to two years. *Drug Chem Toxicol.* 1988;11:225–235.
2. Abou-Samra A, Uneno S, Jüppner H, *et al.* Non-homologous sequences of parathyroid hormone and the parathyroid hormone-related peptide bind to a common receptor on ROS 17/2.8 cells. *Endocrinology.* 1989;125:2215–2217.
3. Abou-Samra A-B, Jüppner H, Force T, *et al.* Expression cloning of a common receptor for parathyroid hormone and parathyroid hormone–related peptide from rat osteoblast-like cells: a single receptor stimulates intracellular accumulation of both cAMP and inositol triphosphates and increases intracellular calcium. *Proc Natl Acad Sci U S A.* 1992;89:2732–2736.
4. Armbrecht HJ, Wongsurawat N, Zenser TV, Davis BB. Differential effects of parathyroid hormone on the renal 125-dihydroxyvitamin D_3 and 24,25-dihydroxyvitamin D_3 production of young and adult rats. *Endocrinology.* 1982;111:1339–1344.
5. Asa SL, Henderson J, Goltzman D, Drucker DJ. Parathyroid hormone-like peptide in normal and neoplastic human endocrine tissues. *J Clin Endocrinol Metab.* 1990;71:1112–1118.
6. Atwal OS. Ultrastructural pathology of ozone-induced experimental parathyroiditis, IV: biphasic activity in the chief cells of regenerating parathyroid glands. *Am J Pathol.* 1979;95:611.
7. Atwal OS, Pemsingh RS. Morphology of microvascular changes and endothelial regeneration in experimental ozone-induced parathyroiditis, III: some pathologic considerations. *Am J Pathol.* 1981;102:297–307.
8. Atwal OS, Wilson T. Parathyroid gland changes following ozone inhalation: a morphologic study. *Arch Environ Health.* 1974;28:91.

9. Atwal OS, Samagh BS, Bhatnagar MK. A possible autoimmune parathyroiditis following ozone inhalation, II: a histopathologic, ultrastructural, and immunofluorescent study. *Am J Pathol.* 1975;80:53.

10. Ayer LM, Szarka RJ, Mortimer ST, *et al.* Analysis of parathyroid hormone in bovine parathyroid cysts. *J Bone Miner Res.* 1989;4:335-340.

11. Barbosa JA, Gill BM, Takiyyuddin MA, O'Connor DT. Chromogranin A: Posttranslational modifications in secretory granules. *Endocrinology.* 1991;128:174–190.

12. Beck N, Singh H, Reed SW, Davis BB. Direct inhibitory effect of hypercalcemia on renal actions of parathyroid hormone. *J Clin Invest.* 1974;53:717–725.

13. Black HE, Capen CC, Arnaud CD. Ultrastructure of parathyroid glands and plasma immunoreactive parathyroid hormone in pregnant cows fed normal and high calcium diets. *Lab Invest.* 1973;29:173–185.

14. Boquist L, Bergdahl L, Andersson Å. Parathyroid adenoma complicated by acute hyperparathyroidism. *Ann Surg.* 1971;173:593–603.

15. Bourdeau AM, Plachot JJ, Gournot-Witmer G, Pointillart A, Balsan S, Sochs C. Parathyroid response to aluminum in vitro: ultrastructural changes and PTH release. *Kidney Int.* 1987;31:15–24.

16. Brandt DW, Burton DW, Gazdar AF, Oie HE, Deftos LJ. All major lung cancer cell types produce parathyroid hormone-like protein: heterogeneity assessed by high performance liquid chromatography. *Endocrinology.* 1991;129:2466–2470.

17. Brown EM. PTH secretion in vivo and in vitro. Regulation by calcium and other secretagogues. *Miner Electrolyte Metab.* 1982; 8:130–150.

18. Burton PBJ, Moniz C, Knight DE. Parathyroid hormone–related peptide can function as an autocrine growth factor in human renal cell carcinoma. *Biochem Biophys Res Commun.* 1990;167:1134–1138.

19. Capen CC. Calcium-regulating hormones and metabolic bone disease. In: Newton CD, Nunamaker DM, eds. *Textbook of Small Animal Orthopaedics.* Philadelphia, Pa: JB Lippincott; 1985:673–722.

20. Capen CC. The endocrine glands. In: Jubb KVF, Kennedy PC, Palmer N, eds. *Pathology of Domestic Animals.* 3rd ed. Orlando, Fla: Academic Press; 1985:238–305.

21. Capen CC. Tumors of the endocrine glands. In: Moulton JE, ed. *Tumors in Domestic Animals.* 3rd ed. Berkeley and Los Angeles, Calif: University of California Press; 1990:553–639.

22. Capen CC, Martin SL. Hyperparathyroidism in animals. In: Kirk RW, ed. *Current Veterinary Therapy, V: Small Animal Practice.* Philadelphia, Pa: WB Saunders, 1974;797–805.

23. Capen CC, Rosol TJ. Calcium regulating hormones and diseases of mineral (calcium, phosphorus, magnesium) metabolism. In: Kaneko JJ, ed. *Clinical Biochemistry of Domestic Animals.* New York, NY: Academic Press; 1989:682–766.

24. Capen CC, Roth SI. Ultrastructural and functional relationships of normal and pathologic parathyroid cells. In: Ioachim HL, ed. *Pathobiology Annual.* New York, NY: Appleton; 1973:129–175.

25. Capen CC, Rowland GN. Ultrastructural evaluation of the parathyroid glands of young cats with experimental hyperparathyroidism. *Z Zellforsch.*

26. Capen CC, Cole CR, Hibbs JW. The influence of vitamin D on calcium metabolism and the parathyroid glands of cattle. *Fed Proc.* 1968;27:142–152.

27. Capen CC, Koestner A, Cole CR. The ultrastructure, histopathology, and histochemistry of the parathyroid glands of pregnant and nonpregnant cows fed a high level of vitamin D. *Lab Invest.* 1965;14:1809–1825.

28. Carillo BJ, Woker NA. Enteque seco: Arteriosclerosis y calcificacion metastasica de origen toxico en animales a pastoreo. *Patologica Animales.* 1967;4:9–11.

29. Caulfield MP, McKee RL, Goldman ME, *et al.* Parathyroid hormone–related protein (PTHrP): studies with synthetic peptides indicate that parathyroid hormone and PTHrP interact with the same receptor. *Nucl Med Biol.* 1990;17:633–637.

30. Chambers TJ. The cellular basis of bone resorption. *Clin Orthop.* 1980;151:283–293.

31. Chambers TJ, Revell PA, Fuller K, Athanasou NA. Resorption of bone by isolated rabbit osteoclasts. *J Cell Sci.* 1984;66:383–399.

32. Chew DJ, Nagode LA, Rosol TJ, Carothers MA, Schenck P. Utility of diagnostic assays in the evaluation of hypercalcemia and hypocalcemia: parathyroid hormone, vitamin D metabolites, parathyroid hormone–related peptide, and ionized calcium. In: Peterson M, ed. *Current Veterinary Therapy, XII: Endocrine and Metabolic Disorders.* Philadelphia, Pa: WB Saunders; 1995:378–383.

33. Chisari FV, Hochstein HD, Kirschstein RL. Parathyroid necrosis and hypocalcemic tetany induced in rabbits by L-asparaginase. *Am J Pathol.* 1972;69:461–476.

34. Cohn DV, Fasciotto BH, Zhang J-X, Gorr, S-U. Chemistry and biology of chromogranin A (secretory protein I) of the parathyroid and other endocrine glands. In: Bilezikian JP, Marcus R, Levine MA, eds. *The Parathyroids: Basic and Clinical Concepts.* New York, NY: Raven Press; 1993:104-119.

35. Cole JA, Eber SL, Poelling RE, Thorne PK, Forte LR. A dual mechanism for regulation of kidney phosphate transport by parathyroid hormone. *Am J Physiol.* 1987;253:E221–E227.
36. Collins WT, Capen CC. Ultrastructural evaluation of parathyroid glands and thyroid C-cells of cattle fed *Solanum malacoxylon. Am J Pathol.* 1977;87:603–614.
37. Cordier AC, Haumont SM. Development of thymus, parathyroids and ultimo branchial bodies in NMRI and nude mice. *Am J Anat.* 1980;157:227–263.
38. Corradino RA, Wasserman RH. 1,25-dihydroxycholecalciferol-like activity of *Solanum malacoxylon* extract on calcium transport. *Nature.* 1974;252:716–720.
39. Danks J, Ebeling P, Hayman J, et al. Parathyroid hormone–related protein: immunohistochemical localization in cancers and in normal skin. *J Bone Miner Res.* 1989;4:273–278.
40. de Vernejoul M-C, Horowitz M, Demignon J, Neff L, Baron R. Bone resorption by isolated chick osteoclasts in culture is stimulated by murine spleen cell supernatant fluids (osteoclast-activating factor) and inhibited by calcitonin and prostaglandin E2. *J Bone Miner Res.* 1988;3:69–80.
41. Dirksen G. Experimental investigations on the etiology of an enzootic calcinosis in cattle. In: Norman AW, Schaffer HG, Grigoleit DV, Herrath ER, eds. *Vitamin D and Problems Related to Uremic Bone Disease.* New York, NY: Walter de Gruyter; 1975:697-698.
42. Döbereiner J, Done SH, Beltran LE. Experimental *Solanum malacoxylon* poisoning in calves. *Br Vet J.* 1975;131:175–185.
43. Döbereiner J, Tokarnia CH, DaCosta JBD, Campos JLE, Dayrell M. "Espichamento", intoxicacao de bovinos por *Solanum malacoxylon,* no pantanal de Mato Gross. *Pesq Agropee Bras (Ser Vet).* 1971;6:91–117.
44. Donahue HJ, Fryer MJ, Eriksen EF, Heath H III. Differential effects of parathyroid hormone and its analogues on cytosolic calcium ion and cAMP levels in cultured rat osteoblast-like cells. *J Biol Chem.* 1988;263:13522–13527.
45. Elliot RL, Arhelger RB. Fine structure of parathyroid adenomas with special reference to annulate lamellae and septate desmosomes. *Arch Pathol Lab Med.* 1966;81:200–212.
46. Ellis HA, Coaker T. Ultrastructure of parathyroid autografts in chronic renal failure including the occurrence of concentric membraneous whorls and intermediate filaments. *Histopathology.* 1989;14:401–407.
47. Faccini JM. Fluoride-induced hyperplasia of the parathyroid glands. *Proc R Soc Med.* 1969;62:241-245.
48. Faccini JM, Care AD. Effect of sodium fluoride on the ultrastructure of the parathryoid glands of the sheep. *Nature.* 1965;207:1399-1401.
49. Farndale RW, Sandy JR, Atkinson SJ, Pennington SR, Meghi S, Meikle MC. Parathyroid hormone and prostaglandin E2 stimulate both inositol phosphates and cyclic AMP accumulation in mouse osteoblast cultures. *Biochem J.* 1988;252:262–268.
50. Fasciotto BH, Gorr S-U, Bourdeau AM, Cohn DV. Autocrine regulation of parathyroid secretion: inhibition of secretion by chromogranin-A (secretory protein-I) and potentiation of secretion by chromogranin-A and pancreastatin antibodies. *Endocrinology.* 1990; 127:1329–1335.
51. Fox J. Regulation of parathyroid hormone secretion by plasma calcium in aging rats. *Am J Physiol 260 (Endocrinol Metab 23)* 1991;E220–E225.
52. Frith CH, Fetters J. Ectopic parathyroid mouse. In: Jones TC, Mohr U, Hunt RD, eds. *Endocrine System.* Berlin, Germany: Springer-Verlag; 1983:263–264.
53. Goltzman D, Hendy GN, Banville D. Parathyroid hormone–like peptide: molecular characterization and biological properties. *Trends Endocrinol Metab.* 1989;1:39–44.
54. Goltzman D, Bennett HPJ, Koutsilieris M, Mitchell J, Rabbani SA, Rouleau MF. Studies of the multiple molecular forms of bioactive parathyroid hormone and parathyroid hormone–like substances. *Recent Prog Horm Res.* 1986;42:665–703.
55. Gröne A, Rosol TJ, Baumgärtner W, Capen CC. Effects of humoral hypercalcemia of malignancy on the parathyroid gland in nude mice. *Vet Pathol.* 1992;29:343–350.
56. Gutierrez GE, Poser JW, Katz MS, Yates AJP, Henry HL, Mundy GR. Mechanisms of hypercalcaemia of malignancy. *Baillières Clin Endocrinol Metab.* 1990;4:119–138.
57. Habener JF. Recent advances in parathyroid hormone research. *Clin Biochem.* 1981;14:223–229.
58. Hanai HM, Ishida M, Liang CT, Sacktor B. Parathyroid hormone increases sodium/calcium exchange activity in renal cells and the blunting of the response in aging. *J Biol Chem.* 1986;261:5419–5425.
59. Haselton PS, Ali HH. The parathyroid in chronic renal failure—a light and electron microscopical study. *J Pathol.* 1980;132:307–323.

60. Haussler MR. 1,25-dihydroxyvitamin D$_3$–glycoside. Identification of a calcinogenic principle of *Solanum malacoxylon*. *Life Sci*. 1976;18:1049–1056.

61. Hayman JA, Danks JA, Ebeling PR, Moseley JM, Kemp BE, Martin TJ. Expression of parathyroid hormone–related protein in normal skin and in tumors of skin and skin appendages. *J Pathol*. 1989;158:293–296.

62. Heath DA, Senior PV, Varley JM, Beck F. Parathyroid hormone–related protein in tumours associated with hypercalcaemia. *Lancet*. Jan 1990;13:66–69.

63. Henderson JE, Shustik C, Kremer R, Rabbani SA, Hendy GN, Goltzman D. Circulating concentrations of parathyroid hormone–like peptide in malignancy and in hyperparathyroidism. *J Bone Miner Res*. 1990;5:105–113.

64. Henry HL. Parathyroid hormone modulation of 25-hydroxyvitamin D$_3$ metabolism by cultured chick kidney cells is mimicked and enhanced by forskolin. *Endocrinology*. 1985;116:503–510.

65. Herrmann-Erlee MPM, van deer Meer JM, Lowik CWGM, van Leeuwen JPTM, Boonekamp PM. Different roles for calcium and cyclic AMP in the action of PTH: studies in bone explants and isolated bone cells. *Bone*. 1988;9:93–100.

66. High WB, Black HE, Capen CC. Histomorphometric evaluation of the effects of low dose parathyroid hormone administration on cortical bone remodeling in adult dogs. *Lab Invest*. 1981;44:449–454.

67. Hruska KA, Moskowitz D, Esbrit P, Civitelli R, Westbrook S, Huskey M. Stimulation of inositol trisphosphate and diacylglycerol production in renal tubular cells by parathyroid hormone. *J Clin Invest*. 1987;79:230–239.

68. Ikeda K, Weir E, Mangin M, *et al*. Expression of messenger ribonucleic acids encoding a parathyroid hormone–like peptide in normal human and animal tissues with abnormal expression in human parathyroid adenomas. *Mol Endocrinol*. 1988;2:1230–1236.

69. Insogna KL. Humoral hypercalcemia of malignancy: the role of parathyroid hormone–related protein. *Endocrinol Metab Clin North Am*. 1989;18:779–794.

70. Isono H, Shoumura S, Ishizaki N, *et al*. Electron microscopic study of the parathyroid gland of the reserpine-treated mouse. *J Clin Electron Microscopy*. 1981;14:113–120.

71. Isono H, Shoumura S, Ishizaki N, *et al*. Effects of glucocorticoid on the ultrastructure of the mouse parathyroid gland. *Arch Histol Jap*. 1983;46:293–305.

72. Isono H, Shoumura S, Ishizaki N, *et al*. Effects of starvation on the ultrastructure of the mouse parathyroid gland. *Acta Anat*. 1985;121:46–52.

73. Jaffe N, Traggis D, Das L, *et al*. Comparison of daily and twice-weekly schedule of L-asparaginase in childhood leukemia. *Pediatrics*. 1972;49:590–595.

74. Jüppner H, Abou-Samra A-B, Freeman M, *et al*. A G protein–linked receptor for parathyroid hormone and parathyroid hormone–related protein. *Science*. 1991;254:1024–1026.

75. Kalu DN, Hardin RR, Murata I, Huber MB, Roos BA. Age-dependent modulation parathyroid hormone action. *Ageing* 1982;5:25–29.

76. Karaplis AC, Yasuda T, Hendy GN, Goltzman D, Banville D. Gene-encoding parathyroid hormone–like peptide: nucleotide sequence of the rat gene and comparison with the human homologue. *Mol Endocrinol*. 1990;4:441–446.

77. Kiebzak GM, Sacktor B. Effect of age on renal conservation of phosphate in the rat. *Am J Physiol 251 (Renal Fluid Electrolyte Physiol 20)*. 1986;F399–F407.

78. Knox FG, Haramati A. Renal regulation of phosphate excretion In: Seldin DW, Giebisch G, eds. *The Kidney: Physiology and Pathophysiology*. New York, NY: Raven Press; 1985.

79. Kramer S, Reynolds FH, Castillo M, Valenzuela DM, Thorikay M, Sorvillo JM. Immunological identification and distribution of parathyroid hormone–like protein polypeptides in normal and malignant tissues. *Endocrinology*. 1991;128:1927–1937.

80. Kronenberg HM, Igarashi T, Freeman MW, *et al*. Structure and expression of the human parathyroid hormone gene. *Recent Prog Horm Res*. 1986;42:641–663.

81. Krook L. Hypercalcemia and calcinosis in Florida horses: implication of the shrub, *Cestrum diurnum*, as the causative agent. *Cornell Vet*. 1975;65:26–56.

82. Kukreja SC, D'Anza JJ, Melton ME, Wimbicus SA, Grill V, Martin TJ. Lack of effects of neutralization of parathyroid hormone–related protein on calcium homeostasis in neonatal mice. *J Bone Miner Res*. 1991;6:1197–1201.

83. Kukreja SC, Rosol TJ, Wimbicus SA, *et al*. Tumor resection and antibodies to parathyroid hormone–related protein cause similar changes on bone histomorphometry in hypercalcemia of cancer. *Endocrinology*. 1990;127:305–310.

84. Kukreja SC, Shevrin DH, Wimbicus SA, *et al*. Antibodies to parathyroid hormone–related protein lower serum calcium in athymic mouse models of malignancy-associated hypercalcemia due to human tumors. *J Clin Invest*. 1988;82:1798–1802.
85. Latta JS, Rutz TJ. Special ultrastructural features of parathyroid cells from Swiss mice bearing Ehrlich's ascites tumor. *Anat Rec*. 1968;160:255–260.
86. Lee DBN, Yanagawa N, Jo O, *et al*. Phosphaturia of aging: studies on mechanisms. *Adv Exp Med Biol*. 1984;178:103–108.
87. Lin HY, Harris TL, Flannery MS, *et al*. Expression cloning of an adenylate cyclase–coupled calcitonin receptor. *Science*. 1991;254:1022–1024.
88. Loveridge N, Dean V, Goltzman D, Hendy GN. Bioactivity of parathyroid hormone and parathyroid hormone–related peptide: agonist and antagonist activities of amino-terminal fragments as assessed by the cytochemical bioassay and in situ hybridization. *Endocrinology*. 1991;128:1938–1946.
89. Lupulescu A, Potorac E, Pop A, *et al*. Experimental investigation on immunology of the parathyroid gland. *Immunology*. 1968;14:475.
90. MacIsaac RJ, Heath JA, Rodda CP, *et al*. Role of the fetal parathyroid glands and parathyroid hormone–related protein in the regulation of placental transport of calcium, magnesium, and inorganic phosphate. *Reprod Fertil Dev*. 1991;3:447–457.
91. Mallette LE. The parathyroid polyhormones: new concepts in the spectrum of peptide hormone action. *Endocr Rev*. 1991;12:110–117.
92. Mangin M, Ikeda K, Broadus AE. Structure of the mouse gene encoding parathyroid hormone–related protein. *Gene*. 1990;95:195–202.
93. Mangin M, Ikeda K, Dreyer BE, Broadus AE. Identification of an up-stream promoter of the human parathyroid hormone–related peptide gene. *Mol Endocrinol*. 1990;4:851–858.
94. Mangin M, Ikeda K, Dreyer BE, Milstone L, Broadus AE. Two distinct tumor-derived, parathyroid hormone–like peptides result from alternative ribonucleic acid splicing. *Mol Endocrinol*. 1988;2:1049–1055.
95. Mangin M, Webb AC, Dreyer BE, *et al*. Identification of a cDNA encoding a parathyroid hormone–like peptide from a human tumor associated with humoral hypercalcemia of malignancy. *Proc Natl Acad Sci U S A*. 1988;85:597–601.
96. Martin TJ. Humoral hypercalcemia of malignancy. *Horm Res*. 1989;32:84–88.
97. Martin TJ, Allan EH, Caple IW, *et al*. Parathyroid hormone–related protein: isolation, molecular cloning, and mechanism of action. *Recent Prog Horm Res*. 1989;45:467–506.
98. Mayer GP, Hurst JG. Comparison of the effects of calcium and magnesium on parathyroid hormone secretion rate in calves. *Endocrinology*. 1978;102:1803–1807.
99. McSheehy PM, Chambers TJ. Osteoblastic cells mediate osteoclastic responsiveness to parathyroid hormone. *Endocrinology*. 1986;118:824–828.
100. Merryman JI, Rosol TJ, Brooks CL, Capen CC. Separation of parathyroid hormone–like activity from transforming growth factor -α and -β in the canine adenocarcinoma (CAC-8) model of humoral hypercalcemia of malignancy. *Endocrinology*. 1989;124:2456–2563.
101. Meuten DJ, Cooper BJ, Capen CC, Chew DJ, Kociba GJ. Hypercalcemia associated with an adenocarcinoma derived from the apocrine glands of the anal sac. *Vet Pathol*. 1981;18:454–471.
102. Meuten DJ, Kociba GJ, Capen CC, *et al*. Hypercalcemia in dogs with lymphosarcoma: biochemical, ultrastructural, and histomorphometric investigations. *Lab Invest*. 1983;49:553–562.
103. Meuten DJ, Segre GV, Capen CC, *et al*. Hypercalcemia in dogs with adenocarcinoma derived from apocrine glands of the anal sac: biochemical and histomorphometric investigations. *Lab Invest*. 1983;48:428–435.
104. Morrissey J, Slatopolsky E. Effect of aluminum on parathryoid hormone secretion. *Kidney Int*. 1986;29:S41–S44.
105. Morrissey J, Rothstein M. Mayor G, Slatopolsky E. Suppression of parathyroid hormone secretion by aluminum. *Kidney Int*. 1983;23:699–704.
106. Moseley JM, Hayman JA, Danks JA, *et al*. Immunohistochemical detection of parathyroid hormone–related protein in human fetal epithelia. *J Clin Endocrinol Metab*. 1991;73:478–484.
107. Moseley JM, Kubota M, Diefenbach-Jagger H, *et al*. Parathyroid hormone–related protein purified from a human lung cancer cell line. *Proc Natl Acad Sci U S A*. 1987;84:5048–5052.
108. Mundy GR. Hypercalcemia of malignancy revisited. *J Clin Invest*. 1988;82:1–6.
109. Mundy GR. Hypercalcemic factors other than parathyroid hormone–related protein. *Endocrinol Metab Clin North Am*. 1989;18:795–806.

110. Mundy GR. Pathophysiology of cancer-associated hypercalcemia. *Semin Oncol.* 1990;17:10–15.

111. Mundy GR, Ibbotson KJ, D'Souza SM, Simpson EL, Jacobs JW, Martin TJ. The hypercalcemia of cancer. Clinical implications and pathogenic mechanisms. *N Engl J Med.* 1984;310:1718–1727.

112. Nemere I, Norman AW. Parathyroid hormone stimulates calcium transport in perfused duodena from normal chicks. Comparison with the rapid (transcaltachic) effect of 1,25-dihydroxyvitamin D_3. *Endocrinology.* 1986;119:1406–1408.

113. Oettgen HF, *et al.* Toxicity of E. coli L-asparaginase in man. *Cancer.* 1970;25:253–278.

114. Orloff JJ, Wu TL, Stewart AF. Parathyroid hormone–like proteins: biochemical responses and receptor interactions. *Endocr Rev.* 1989;10:476–494.

115. Oslapas R, Prinz R, Ernst K, *et al.* Incidence of radiation-induced parathyroid tumors in male and female rats. *Clin Res.* 1981;29:734A.

116. Oslapas R, Shah KH, Hoffman C, *et al.* Effect of gonadectomy on the incidence of radiation-induced parathyroid tumors in male and female rats. *Clin Res.* 1982;30:401A.

117. Pliam NB, Nyiredy KO, Arnaud CD. Parathyroid hormone receptors in avian bone cells. *Proc Natl Acad Sci U S A.* 1982;79:2061–2063.

118. Pour PM, Qureshi SR, Salmasi S. Anatomy, histology, ultrastructure, parathyroid, mouse. In: Jones TC, Mohr U, Hunt RD, eds. *Endocrine System.* Berlin, Germany: Springer-Verlag; 1983;252–257.

119. Proscal DA. 1,25-dihydroxyvitamin D_3–like component present in the plant *Solanum glaucophyllum*. *Endocrinology.* 1976;99:437–444.

120. Rabbani SA, Mitchell J, Roy DR, Hendy GN, Goltzman D. Influence of the amino-terminus on in vitro and in vivo biological activity of synthetic parathyroid hormone–like peptides of malignancy. *Endocrinology.* 1988;123:2709–2716.

121. Raisz LG, Kream BE. Regulation of bone formation. *New Engl J Med.* 1983;309:83–89.

122. Ratcliffe WA, Norbury S, Stott RA, Heath DA, Ratcliffe JG. Immunoreactivity of plasma parathyrin–related peptide: three region-specific radioimmunoassays and a two-site immunoradiometric assay compared. *Clin Chem.* 1991;37:1781–1787.

123. Ream LJ, Principato R. Glycogen accumulation in the parathyroid gland of the rat after fluoride ingestion. *Cell Tissue Res.* 1981;220:125–130.

124. Rijnberk A, Elsinghorst AM, Koeman JP, Hackeng WHL, Lequin RM. Pseudohyperparathyroidism associated with perirectal adenocarcinomas in elderly female dogs. *Tijdschr Diergeneeskd.* 1978;103:1069–1075.

125. Rodan GA, Martin TJ. Role of osteoblasts in hormonal control of bone resorption—a hypothesis. *Calcif Tissue Int.* 1981;33:349–351.

126. Rosol TJ, Capen CC. The effect of low calcium diet, mithramycin, and dichlorodimethylene bisphosphonate on humoral hypercalcemia of malignancy in nude mice transplanted with the canine adenocarcinoma tumor line (CAC-8). *J Bone Miner Res.* 1987;2:395–405.

127. Rosol TJ, Capen CC. Inhibition of in vitro bone resorption by a parathyroid hormone receptor antagonist in the canine adenocarcinoma model of humoral hypercalcemia of malignancy. *Endocrinology.* 1988;122:2098–2102.

128. Rosol TJ, Capen CC. Biology of disease: mechanisms of cancer-induced hypercalcemia. *Lab Invest.* 1992;67:680–702.

129. Rosol TJ, Capen CC, Brooks CL. Bone and kidney adenylate cyclase–stimulating activity produced by a hypercalcemic canine adenocarcinoma line (CAC-8) maintained in nude mice. *Cancer Res.* 1987;47:690–695.

130. Rosol TJ, Capen CC, Horst RL. Effects of infusion of human parathyroid hormone–related protein (1-40) in nude mice: histomorphometric and biochemical investigations. *J Bone Miner Res.* 1988;3:699–706.

131. Rosol TJ, Capen CC, Deftos LJ, Horst RL. Nude mouse model (CAC-8) of humoral hypercalcemia of malignancy with increased serum levels of 1,25-dihyroxycholecalciferol: in vivo and in vitro studies. In: Norman AW, Schaefer K, Grigoleit HG, Herrath DV, eds. *Vitamin D–1988: Molecular, Cellular and Clinical Endocrinology.* Berlin, Germany: Walter de Gruyter; 1988;867–868.

132. Rosol TJ, Capen CC, Weisbrode SE, Horst RL. Humoral hypercalcemia of malignancy in nude mouse model of a canine adenocarcinoma derived from apocrine glands of the anal sac. *Lab Invest.* 1986;54:679–688.

133. Rosol TJ, Capen CC, Danks JA, *et al.* Identification of parathyroid hormone–related protein in canine apocrine adenocarcinoma of the anal sac. *Vet Pathol.* 1990;27:89–95.

134. Rosol TJ, Nagode LA, Couto CG, *et al.* Parathyroid hormone (PTH)–related protein, PTH, and 1,25-dihydroxyvitamin D in dogs with cancer-associated hypercalcemia. *Endocrinology.* 1992; 131:1157–1164.

135. Roth SI, Raisz LG. Effect of calcium concentration on the ultrastructure of rat parathyroid in organ culture. *Lab Invest.* 1964;13:331–345.

136. Schermer DT, Chan SDH, Bruce R, Nissenson RA, Wood WI, Strewler GJ. Chicken parathyroid hormone–related protein and its expression during embryologic development. *J Bone Miner Res.* 1991;6:149–155.

137. Selvanayagam P, Graves K, Cooper C, Rajaraman S. Expression of the parathyroid hormone–related peptide gene in rat tissues. *Lab Invest.* 1991;64:713–717.

138. Shaw AJ, Mughal MZ, Maresh MJA, Sibley CP. Effects of two synthetic parathyroid hormone–related protein fragments on maternofetal transfer of calcium and magnesium and release of cyclic AMP by the in-situ perfused rat placenta. *J Endocrinol.* 1991;129:399–404.

139. Silve CM, Hradek GT, Jones AL, Arnaud CD. Parathyroid hormone receptor in intact embryonic chicken bone: characterization and cellular localization. *J Cell Biol.* 1982;94:379–386.

140. Smith C, Clifford CP. Histochemical study of aberrant parathyroids associated with the thymus of the mouse. *Anat Rec.* 1962;143:229–237.

141. Solleveld HA, Haseman JK, McConnell EE. National history of body weight gain, survival and neoplasia in the F344 rat. *J Natl Cancer Inst.* 1984;72:929-940.

142. Stewart AF, Broadus AE. Clinical review 16: parathyroid hormone–related proteins: coming of age in the 1990's. *J Clin Endocrinol Metab.* 1990;71:1410–1414.

143. Strewler GJ, Nissenson RA. Nonparathyroid hypercalcemia. *Adv Intern Med.* 1987;32:235–258.

144. Strewler GJ, Stern PH, Jacobs JW, *et al.* Parathyroid hormonelike protein from human renal carcinoma cells: structural and functional homology with parathyroid hormone. *J Clin Invest.* 1987;80:1803–1807.

145. Sutton RAL, Dirks JH. Renal handling of calcium. *Fed Proc.* 1978;37:2112–2119.

146. Suva LJ, Mather KA, Gillespie MT, *et al.*. Structure of the 5' flanking region of the gene encoding human parathyroid-hormone–related protein (PTHrP). *Gene.* 1989;77:95–105.

147. Suva LJ, Winslow GA, Wettenhall REH, *et al.* A parathyroid hormone–related protein implicated in malignant hypercalcemia: cloning and expression. *Science.* 1987;237:893–896.

148. Teotia SPS, Teotia M. Secondary hyperparathyroidism in patients with endemic fluorosis. *Br Med J.* 1973;1:637-640.

149. Tettenborn D, Hobik HP, Luckhaus G. Hypoparathyroidismus beim Kaninchen nach Verabreichung von L-asparaginase. *Arzneimittelforschung.* 1970;20:1753–1755.

150. Thiede MA, Strewler GJ, Nissenson RA, Rosenblatt M, Rodan GA. Human renal carcinoma expresses two messages encoding a parathyroid hormone–like peptide: evidence for the alternative splicing of a single copy gene. *Proc Natl Acad Sci U S A.* 1988;85:4605–4609.

151. Thiede MA, Daifotis AG, Weir EC, *et al.* Intrauterine occupancy controls expression of the parthyroid hormone–related peptide gene in preterm rat myometrium. *Proc Natl Acad Sci U S A.* 1990;87:6969–6973.

152. Thurston AW, Cole JA, Hillman LS, *et al.* Purification and properties of parathyroid hormone–related peptide isolated from milk. *Endocrinology.* 1990;126:1183–1190.

153. Uden P, Halloran B, Daly R, Duh Q-Y, Clark O. Set-point for parathyroid hormone release increases with postmaturational aging in the rat. *Endocrinology.* 1992;131:2251–2256.

154. Vaes G. Cellular biology and biochemical mechanism of bone resorption: a review of recent developments on the formation, activation, and mode of action of osteoclasts. *Clin Orthop.* 1988;231:239–271.

155. Wada L, Daly R, Kern D, Halloran B. Kinetics of 1,25-dihydroxyvitamin D metabolism in the aging rat. *Am J Physiol 262 (Endocrinol Metab 25)* 1992;E906–E910.

156. Wasserman MR. Calcinogenic factor in *Solanum malacoxylon: evidence that it is a 1,25-dihydroxyvitamin D₃-glycoside. Science.* 1976;194:853–855.

157. Wasserman RH. Active vitamin D–like substances in *Solanum malacoxylon* and other calcinogenic plants. *Nutr Rev.* 1975;33:1–5.

158. Wasserman RH, Corradino RA, Krook L. *Cestrum diurnum: a domestic plant with 1,25-dihydroxycholecalciferol-like activity.* Biochem Biophys Res Commun. 1975;62:85–91.

159. Weir EC, Norrdin RW, Matus RE, *et al.* Humoral hypercalcemia of malignancy in canine lymphosarcoma. *Endocrinology.* 1988;122:602–608.

160. Wild P, Gloor S, Vetsch E. Quantitative aspects of membrane behavior in rat parathyroid cells after depression or elevation of serum calcium. *Lab Invest.* 1985;52:490–496.

161. Wong GL. Skeletal effects of parathyroid hormone. In: Peck WA, ed. *Bone and Mineral Research.* 4th ed. Amsterdam, the Netherlands: Elsevier Science Publishers; 1986:103–129.

162. Wongsurawat N, Armbrecht HJ. Comparison of calcium effect on in vitro calcitonin and parathyroid hormone release by young and aged thyroparathyroid glands. *Exp Gerontol.* 1987;22:263–269.

163. Wynford-Thomas V, Wynford-Thomas D, Williams ED. Experimental induction of parathyroid adenomas in the rat. *J Natl Cancer Inst.* 1982;70:127–134.

164. Yamaguchi DT, Kleeman CR, Muallem S. Protein kinase C–activated calcium channel in the osteoblast-like clonal osteosarcoma cell line UMR-106. *J Biol Chem.* 1987;262:14967–14973.

165. Yamamoto M, Fisher JE, Thiede MA, Caulfield MP, Rosenblatt M, Duong LT. Concentrations of parathyroid hormone–related protein in rat milk change with duration of lactation and interval from previous suckling, but not with milk calcium. *Endocrinology.* 1992;130:741–747.

166. Yamamoto M, Duong LT, Fisher JE, et al. Suckling-mediated increases in urinary phosphate and 3',5'-cyclic adenosine monophosphate excretion in lactating rats: possible systemic effects in parathyroid hormone–related protein. *Endocrinology.* 1991;129:2614–2622.

167. Yasuda T, Banville D, Rabbani S, Hendy G, Goltzman D. Rat parathyroid hormone–like peptide: comparison with the human homologue and expression in malignant and normal tissue. *Mol Endocrinol.* 1989;3:518–525.

168. Young DM, Olson HM, Prieur DJ, Cooney DA, Reagan RL. Clinicopathologic and ultrastructural studies of L-asparaginase–induced hypocalcemia in rabbits: an experimental animal model of acute hypoparathyroidism. *Lab Invest.* 1973;29:374–386.

Endocrine Toxicology, 2nd ed.,
Edited by J. A. Thomas and H. D. Colby
Copyright © 1997 Taylor & Francis

2

Physiology of the Thyroid Gland and Agents Affecting Its Secretion

John M. Connors

Department of Physiology, West Virginia University
Robert C. Byrd Health Sciences Center, Morgantown, West Virginia 26506-9229

THYROID GLAND AND THYROID HORMONES

The thyroid gland of mammals synthesizes and releases three hormones: thyroxine (tetraiodothyronine [T_4]), triiodothyronine (T_3), and calcitonin. Structurally related and iodine-containing, T_4 and T_3 are the products of epithelial cells that make up the spherical thyroid follicles. These hormones influence the metabolic level in most tissues and are required for normal growth and differentiation. The single-chain polypeptide calcitonin, the product of the parafollicular C cells of the thyroid gland, is involved in the regulation of serum calcium homeostasis. The focus of this chapter will be on the physiology of thyroid gland secretion of T_4 and T_3 and common disorders affecting the thyroid gland.

Both T_4 and T_3 are amino acids with a unique diphenyl ether structure that contains the element iodine (Fig. 1). Thus, the long-term maintenance of the synthesis of T_4 and T_3 requires a dietary source of iodine. These iodinated hormones are stored within the thyroid follicles as integral amino acid units within the large protein thyroglobulin but exist in the blood noncovalently bound to plasma proteins. Under normal conditions, T_4 is synthesized and secreted from the thyroid gland in greater quantities than T_3. Although T_3 is also secreted in significant quantities by the thyroid gland, the majority of the circulating T_3 arises from the extrathyroidal monodeiodination of T_4.

T_4 and T_3 exert important, but not necessarily identical, effects on most tissues in the body. They appear to be required for the optimal functioning of several other hormones, including the catecholamines, corticosteroids, and antidiuretic hormone (vasopressin). Inadequate or excessive circulating levels of these thyroid hormones result in the conditions of hypothyroidism or hyperthyroidism, respectively. Thyroid dysfunction can produce dramatic changes in cardiovascular, gastrointestinal, skeletal, neuromuscular, and reproductive systems, as well as alterations in the pattern of growth and development.

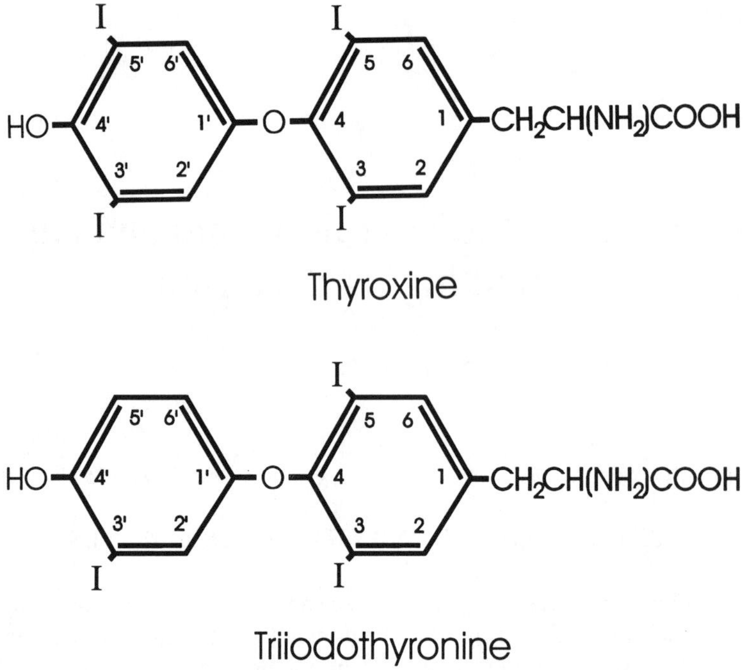

Thyroxine

Triiodothyronine

FIG 1. Structure of thyroxine (T_4) and triiodothyronine (T_3)

Biosynthesis, Storage, and Secretion of Thyroid Hormones

The functional unit of the thyroid gland is the thyroid follicle (see below). The thyroid follicular cells synthesize thyroid hormones by iodinating tyrosyl residues contained within the large glycoprotein thyroglobulin to form iodotyrosyl residues (monoiodotyrosine and diiodotyrosine) and then by coupling two iodotyrosyl residues to yield the iodothyronine hormones, T_4 and T_3. The requirement for iodide for thyroid hormone synthesis makes an adequate dietary intake of iodine necessary. Dietary iodine (I_2) is reduced to the oxidative level of iodide (I-) before virtually complete absorption in the small intestine.

The synthesis and secretion of thyroid hormones involve a series of biochemical steps in thyroid follicles that include the following:

1. Active transport of iodine across the follicular epithelium and concentration in the follicular lumen.
2. Thyroglobulin synthesis within the follicle cells and secretion into the follicular lumen.
3. Synthesis of the enzyme thyroperoxidase, generation of hydrogen peroxide (H_2O_2), and translocation to the apical cell membrane (facing the follicular lumen).

4. Oxidation of iodide and iodination of tyrosyl residues of thyroglobulin to form iodotyrosyl residues at the apical cell membrane.
5. Coupling of iodotyrosyl residues of thyroglobulin to form the iodothyronines T_4 and T_3 within the follicle.
6. Uptake of thyroglobulin from the follicular lumen into the follicle cells and the proteolysis of thyroglobulin to release free iodotyrosines and iodothyronines.
7. Secretion of T_4 and T_3 across the basal membrane and into the blood.

Each of these steps is stimulated by thyrotropin (thyroid stimulating hormone [TSH]) from the anterior pituitary gland. These steps may be compromised by iodine deficiency or disease and can also be blocked selectively by a variety of chemicals and drugs.

Biosynthetic Pathway

Iodide Transport

A characteristic feature of the thyroid gland is the organization of epithelial cells into follicles. Each follicle is a spherical, cyst-like structure composed of a single layer of epithelial cells enclosing the follicular lumen. The follicular lumen is filled with a proteinaceous solution, the follicular colloid. Adjacent follicle cells are connected by tight junctions (zonulae occludentes) that bind the cells together and make the epithelium a tight monolayer separating the follicular lumen from the extrafollicular space. These follicular epithelial cells are polarized; that is, the apical plasma membrane (facing the follicular lumen) and the basolateral membrane differ. Structurally, only the apical membrane displays microvilli and pseudopods that extend into the follicular lumen. In addition, the apical and basolateral membranes differ in their enzyme components; thyroperoxidase, aminopeptidase, and H_2O_2-generating activities occur only at the apical membrane, while an iodide-carrier protein and Na^+-K^+ adenosine triphosphatase (ATP-ase) are located only at the basolateral membrane.

The thyroid gland has the ability to take up iodide (I-) from the circulation and to concentrate it within the thyroid follicles. The iodide that accumulates within the follicular lumen is rapidly bound to proteins and to a lesser extent to lipids; accordingly, it exists in the follicular lumen as both inorganic iodide and organically bound iodine. The iodide-concentrating mechanism of the thyroid includes two major processes: the influx of iodide across the basal membrane of the thyroid follicular cell and the efflux of the iodide across the apical membrane into the follicular lumen. Although iodide accumulates within the cells prior to its entry into the follicular lumen (2,50), the concentration of iodide in the lumen is higher than in the follicle cells (14). Iodide moves down an electrical gradient from the cell to the follicular lumen. The potential difference across the basal plasma membrane of the follicular cell is −40 to −60 mV, with the interior of the cell negative, and a potential difference between the extracellular space and the follicular lumen is 0 to -10 mV (69,79).

The follicular architecture is not a prerequisite for iodide transport into the thyroid cell, and iodide accumulates within thyroid cells against a chemical and electrical gradient; energy is required for the transport. The active transport of iodide across the basal plasma membrane ("iodide trapping") appears to be accomplished by "Na^+-dependent secondary active transport" involving a carrier of iodide and a Na^+-K^+ ATPase pump in the plasma membrane (66). In this model, the plasma membrane carrier forms a binary complex with Na^+ on the external surface of the cell and then a ternary complex with iodide or another anion. The complex is translocated across the cell membrane and both Na^+ and iodide may diffuse off the carrier inside the cell. The Na^+-K^+ ATPase located in the basal membrane extrudes the Na^+, which enters the cell and establishes and maintains a very high Na^+ gradient, trapping the iodide inside the cell. It has been suggested that the carrier requires two Na^+ ions to transport one anion (I-) into the cell (53).

After the accumulation of iodide within the thyroid follicle cell, the cell's apical membrane acts as a permeability barrier to the movement of iodide down its electrical gradient into the follicular lumen. The iodide concentration in the follicular lumen is higher than that in the thyroid cells. The permeability of the apical membrane may be modulated by TSH and autoregulatory processes.

TSH is an important regulating variable for iodide transport. It appears to stimulate iodide accumulation by the induction of a carrier or an enzyme required in the energy-dependent iodide transport (36,78) across the basal plasma membrane. The permeability of the apical membrane to iodide may also be influenced by TSH. Andros and Wollman (2) suggest that the diffusion rate across this membrane may be a function of the level of TSH stimulation. TSH also induces a decrease in the transepithelial potential difference, facilitating the movement of iodide across the thyroid follicle cell into the follicular lumen (80,84). A similar effect is observed in response to low dietary iodine (37).

According to Wolff (81), inhibitors of iodide transport can be divided into three categories: (1) metabolic, (2) transport, and (3) competitive.

Metabolic inhibitors include inhibitors of the respiratory chain (rotenone, amobarbitol [Amytal], oligomycin, citrinin [Antimycin]) and of oxidative processes (CN^-, azide), as well as uncouplers of oxidative phosphorylation (2,4-dinitrophenol, dicumarol), SH reagents, and numerous quinones. These agents lower the cellular ATP concentration and are effective inhibitors of iodide accumulation (81).

Ouabain and other cardiac glycosides are classified as transport inhibitors because of their inhibitory effect on Na^+-K^+ ATPase. In the presence of ouabain, the intracellular Na^+ concentration increases and interferes with the unloading of iodide from the membrane carrier or enhances its efflux across the basal membrane (83).

Anions that competitively inhibit iodide accumulation in the thyroid include halides (bromide, Br^-), pseudohalides (cyanate, OCN^-; thiocyanate, SCN^-; selenocyanate, $SeCN^-$), and complex anions (perchlorate, ClO_4^-; pertechnetate, TcO_4^-; perrhenate, ReO_4^-).

Synthesis of Thyroglobulin

TSH regulates the expression of the thyroglobulin gene (1,6,8,76). Thyroglobulin is synthesized in the rough endoplasmic reticulum of the follicle cells and transported via the Golgi complex to exocytic vesicles. During its intracellular transport in an apical direction, thyroglobulin undergoes several post-translational modifications, including glycosylation, phosphorylation, and sulfation; however, it contains no hormones. It is released from the exocytotic vesicles across the apical membrane into the follicular lumen. The thyroid hormones are formed in the follicular lumen in close association with the apical plasma membrane. Formation occurs by the binding of iodine to tyrosyl residues in the thyroglobulin and the coupling of iodotyrosyls to form T_4 and T_3.

Oxidation of Iodide, Iodination of Thyroglobulin, and Coupling of Iodotyrosyls to Form T_4 and T_3

The binding of iodine to thyroglobulin and the subsequent formation of thyroid hormones can be considered to represent the last post-translational modifications of the thyroglobulin molecule. Both the iodination of tyrosyl residues and the coupling reactions are oxidative, catalyzed by thyroperoxidase (TPO) in the presence of H_2O_2. TPO is synthesized on attached ribosomes, inserted in the rough endoplasmic reticulum membrane facing the lumen, and transferred to the apical cell surface via the Golgi complex and exocytic vesicles. The fusion of the exocytic vesicles with the apical plasma membrane in the process of exocytosis results in the orientation of TPO toward the external surface of the apical plasma membrane (ie, the surface facing the follicular lumen). The thyroid follicle cells also have the ability to generate the required H_2O_2 by utilizing an NADPH oxidase located in the apical plasma membrane.

The iodide entering the follicular lumen must be oxidized before it is linked to tyrosyl residues present in thyroglobulin. This oxidation to a higher oxidation state is catalyzed by TPO in the presence of H_2O_2 (which serves as an electron acceptor) to yield the iodinating intermediate, TPO-I_{ox}. Iodide is oxidized in a one- or two-electron transfer process. However, at this time it is not yet clear to which oxidation state iodide is oxidized in vivo. Four different oxidized iodine species are considered possible iodinating species: (1) molecular iodine (I_2), (2) iodine free radical (I^*), (3) iodinium ion (I^-), and (4) hypoiodite (IO^-). Therefore, at least four mechanisms for iodination must be considered.

In reactions with peroxidases, two compounds (I and II) are obligatory intermediates (76). In the presence of H_2O_2, TPO forms the following:

$$TPO + H_2O_2 \rightarrow Compound\ I.$$

Compound I contains two equivalents of oxidation and is able to oxidize either two monoelectron (or monohydrogen) donors

$$\text{Compound I} + X^n \rightarrow \text{Compound II} + X^{n+1}$$
$$\text{Compound II} + X^n \rightarrow \text{TPO} + X^{n+1}$$

or one dihydrogen (or dielectron) donor

$$\text{Compound I} + XH_2 \rightarrow \text{Compound II } XH^*$$
$$\text{Compound II } XH^* \rightarrow \text{TPO} + X.$$

TPO may catalyze the oxidation of iodide to I_2 in a one-electron transfer, in which I^* is formed, or in a two electron transfer, in which I^- is formed. Either I^* or I^- can then form I_2. I_2 can be utilized to iodinate tyrosine and tyrosine residues in proteins in vitro. It was long believed to be involved in the iodination of tyrosyl residues in thyroglobulin in a chemical iodination reaction, with the only role for TPO being to produce I_2. However, this reaction is unlikely to occur under in vivo conditions because I_2 reacts only with the phenoxide form of tyrosine, which requires an alkaline pH for its formation (44). It has also been demonstrated that a competition exists between I_2 formation and iodination, making it unlikely that I_2 is the iodinating species (57,72).

If I^* is the oxidizing species, tyrosine must also be oxidized in a one-electron transfer process, resulting in a tyrosine radical (Tyr*). It is hypothesized that both iodide and tyrosine (or tyrosyl residues in thyroglobulin) bind to TPO to form a intermediary ternary complex to accomplish the oxidation and binding to form iodotyrosines (eg, monoiodotyrosine [MIT] and diiodotyrosine [DIT]) (35):

$$\text{Compound I} + I^- + \text{Tyr} \rightarrow \text{TPO-Tyr}^*\text{-I}^* \text{ complex} \rightarrow \text{TPO} + \text{MIT}.$$

If the iodinium ion (I^-) is the iodinating species, then it may react at neutral pH with nonoxidized tyrosine (47). In this scenario, iodide may be oxidized in a two-electron transfer process to I^- bound to TPO without any detectable production of compound II (5,62):

$$\text{Compound I} + I^- + \text{Tyr} \rightarrow \text{TPO-I}^* \text{ complex} + \text{Tyr} \rightarrow \text{TPO} + \text{MIT}.$$

Another possible iodination mechanism has been suggested in which iodide is oxidized by an iodine compound to form an enzyme-bound hypoiodite (IO^-), in which iodine is present in an oxidation state equivalent to I^+ and can (a) react with H_2O_2, (b) be involved in iodination of tyrosine, or (c) take part in oxidation of iodide to I_2 (43):

$$\text{(a) Compound I} + I^- + H_2O_2 \rightarrow \text{Compound I-I}^- \text{ complex}$$
$$+ H_2O_2 \rightarrow O_2 + H_2O + I^- + \text{TPO}$$

$$\text{(b) Compound I} + I^- + \text{Tyr} \rightarrow \text{Compound I-I}^- \text{ complex}$$
$$+ \text{Tyr} \rightarrow \text{MIT} + OH^- + \text{TPO}$$

$$\text{(c) Compound I} + 2I^- + H_2O \rightarrow \text{Compound I-I}^- \text{ complex}$$
$$+ I^- + H_2O \rightarrow I_2 + 2OH^- + \text{TPO}$$

Within the thyroid gland, coupling of iodotyrosines (MIT and DIT) of thyroglobulin to form the thyroid hormones (T_4 and T_3) is also catalyzed by TPO. As first proposed by Johnson and Tewkesbury (34), it is most likely that this involves an intramolecular, free radical mechanism. Taurog (73) extended this hypothesis to be compatible with TPO-catalyzed iodination. The proposed coupling reaction is composed of three steps: (1) oxidation of iodotyrosyl residues to an activated form by TPO; (2) coupling of activated iodotyrosyl residues within the same thyroglobulin molecule to form a quinol ether intermediate; and (3) splitting of the quinol ether to form an iodothyronine residue.

In the first step of the coupling reaction, iodotyrosyl residues in thyroglobulin are activated by TPO. As in the case of iodination of tyrosyl residues, this may occur by univalent or divalent oxidation. With univalent oxidation, two hormonogenic iodotyrosine residues are oxidized to iodotyrosyl free radicals:

$$\text{Compound I} + \text{iodo-Tyr}^- \rightarrow \text{Compound II} + \text{iodo-Tyr}^*$$
$$\text{Compound II} + \text{iodo-Tyr}^- \rightarrow \text{TPO} + \text{iodo-Tyr}^*$$

These two iodotyrosyl radicals form a hormone residue:

$$\text{Iodo-Tyr}^* + \text{iodo-Tyr}^* \rightarrow \text{iodothyronine}.$$

In the divalent oxidation, a single iodotyrosyl residue is oxidized to a cation:

$$\text{Compound I} + \text{iodo-Tyr}^- \rightarrow \text{TPO} + \text{iodo-Tyr}^+.$$

This cation may form a hormone residue by combining with an unoxidized iodotyrosyl residue

$$\text{Iodo-Tyr}^+ + \text{iodo-Tyr}^- \rightarrow \text{iodothyronine}.$$

For both types of reaction, two equivalents of oxidation are probably required, as is the case for the iodination of tyrosyl residues.

Thyroglobulin is a large dimeric protein composed of two identical glycosylated peptides of approximately 300 kd each. Each polypeptide chain contains about 70 tyrosyl residues, a number that does not differ significantly from the average tyrosine content of all proteins observed in a protein data bank (45). Of the 140 tyrosyl residues per molecule of thyroglobulin, only about 40 may be iodinated. Only a few of the iodinated tyrosyl residues in each of the peptide chains are actually involved in hormone synthesis. Within each of the chains, a single T_3 site is located at the carboxyl end; a single T_4 site is located at the amino end, and two additional T_4 sites are located around position 2500. In the coupling of two iodotyrosyl residues, one iodotyrosyl is the acceptor of the iodophenyl group to form the outer ring of the iodothyronine in hormone synthesis, and the other is the donor. Loss of the iodophenyl group converts the iodotyrosyl residue into an alanine, which is converted to dehydroalanine and remains within the thyroglobulin structure. Whereas all the acceptor tyrosines are identified in the primary structure, little is known about the donor tyrosines.

TSH increases the rate of thyroglobulin iodination and hormone formation by increasing the presence of all four components required for thyroglobulin iodination and coupling at the apical cell surface. Namely, it increases (1) the NADPH-dependent generation of H_2O_2 at the apical plasma membrane; (2) the accumulation of iodide in the follicular lumen; (3) the activity of TPO at the apical plasma membrane; and (4) the synthesis and secretion of thyroglobulin across the apical membrane into the follicular lumen. Thus, hormone synthesis is also increased.

Inhibitors of TPO-catalyzed iodination of thyroglobulin and the coupling of iodotyrosyl residues have proven to be clinically useful antithyroid compounds. The most potent inhibitors are the thionamides,

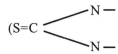

which have no effect on the iodide trap or on thyroid hormone release. Of the thionamides, the thioureylenes

$$(S{=}C \diagup\diagdown \begin{matrix} N- \\ N- \end{matrix}$$

have been found to be the most useful clinically. In particular, two heterocyclic derivatives of thiourea, propylthiouracil (6-propyl-2-thiouracil) and methimazole (1-methyl-2-mercaptoimidazole), are widely used to treat hyperthyroidism. Another drug, carbimazole (1-methyl-2-mercapto-3-carbethoxyimidazole), used mainly in Europe, is metabolized to methimazole in vivo. Goitrin (L-5-vinyl-2-thiooxazolidone), found in plant species of the cabbage family (*Brassica*), also inhibits organification of iodide and coupling of iodotyrosyl residues and may cause hypothyroidism if ingested in sufficient quantities. These agents are thought to serve as substrates for the iodinating intermediate, TPO-I_{ox}, and are themselves oxidized and ultimately metabolized (11,17). In the process, TPO-I_{ox} is depleted and less is available for tyrosine iodination and hormone biosynthesis (74).

Resorcinol (1,3-dihydroxybenzene) is the prototype of a number of phenolic compounds that also inhibit TPO-catalyzed iodination (see ref. 23 for review). These compounds may be present in community water supplies, particularly in coal-rich areas of the world, and serve as an environmental goitrogen. Phthalate esters and phthalaitic acids are also common industrial water pollutants that undergo biodegradation to form dihydroxybenzoic acid derivatives that also inhibit TPO.

Hormone Storage

The thyroid gland is unique among endocrine glands in its ability to store large quantities of hormone and iodine. T_4, T_3, and iodine (in the form of MIT and DIT) are stored in peptide linkage within the structure of thyroglobulin in the follicular lumen. Thyroglobulin is the major component of the colloid filling the lumen of the follicle.

Secretory Pathway

T_4 and T_3, stored within the thyroglobulin in the follicular lumen, are released across the basolateral membrane of the thyroid follicle cell as individual T_4 and T_3 molecules. The release of hormone from the thyroid involves the uptake of thyroglobulin from the follicular colloid by endocytosis and the proteolysis of the thyroglobulin to release the T_4 and T_3 held in peptide linkage.

Endocytosis

The first step in the release of thyroid hormones from the thyroid gland is endocytosis of colloid from the follicular lumen into the follicle cells (for reviews see refs. 18,19,22). Endocytosis of colloid may occur by macropinocytosis and micropinocytosis. Both processes are stimulated by TSH and result in the uptake of macro- or micropinocytotic vesicles limited by a single membrane and filled with colloid inclusions (colloid droplets).

Thyroglobulin Hydrolysis and Secretion of Thyroid Hormones

Within a few minutes of their formation, the colloid droplets become surrounded by lysosomes, which eventually fuse with the droplets. These lysosomes contain glycoside hydrolases and proteases that degrade thyroglobulin to peptide fragments, iodoamino acids (MIT, DIT), iodothyronines (T_4 and T_3), and other free amino acids. Almost all of the MIT and DIT is deiodinated within the follicle cells by a microsomal iodotyrosine dehalogenase and the iodide released contributes to the intracellular iodide pool and can be reutilized (64). Exit of free T_4 and T_3 across the basolateral membrane is thought to be by passive diffusion.

Thyroid Hormone Transport and Metabolism

Plasma Transport Proteins

Thyroid hormones exhibit low solubility in aqueous solutions. As they enter the blood, they are bound to carrier proteins and only a small fraction (<1%) exist in the "free" or unbound form. The three major thyroid hormone–binding proteins are thyroxine-binding globulin (TBG), transthyretin (formerly known as thyroxine-binding prealbumin [TBPA]), and albumin.

TBG is synthesized by the liver and is the principal thyroid hormone–binding protein in humans. T_4 and T_3 compete for the single binding site on the glycosylated single polypeptide chain that makes up TBG molecule. The apparent affinity constant (K_a) for binding of T_4 is 1.0 x 10^{10} M^{-1} and that for T_3 is 5 x 10^8 M^{-1}, at pH 7.4 and 37∞C (61). Despite the relatively high affinity for T_4, dissociation from the TBG binding site is rapid. The $t_Ω$ value for T_4 dissociation from TBG under physiologic conditions is 39 seconds (28), and for T_3, 4 seconds (29). The normal plasma concentration of TBG ranges from approximately 280 to 510 nM (1.5–3.0 mg/dL), and it binds approximately 70% of the circulating T_4 (59).

Transthyretin, also synthesized by the liver, is a 55 kd tetramer composed of four identical 127 amino acid subunits. It possesses two identical binding sites for iodothyronines. However, the K_a values for T_4 are 7 x 10^7 and 7 x 10^5 M^{-1} and for T_3 are 1 x 10^7 and 6 x 10^5 M^{-1}, at pH 7.4 and 37∞C. Despite the identity of the two binding sites, the affinity of the "second" site is two orders of magnitude lower than that of the "first" binding site because interaction of T_4 or T_3 with one binding site causes a conformational change, resulting in negative cooperativity with regard to the other binding site (33). As with TBG, the dissociation of T_4 and T_3 is rapid; 1/2 values for dissociation are 7.4 seconds and 1.0 seconds, respectively (28,29). The normal concentration of transthyretin in human plasma varies between 2250 and 4300 nM (12–24 mg/dL), and it binds approximately 10% of the circulating T_4.

Albumin has a molecular weight of 66 kd and is known to bind many compounds, including thyroid hormones, calcium, and bilirubin. It is composed of a single unglycosylated peptide chain of 584 residues. It possesses several binding sites for thyroid hormones. One binding site binds T_4 or T_3 with K_a values of 5 x 10^5 and 1 x 10^5 M^{-1}, respectively (59). Two to six additional sites may bind T_4 or T_3 with K_a values of 5 x 10^4 and 5 x 10^3 M^{-1}. Finally, there is a T_4 binding site with a K_a of 0.7 x 10^7 M^{-1} (12). Albumin normally binds approximately 20% of the circulating T_4.

The Role of Transport Proteins in the Delivery of Thyroid Hormones to Tissues

Protein-bound hormone and free hormone are in dynamic equilibrium. Thus, the serum binding proteins may play not only a carrier but also a storage function; protein-bound T_4 and T_3 may act as a reservoir of hormone. According to the "free hormone hypothesis," originally proposed by Robbins and Rall (60), only the free hormone pool is available for delivery to the cell. Therefore, the concentration of free hormone would determine the amount of hormone available to cellular receptors and, ultimately, the degree of hormone action. Perturbations of this equilibrium resulting in alteration of the free hormone concentration might be expected to alter the effectiveness of the circulating hormone.

Free T_4 + binding protein $\rightleftharpoons T_4$-binding protein complex

Only transient alterations in the concentrations of free T_4 and free T_3 normally result from the perturbations of the equilibrium between protein-bound and free hormone levels. This is due to the workings of a negative feed-back system, involving the hypothalamus, the anterior pituitary, and the thyroid gland (the hypothalamic–pituitary–thyroid axis [HPTA]), which acts to regulate the concentrations of free T_4 and free T_3 (ie, keeping the free T_4 and T_3 concentrations near a set point). Through the regulatory function of the HPTA, the secretion of T_4 and T_3 by the thyroid gland would be adjusted appropriately to minimize the effects of any perturbation in the free hormone concentrations.

A common example of the workings of this system is the response to the estrogen-induced increase in TBG resulting from elevated plasma estrogen levels (due to pregnancy or exogenous estrogen therapy). As a consequence, more thyroid hormone–binding sites are available on TBG and the above equation is driven to the right, reducing free T_4. The HPTA responds with an increase in secretion of thyroid hormones to restore the free hormone concentrations. The result is little alteration in the free hormone concentrations, but an increase in the amount of hormone bound to TBG. Thus, the total hormone concentration in serum (eg, free T_4 + T_4-binding protein complex) would be increased. This adjustment by the HPTA will result in the maintenance of euthyroidism, since the free hormone concentration is unchanged.

Conversely, addition of free T_4 to the circulation would increase the plasma total T_4, bound T_4, and free T_4, resulting in an increase in the effects of T_4. The elevation of the plasma free T_4 would evoke a response from the HPTA inhibiting endogenous thyroid hormone secretion by the thyroid gland in an effort to return the free T_4 to its set point.

The HPTA will be described in more detail in a subsequent section.

Cellular Uptake of Thyroid Hormones

Transport of free thyroid hormones across the plasma and nuclear membranes is necessary in order to gain access to receptors located in the cell nucleus. T_4 and T_3 appear to traverse the plasma membrane into the cell by utilizing an energy-dependent, saturable process (7,13,48,58,75). Several therapeutic and diagnostic agents have been shown to interfere with the transport of T_4 and T_3 into hepatocytes and other cell types (38). These include iodinated substances such as radiocontrast agents and amiodarone (38). Noniodinated substances include nonsteroidal antiinflammatory drugs (75), ploretin (48), cytochalasin B (25), dansycladavarine (25), chloroquine (25), and 5,5'-diphenyl-hydantoin (68).

Thyroid Hormone Metabolism

In humans, T_4 and T_3 have relatively long half-lives compared to other hormones. The half-life of T_4 is approximately 6.5 days, while that of T_3 is approximately 1 day. These extremely long half-lives may be attributed to the large proportion of these hormones that are protein bound and not subject to the metabolic reactions described below.

Deiodination

In humans, deiodination is the most important metabolic pathway of thyroid hormones not only in quantitative terms but also because of its dual role in the activation and inactivation of T_4.

Deiodination of T_4 by 5'- or 5-monodeiodination to yield T_3 or reverse T_3 (rT_3), respectively, accounts for about 80% of the total T_4 turnover (16,26). Subsequent deiodinations are also important in the elimination of T_3 and rT_3 to yield diiodothyronines (T_2), monoiodothyronines (T_1), and thyronine (T_0). This cascade of reactions, beginning with the fully iodinated thyronine (T_4), is depicted in Figure 2. There is general agreement that there are at least three enzymes that catalyze the iodothyronine deiodinating reactions, two that catalyze 5'-deiodination, and one that catalyzes 5-deiodination. According to currently accepted nomenclature, the two enzymes catalyzing 5' deiodination are referred to as type I 5'-deiodinase and type II 5'-deiodinase; the enzyme catalyzing 5-deiodination is referred to as tyrosyl-ring deiodinase.

Usually, the metabolism of a hormone involves the conversion of an active hormone to an inactive metabolite. T_4 may undergo monodeiodination to produce substances that may be either more or less active than the parent compound, depending on which iodine is removed.

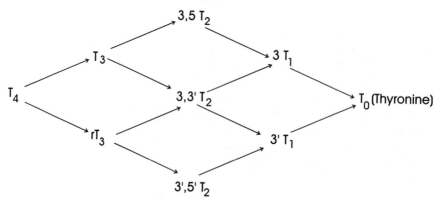

FIG 2. Iodothyronine deiodination cascade.

Although T_4 is the predominant product secreted by the normal thyroid gland, it is T_3 that binds with highest affinity to the receptors in the nucleus of cells. The intracellular 5'-monodeiodination of T_4 to yield T_3 thus results in the production of a more active metabolite. Via an alternative deiodination (ie, 5-monodeiodination), T_4 is converted to the inactive metabolite 3,3',5'-triiodothyronine (rT_3) that has very low affinity for the thyroid hormone receptor. As described above, both T_3 and rT_3 may be degraded to thyronine by sequential monodeiodinations; none of the intervening diiodothyronines or monoiodothyronines are thought to have physiologically significant biological activities.

Side Chain Modification

A minor metabolic pathway involves the oxidative deamination and decarboxylation of iodothyronines. Approximately 2% of the T_4 turnover is accounted for by conversion to tetraiodothyroacetic acid (tetrac), and about 14% of T_3 metabolism occurs by transformation into triiodothyroacetic acid (triac) (16).

Ether Bond Cleavage

Cleavage of the ether bridge connecting the phenolic rings of iodothyronines to yield iodotyrosines (eg, MIT, DIT) is the least important metabolic reaction involving thyroid hormones in humans (16).

Conjugation and Biliary Clearance

T_4, T_3, and their metabolites can undergo glucuronidation or sulfation in the liver and be secreted into bile. The exact role of these processes and the possible enterohepatic circulation of thyroid hormones on the clearance of T_4 and T_3 in humans remains to be determined.

Mechanism of Thyroid Hormone Action

Thyroid hormones exert their effects in cells and tissues by stimulating or inhibiting the accumulation of mRNAs that code for specific proteins. Abundant evidence exists to indicate that most, if not all, significant cellular responses regulated by thyroid hormones are mediated by a cellular receptor (thyroid hormone receptor [TR]) localized to the cell nucleus (54,65). The TRs are ligand-dependent transcription factors that belong to a large superfamily of nuclear hormone receptors, including receptors for steroid hormone, vitamin D, and retinoic acid (3,20). There are at least two isoforms of TR, TR α and TR β, encoded on separate genes, that bind T_3 with high affinity (20,40). These isoforms of TR influence the expression of many genes by binding to thyroid hormone–response elements (TREs) in the promotor region of target genes. The TR isoforms bind to the TREs as monomers or homodimers (21,31,41). Furthermore, TRs may heterodimerize with other similar nuclear proteins known as T_3-receptor auxiliary proteins (TRAPs) (49,85). Retinoid-X receptors, members of the same nuclear hormone receptor superfamily which bind 9-*cis* retinoic acid, may heterodimerize with a TR monomer and enhance overall TR binding to TREs (27,42). Heteroimerization may augment the ligand-regulated transcriptional activity with T_3 alone or, in some cases, T_3 and 9-*cis* retinoic acid may act to regulate transcriptional activity (24,63,86).

The effects of T_3 on the level of mRNAs appear to be tissue-specific, correlating with the presence of nuclear TRs in thyroid hormone–responsive tissues. Through this mechanism, T_3 can have either a positive or a negative effect on the production of specific RNAs. The magnitude of the effect of T_3 is related to the nuclear T_3 concentration, cell type, concentration and composition of TRs, the specific TRE involved, and, perhaps, the abundance of unliganded receptors for other hormones.

Physiologic Effects of Thyroid Hormones

By stimulating or inhibiting the accumulation of mRNAs that code for specific proteins, thyroid hormones exert a wide range of actions, including specific actions on protein, carbohydrate, and lipid metabolism. Virtually every tissue in the body is affected in some way by the thyroid hormones. They influence growth and development and are involved in the maintenance of reproductive, cardiac, gastrointestinal, and hematopoietic functions. In accomplishing their wide range of activities, thyroid hormones also interact with various other hormones. The actions of thyroid hormones are understood largely in terms of the metabolic alterations that occur in the hypothyroid and hyperthyroid state.

Calorigenic Effect

One of the long-known effects of thyroid hormones is a thermogenic or calorigenic action in which oxygen consumption and heat production are stimulated. This calorigenic effect is the consequence of the additive effects of small changes in the levels of numerous rate-limiting enzymes involved in oxidative metabolism. Thus, thyroid hormones stimulate the overall metabolic rate.

Fuel Metabolism

Overall the effects of thyroid hormones on fuel metabolism favor the consumption of body fuel stores rather than the storage of fuel. At normal euthyroid levels, a balance exists, but the balance shifts toward fuel storage at low thyroid hormone levels and toward fuel mobilization and utilization at high thyroid hormone levels.

Thyroid hormones increase the rate of intestinal glucose absorption and its subsequent entry into tissues such as muscle and fat. The tissue uptake of glucose is also enhanced by potentiation of the effects of insulin on glucose uptake in these tissues. Thyroid hormones stimulate glycogenolysis, that is, the breakdown of tissue glycogen stores. High circulating thyroid hormone levels in hyperthyroid patients may lead to depletion of liver glycogen; low levels enhance the storage of glycogen.

All aspects of lipid metabolism are stimulated by thyroid hormones, including lipogenesis, tissue uptake of lipoproteins, and lipolysis. Increasing levels of thyroid hormones stimulate the utilization of lipids as energy sources while enhancing lipolysis and tissue uptake of low density lipoproteins. The net effect favors the lowering of plasma cholesterol and the depletion of tissue fat stores.

Protein synthesis required for normal somatic growth requires adequate amounts of thyroid hormones. However, high circulating levels of thyroid hormones produce catabolic effects on protein metabolism with mobilization of amino acids from protein and use in energy production.

Sympathomimetic Effect

Many of the symptoms of hyperthyroidism are similar to those observed with activation of the sympathetic nervous system. It is generally accepted that an interaction exists between thyroid hormones and catecholamines (eg, epinephrine, norepinephrine). T_3 does not appear to alter the production or the concentration of catecholamines, but it does induce the synthesis of β-adrenergic receptors in target tissues. The increase in the number of β-adrenergic receptors enhances the effects of catecholamines. Thus, at high circulating thyroid hormone levels, many of the signs and symptoms of hyperthyroidism (eg, tachycardia, increased cardiac output, peripheral vasodilation, diffuse anxiety, eyelid retraction, increased motor activity) reflect increased β-adrenergic activity. Consequently, many of the symptoms of hyperthyroidism may be reduced or abolished by β-adrenergic receptor blockade. At the other end of the continuum, low thyroid hormone levels result in impaired β-adrenergic receptor synthesis, and α-adrenergic activity may predominate, resulting in peripheral vasoconstriction and increased blood pressure.

Cardiovascular System

In addition to the effects on the heart mediated by effects on adrenergic receptors, thyroid hormones are involved in the maintenance of myocardial contractility, in part through modulating the expression of the most active isoenzyme of myosin ATPase (30). In hypothyroidism, a less active isoenzyme predominates; administration of thyroid hormone restores the normal isoenzyme activity.

Nervous System

Thyroid hormones play a crucial role in the development and growth of the nervous system. In the hypothyroid neonate, central nervous system development is impeded and permanent mental retardation may result if the condition is not recognized and treated promptly.

The effects of thyroid hormones on the adult central nervous system are illustrated by the behavioral changes associated with thyroid disease. In general, hyperthyroid patients are mentally quick and often irritable and anxious; hypothyroid patients are mentally slow and lethargic.

FEEDBACK CONTROL OF THYROID GLAND ACTIVITY

Hypothalamic–Pituitary–Thyroid Axis

The activity of the thyroid gland is regulated by two negative feedback systems. One system, the HPTA, acts to keep the levels of plasma free T_4 and free T_3 close to the normal operating level, or set point. The second, the thyroid autoregulatory system, acts independently of thyrotropin (thyroid-stimulating hormone [TSH]) to maintain an intrathyroidal pool of iodine and the ability of the gland to synthesize the thyroid hormones.

The HPTA responds to perturbations of the plasma free T_4 or free T_3 from the normal operating point with the appropriate adjustment in hormone secretion by the thyroid gland to minimize the effect of the perturbation on the plasma concentrations of free hormone. Adjustments in the rate of secretion of thyroid hormones are effected by alterations in the pituitary secretion of TSH, which stimulates both the synthesis and secretion of thyroid hormones. The hypothalamus exerts a net stimulatory influence on pituitary TSH synthesis and secretion primarily through the release of thyrotropin-releasing hormone (TRH). The negative feedback loop is completed by the negative feedback inhibition exerted by thyroid hormones on both TSH and TRH secretion.

The normal steady-state activity of the HPTA is driven by the peripheral consumption (metabolism) of thyroid hormones. The loss of thyroid hormones due to metabolism results in a decrease in the negative feedback inhibition of TRH and TSH secretion, increased secretion of TSH, and stimulation of the thyroid gland to synthesize and secrete hormone to replace what was lost. Thus, in the normal steady-state, the rate of thyroid gland hormone secretion equals the rate of disappearance of thyroid hormones. Any decrease in the plasma free T_4 or free T_3 below the operating point would induce a further elevation in the plasma TSH and increased stimulation of the thyroid gland. Conversely, if the free T_4 or free T_3 is elevated above the normal set point, then the TSH-stimulated secretion of thyroid hormones by the thyroid gland is decreased.

T_4 and T_3 exert their negative feedback effects by directly inhibiting the transcription of genes for both the α- and β-TSH subunits in the pituitary thyrotroph.

The thyroid hormones may also indirectly inhibit TSH secretion by inhibiting the transcription of pre-proTRH in neurons of the paraventricular nucleus of the hypothalamus responsible for the release of TRH into the hypophysial-portal blood.

Thyroid Autoregulation

The second major influence on thyroid activity involves iodine and an additional negative feedback loop integral to the thyroid gland itself. The rate-limiting commodity in the biosynthesis of thyroid hormones is iodide. The biosynthesis of thyroid hormones depends on an adequate supply of iodide, and the thyroid has the ability to take up and concentrate iodide from the circulation. The availability of iodide has complex and varied effects on thyroid function. The thyroid gland has the intrinsic ability to autoregulate many of its functions in response to alterations in the availability of iodide (ie, plasma iodide) for uptake and the synthesis of thyroid hormones. Autoregulated functions include iodide trapping, cell proliferation, thyroid blood flow, organification of iodide, and thyroid hormone secretion. The thyroidal autoregulatory negative feedback loop acts to maintain the concentration of some internal pool of organified iodine close to the normal value (set point) and, in the process, assures that an adequate supply of iodide is also available for thyroid hormone synthesis. Autoregulatory adjustments in the efficiency by which the thyroid cells extract iodide from the blood, the number of thyroid cells, and even thyroid blood flow make it possible for the thyroid gland to accommodate a wide range of dietary iodine intake and maintain thyroid hormone synthesis and secretion. By definition, these autoregulatory adjustments occur without invoking a response in the HPTA negative feedback system or alterations in plasma TSH.

Iodide Clearance

In response to restricted dietary iodine intake, autoregulatory mechanisms increase the rate of thyroidal iodide clearance from the blood in order to maintain the rate of absolute iodide uptake.

Absolute I⁻ uptake = I⁻ clearance x plasma I⁻
(mass/time) (volume/time) (mass/volume)

Enhanced activity of the thyroid iodide-trapping mechanism (increased iodide trapping per cell or an increase in the number of thyroid cells) may increase the iodide-extraction efficiency as the plasma iodide is decreased (71). However, at a given plasma iodide, the rate of iodide delivery to the gland may become a limiting factor for thyroid iodine uptake.

I⁻ clearance = I⁻ extraction efficiency x thyroid blood flow
(volume/time) (thyroid I⁻:plasma I⁻ratio) (volume/time)

Thyroidal uptake of iodide may be maintained under these circumstances by an autoregulatory increase in thyroid blood flow.

Conversely, high levels of dietary iodine intake are associated with decreased iodide-trapping activity (32,51,52) and thyroid blood flow (9,46). It appears that the decrease in iodide trapping is induced by iodide only when it has become organified, suggesting that an iodoprotein is necessary for the effect (67). Acute administration of iodide has been used clinically to inhibit thyroid gland uptake of radioactive iodide before the administration of ^{131}I-containing radioisotopes used in medical imaging or after accidental release of radioiodine isotopes into the atmosphere (eg, the Chernobyl disaster) (4).

Iodide Organification

Unless dietary iodide intake is very low, absolute iodide uptake is maintained by autoregulatory mechanisms, and hormone synthesis may be maintained. With very high levels of dietary iodide intake (8–10 mg/day in humans), there is a dramatic fall in the rate of iodide organification (the Wolff–Chaikoff effect) (82) in addition to the effects on iodide uptake (see above). Although the precise mechanism is not clearly understood, it appears that as plasma iodide levels rise to high levels, increasing amounts of iodide are trapped and organified. At a critical point, the binding of iodide to tyrosyl residues within thyroglobulin falls dramatically, with a consequent decline in hormone synthesis. Several possible mechanisms have been suggested and include (1) inhibition of thyroperoxidase (TPO) function by iodide (72); (2) formation of iodine species that are inefficient iodinators (72); and (3) inhibition of H_2O_2 generation (10). In normal individuals, despite continued administration of high levels of iodide, "escape" occurs from the Wolff–Chaikoff effect due to the decline in intrathyroidal iodide caused by the inhibition of iodide uptake and the decreased generation of an inhibitory iodoprotein (67).

Inhibition of Thyroid Hormone Secretion by High Iodide

An additional aspect of the Wolf–Chaikoff effect induced by high iodine is the inhibition of thyroid hormone release (77). In the clinical setting, the most important effect of iodide is its ability in pharmacologic doses to promptly induce an inhibition of thyroid hormone release. This appears to be an autoregulatory response since the effect does not depend on decreased TSH stimulation or inhibition of cyclic adenosine monophosphate (cAMP) generation (56). Excess iodide may inhibit intrathyroidal lysosomal activity involved in the hydrolysis of thyroglobulin and the release of thyroid hormones (70). It is also known that the more extensively thyroglobulin is iodinated, the more resistant it is to thyroidal proteases (39,55). This rapid effect of iodide on thyroid hormone release make iodide an ideal agent for treating severe thyrotoxicosis ("thyroid storm") when administered with antithyroid drugs. Iodide alone is a poor candidate for long-term therapy because of escape from the autoregulatory effects and the induction of hyperthyroidism in most patients within days or weeks (15).

DISORDERS OF THE THYROID GLAND

Thyroid disease is manifested as a decrease in endocrine activity of the gland (hypothyroidism), an excessive activity (hyperthyroidism), or structural and morphologic changes that do not necessarily result in a change in thyroid hormone status (euthyroidism).

Goiter

A goiter is an enlargement of the thyroid gland. Most often this enlargement is of a diffuse nature, but it may take the form of discrete nodules. In most instances, the growth of the thyroid gland can be viewed as a homeostatic compensatory mechanism that maintains thyroid hormone synthesis and secretion. This growth may be part of an autoregulatory response to low dietary iodine intake, or it may be induced by elevated pituitary TSH secretion in response to a fall in thyroid hormone secretion due to a primary defect in thyroid gland. If the compensatory growth of the thyroid gland is adequate, then the total thyroid hormone synthesis and secretion will be maintained at near normal levels, and the person will be euthyroid. In some instances, however, despite the autoregulatory or HPTA adjustments, hypothyroidism may result.

Regardless of the cause, specific problems can result from the development of a goiter. The goiter may become large enough to constrict the neck and interfere with breathing and eating. In addition, the cosmetic effect may also present a problem.

Endemic Goiter

Endemic goiter is common in many areas in which the soil is deficient in iodine. The resultant low dietary iodine intake may result in the development of a euthyroid goiter or, if the deficiency is severe enough, of a hypothyroid goiter. Other predisposing factors may contribute to the development of endemic goiter in individuals. These include genetic factors, the presence of antithyroid substances in the diet, and bacterial contamination of the drinking water. Whatever the precise cause of the disease, it can be prevented and cured by the administration of iodine. When iodide is administered, the goiter ceases to enlarge and will often regress. Treatment with thyroxine will often cause the goiter to disappear, but the response is not invariable.

A tragic consequence of the hypothyroidism that may develop in endemic-goiter regions is the occurrence of endemic cretinism (see below), which may not fully respond to postnatal hormonal thyroid hormone therapy. Most of the neural effects and mental retardation accompanying cretinism are determined prenatally. The sooner the disease is identified postnatally, the more successful outcome can be expected to be.

Sporadic or "Simple" Goiter

Goiter may also occur in less well-defined situations (sporadic goiter) as a result of genetic and other causes that may influence the requirements and availability of iodide. Dietary iodine intake may be adequate under normal situations, but for some reason the thyroid gland can only gain or utilize a limited amount of it. One cause that may contribute to the development of simple goiter in regions of marginally adequate dietary iodine intake may be the consumption of naturally occurring goitrogens. Many plants of the *Brassica* group (eg, cabbage, kale, cauliflower, and turnips) contain thiocyanate (SCN^-), which prevents iodide trapping by the thyroid gland, or goitrins (eg, L-5-vinyl-2-thiooxazolidone), which inhibit organification of iodide.

Hypothyroidism

Hypothyroidism refers to the exposure of body tissues to a subnormal amount of thyroid hormone resulting from undersecretion of thyroid hormones by the thyroid gland. In the United States, the most common cause of primary hypothyroidism (ie, inability of the thyroid gland itself to produce sufficient hormone) is chronic autoimmune thyroiditis (Hashimoto's thyroiditis). Iodine deficiency is a major cause of hypothyroidism in many underdeveloped countries. Other causes of primary hypothyroidism include surgical removal of the thyroid gland, thyroid gland ablation with radioactive iodine, external irradiation, and iodine organification defects. Secondary hypothyroidism is less common than primary hypothyroidism and may result from pituitary or hypothalamic disease that interferes with pituitary TSH secretion.

The symptoms and signs of hypothyroidism are generally related to the duration and severity of the thyroid hormone deficit, the rapidity with which hypothyroidism occurs, and the psychological characteristics of the patient. In adults, the signs and symptoms can include one or more of the following: fatigue, weight gain, dry skin and cold intolerance, yellow skin, coarseness or loss of hair, hoarseness, goiter, relaxation phase reflex delay, ataxia, constipation, memory and mental impairment, decreased concentration, depression, irregular or heavy menses and infertility, myalgias, hyperlipidemia, bradycardia and hypothermia, and myxedema (fluid infiltration of tissues). In infants, the most serious consequences of thyroid hormone deficiency involve mental and physical development. If uncorrected, deficiency causes progressive impairment of mental development and neurological disturbances. Brain growth and myelination of nerves are impaired, as are linear body growth and skeletal development. The result is cretinism, that is, an infant with myxedema and neurologic, mental, and physical retardation.

Hypothyroidism may also result from chronic exposure to compounds that inhibit thyroid hormone biosynthesis and secretion. As mentioned earlier, a number of monovalent cations (eg, SCN^-, perchlorate [ClO_4^-], and pertechnetate [TcO_4^-]) may act as competitive inhibitors of the iodide-trapping mechanism. Several agents inhibit thyroid hormone synthesis by blocking iodide organification and the coupling of iodotyrosines within thyroglobulin. Thionamides (eg, propylthiouracil, methimazole, and carbimazole), some phenolic compounds (eg, resorcinol), and amino-substituted benzene derivatives (eg, sulfonamides, p-aminobenzoic acid, and p-aminosalicylic acid) fall into this class. Chronic exposure to high dietary intake of lithium may also result in hypothyroidism by inhibiting thyroid hormone release at a step distal to cAMP formation. Many of these drugs have been used to treat hyperthyroidism because of their antithyroid effects.

Hyperthyroidism

Hyperthyroidism refers to any condition in which the body tissues are exposed to supraphysiologic amounts of thyroid hormones and excessive thyroid hormone action. The two most common causes of hyperthyroidism are toxic diffuse goiter (Graves' disease) and toxic adenoma. Less common causes include toxic multinodular goiter, painful subacute thyroiditis, excessive pituitary TSH secretion, exposure to high dietary iodine with "escape" from its inhibitory effects (see above), and excessive ingestion of exogenous thyroid hormones.

The symptoms and signs of hyperthyroidism are secondary to the effects of excess thyroid hormone in the circulation and may be related to the duration of the illness, the magnitude of the hormone excess, and the age of the patient. The spectrum of possible signs and symptoms associated with hyperthyroidism include the following: nervousness and irritability, palpitations and tachycardia, heat intolerance and increased sweating, tremor, weight loss, alterations in appetite, frequent bowel movements, fatigue and muscle weakness, exertional intolerance and dyspnea, menstrual disturbance (decreased flow), impaired fertility, mental disturbances, sleep disturbances (including insomnia), changes in vision (photophobia, eye irritation, diplopia, or exophthalmos), dependent lower extremity edema, pretibial myxedema (with Graves' disease), and thyroid enlargement (depending on the cause). A patient need not have all of these symptoms of hyperthyroidism.

Treatment of hyperthyroidism is directed at reducing the excessive secretion of thyroid hormones. This may be accomplished by reducing the amount of functional thyroid tissue by subtotal thyroidectomy or ablation of thyroid tissue with radioiodine (^{131}I). It may also be achieved by inhibiting thyroid hormone synthesis and secretion through the use of antithyroid drugs. Since many of the signs and symptoms of hyperthyroidism reflect increased cellular sensitivity to adrenergic stimulation, a β-adrenergic antagonist (eg, propranolol) is often used adjunctively.

Treatment with either subtotal thyroidectomy or radioiodine ablation of the thyroid gland often results in the development of hypothyroidism. This fact constitutes the major argument for the use of such antithyroid drugs as propylthiouracil and methimazole. However, only a small proportion of patients treated with antithyroid drugs obtain long-term remission of their hyperthyroidism.

If the hyperthyroidism is due to the ingestion of high dietary iodine or thyroid hormones themselves, then the elimination of these dietary causes of the high circulating thyroid hormone levels will ameliorate the problem.

REFERENCES

1. André J, Van Herle MD, Vassart G, Dumont JE. Control of thyroglobulin synthesis and secretion. *N Engl J Med.* 1979;301:239–249.
2. Andros G, Wollman SH. Autoradiographic localization of radioiodide in the thyroid gland of the mouse. *Am J Physiol.* 1967;213:198–208.
3. Beato M. Gene regulation by thyroid hormones. *Cell.* 1989;56:335–344.
4. Becker DV. Reactor accidents: public health strategies and their medical implications. *JAMA.* 1987;258:649–654.
5. Bjökstén F. The horseradish peroxidase–catalyzed oxidation of iodide. Outline of the mechanism. *Biochim Biophys Acta.* 1970;212:396–406.
6. Bone E, Kohn LD, Chomczynski P. Thyroglobulin gene activation by thyrotropin and cAMP in hormonally-depleted FRTL-5 thyroid cells. *Biochem Biophys Res Commun.* 1986;141:1261–1266.
7. Centanni M, Mancini G, Andreoli M. Carrier-mediated [^{125}I]-T$_3$ uptake by mouse thymocytes. *Endocrinology.* 1989;124:2443–2448.
8. Chabaud O, Chambard M, Gaudry N, Mauchamp P. Thyrotropin and cyclic AMP regulation of thyroglobulin gene expression in cultured porcine thyroid cells. *J Endocrinol.* 1988;116:25–33.
9. Chang DCS, Wheeler MH, Woodcock JP, et al. The effect of pre-operative Lugol's iodine on thyroid blood flow in patients with Graves' hyperthyroidism. *Surgery.* 1987;102:1055–1061.
10. Chiraseveenuprapund P, Rosenberg IN. Effects of hydrogen peroxide–generating systems on the Wolff–Dhaikorr effect. *Endocrinology.* 1981;109:2095–2101.
11. Davidson B, Soodak M, Neary JT, et al. The irreversible inactivation of thyroid peroxidase by methylmercaptoimidazole, thiouracil, and propylthiouracil in vitro and its relationship to in vivo findings. *Endocrinology.* 1978;103:871–882.
12. Docter R, Bos G, Krenning EP, Hennemann G. Specific thyroxine binding albumin is constituent of normal human serum. *Lancet.* 1984;1:50.
13. Docter R, Krenning EP, Bernard HF, Hennemann G. Active transport of iodothyronines into human cultured fibroblasts. *J Clin Endocrinol Metab.* 1987;65:624–628.
14. Doniach I, Legothetopoulos JH. Radioautography of inorganic iodide in the thyroid. *J Endocrinol.* 1955;13:65–69.
15. Emerson CH, Anderson AJ, Howard WJ, Utiger RD. Serum thyroxine and triiodothyronine concentration during iodide treatment of hyperthyroidism. *J Clin Endocrinol Metab.* 1975;40:33–36.
16. Engler D, Burger AG. The deiodination of iodothyronines and of their derivatives in man. *Endocr Rev.* 1984;5:151–184.
17. Engler H, Taurog A, Luthy C, Dorris ML. Reversible and irreversible inhibition of thyroid peroxidase–catalyzed iodination by thioureylene drugs. *Endocrinology.* 1983;112:86–95.
18. Ericson, LE. Exocytosis and endocytosis in the thyroid follicle cell. *Mol Cell Endocrinol.* 1981;22:1–24.
19. Ericson LE. Ultrastructural aspects of iodination and hormone secretion in the thyroid gland. *J Endocrinol Invest.* 1983;6:311–324.
20. Evans RM. The steroid and thyroid hormone receptor superfamily. *Science.* 1988;240:889–895.

21. Forman BM, Samuels HH. Dimerization among nuclear hormone receptors. *New Biology* 1990;2:587–594.
22. Fujita H. Fine structure of the thyroid gland. *Int Rev Cytol.* 1975;40:197–280.
23. Gaitan E. Environmental goitrogens. In: Van Middlesworth L, ed. *The Thyroid Gland. A Practical Clinical Treatise.* Chicago, Ill: Year Book; 1986:263–280.
24. Hallenbeck PL, Phyillaier M, Nikodem VM. Divergent effects of 9-*cis*-retinoic acid receptor on positive and negative thyroid hormone receptor–dependent gene expression. *J Biol Chem.* 1993;268:3825–3828.
25. Halpern J, Hinkle PM. Evidence for an active step in thyroid hormone transport to nuclei: drug inhibition of L-^{125}I-triiodothyronine binding to nuclear receptors in rat pituitary tumor cells. *Endocrinology.* 1982;110:1070–1072.
26. Hennemann G, ed. *Thyroid Hormone Metabolism.* New York, NY: Marcel Dekker; 1986.
27. Heyman RA, Mangelsdorf DJ, Dyk JA, et al. 9-*Cis* retinoic acid is a high affinity ligand for the retinoid X receptor. *Cell.* 1992;68:397–361.
28. Hiller AP. Human thyroxine-binding globulin and thyroxine-binding prealbumin dissociation rates. *J Physiol (Lond).* 1971;217:625–634.
29. Hiller AP. The rate of triiodothyronine dissociation from binding sites in human plasma. *Acta Endocrinologica (Copenhagen).* 1975;80:49–57.
30. Hjalmarson AC, Whitfield CF, Morgan HE. Hormonal control of heart function and myosin ATPase activity. *Biochem Biophys Res Commun.* 1970;41:1584–1589.
31. Holloway JM, Glass CK, Adler S, Nelson CA, Rosenfeld MG. The C'-terminal interaction domain of the thyroid hormone receptors confers the ability of the DNA site to dictate positive or negative transcriptional activity. *Proc Natl Acad Sci U S A.* 1990;87:8160–8164.
32. Ingbar SH. Autoregulation of the thyroid: response to iodide excess and depletion. *Mayo Clinic Proc.* 1972;47:814–823.
33. Irace G, Edelhoch H. Thyroxine-induced confirmational changes in prealbumin. *Biochemistry.* 1978;17:5729–5733.
34. Johnson TB, Tewkesbury LB. The oxidation of 3,5-diiodotyrosine to thyroxine. *Proc Natl Acad Sci USA.* 1942;28:73–77.
35. Klebanoff SJ, Yip C, Kessler DK. The iodination of tyrosine by beef thyroid preparations. *Biochim Biophys Acta.* 1962;58:563–574.
36. Knopp J, Stolc V, Tong W. Evidence for the induction of iodide transport on bovine thyroid cells treated with thyroid-stimulating hormone or dibutyryl cyclic adenosine 3',5'-monophosphate. *J Biol Chem.* 1970;245:4403–4408.
37. Konno N, McKenzie JM. In vitro influence of thyrotropin or long-acting thyroid stimulator on mouse thyroid membrane potential. *Metabolism.* 1970;19:724–734.
38. Krenning EP, Docter R. Plasma membrane transport. In: Hennemann G, ed. *Thyroid Hormone Metabolism.* New York, NY: Marcel Dekker; 1986:107–131.
39. Lamas L, Ingbar SH. The effect of varying iodine content on the susceptibility of thyroglobulin to nydrolysis by thyroid acid protease. *Endocrinology.* 1978;102:188–197.
40. Lazar MA, Chin WW. Nuclear thyroid hormone receptors. *J Clin Invest.* 1990;86:1777–1782.
41. Lazar MA, Berrodin TJ, Harding HH. Differential DNA binding by monomeric, homodimeric, and potentially heterodimeric forms of the thyroid hormone receptor. *Mol Cell Biol.* 1991;11:5005–5015.
42. Levin AA, Sturzenbecker LJ, Kazmer S, et al. 9-*Cis* retinoic acid stereoisomer binds and activates the nuclear receptor RXR$_\alpha$. *Nature.* 1992;355:359–361.
43. Magnusson RP, Taurog A. Iodide-dependent catalytic activity of thyroid peroxidase and lactoperoxidase. *Biochem Biophys Res Commun.* 1983;112:475–481.
44. Mayberry WE, Rall JE, Bertoli D. Kinetics of iodination, I: a comparison of the kinetics of iodination of *N*-acetyl-L-tyrosine and *N*-acetyl-3-iodo-L-tyrosine. *J Am Chem Soc.* 1964;86:5302–5307.
45. Mercken L, Simons M-J, Swillens S, Massaer M, Vassart G. Primary structure of bovine thyroglobulin deduced from the sequence of its 8431 base complementary DNA. *Nature.* 1985;316:647–651.
46. Michalkiewicz M, Huffman LJ, Connors JM, Hedge GA. Alterations of thyroid blood flow induced by varying levels of iodine intake in the rat. *Endocrinology.* 1989;125:54–60.
47. Morris DR, Hager LP. Mechanism of the inhibition of enzymatic halogenation by anti-thyroid drugs. *J Biol Chem.* 1966;241:3582–3589.
48. Movius EG, Phyillaier MM, Robbins J. Phloretin inhibits cellular uptake and nuclear receptor binding of triiodothyronine in human HepG2 hepatocarcinoma cells. *Endocrinology.* 1989;124:1988–1997.
49. Murray MB, Towle HC. Identification of nuclear factors that enhance binding of the thyroid hormone receptor to a thyroid hormone response element. *Mol Endocrinol.* 1989;3:1434–1442.

50. Nadler NJ, Benard B, Fitzsimmons G, Leblond CP. An autoradiographic technique to demonstrate inorganic radioiodide in the thyroid gland. In: Roth LJ, Stumpf WD, eds. *Autoradiography of Diffusible Substances*. Orlando, Fla: Academic Press; 1969:121–130.

51. Nagataki S, Ingbar SH. Relation between qualitative and quantitative alteration in thyroid hormone synthesis induced by varying doses of iodide. *Endocrinology*. 1964;74:731–736.

52. Nagataki S, Shizume K, Nakao K. Effect of chronic graded doses of iodide on thyroid hormone synthesis. *Endocrinology*. 1966;79:667–674.

53. Nakamura Y, Ohtake,S, Yamazaki I. Molecular mechanism of iodide transport by thyroid plasmalemmal vesicles: cooperative sodium activation and asymetrical affinities of ions on the outside and inside of vesicles. *J Biochem*. 1985;104:544–549.

54. Oppenheimer JH. The nuclear receptor–triiodothyronine complex: relationship of thyroid hormone distribution, metabolism, and biological action. In: Oppenheimer JH, Samuels HH, eds. *Molecular Basis of Thyroid Hormone Action*. Orlando, Fla: Academic Press, 1983;1–35.

55. Pilar P, Lamas L. The effect of varying iodine content on the proteolytic activity of rat thyroid lysosomes. *Acta Endocrinol (Copenh)*. 1981;98:556–563.

56. Pisarev MA, DeGroot LJ, Hati R. KI and imidazole inhibition of TSH and cAMP induced thyroidal iodine secretion. *Endocrinology*. 1971;88:1217–1221.

57. Pommier J, Dème D, Nunez J. Effect of iodide concentration on thyroxine synthesis catalyzed by thyroid peroxidase. *Eur J Biochem*. 1973;37:406–414.

58. Rao GS, Eckel J, Rao ML, Breuer H. Uptake of thyroid hormone by isolated rat liver cells. *Biochem Biophys Res Commun*. 1976;73:98–104.

59. Robbins J, Bartalena L. Plasma transport of thyroid hormones. In: Hennemann G, ed. *Thyroid Hormone Metabolism*. New York, NY: Marcel Dekker; 1986:3–38.

60. Robbins J, Rall JE. The interaction of thyroid hormones and protein in biological fluids. *Recent Progr Horm Res*. 1957;13:161–208.

61. Robbins J, Rall JE. The iodine-containing hormones: thyroid hormone transport in blood and extravascular fluids. In: Gray CH, James VHT, eds. *Hormones in Blood*. London, UK: Academic Press; 1979;1:576–688.

62. Roman R, Dunford HB. pH Dependence of the oxidation of iodide by compound I of horseradish peroxidase. *Biochemistry*. 1972;11:2076–2082.

63. Rosen ED, O'Donnell AL, Koenig RJ. Ligand-dependent synergy of thyroid hormone and retinoid X receptors. *J Biol Chem*. 1992;267:22010–22013.

64. Rosenberg IN, Gorwanni A. Purification and characterization of a flavoprotein from bovine thyroid with iodotyrosine deiodinase activity. *J Biol Chem*. 1979;254:12318–12325.

65. Samuels HH. Identification and characterization of thyroid hormone receptors and action using cell culture techniques. In: Oppenheimer JH, Samuels HH, eds. *Molecular Basis of Thyroid Hormone Action*. Orlando, Fla: Academic Press; 1983:35–64.

66. Schultz SG, Curran PF. Coupled transport of sodium and organic solutes. *Physiol Rev*. 1970;50:637–718.

67. Sherwin JR, Price DJ. Autoregulation of thyroid iodide transport: evidence for the mediation of protein synthesis in idodide-induced suppression of iodide transport. *Endocrinology*. 1986;119:2553–2559.

68. Smith PJ, Surks MI. 5,5'-Diphenylhydantoin (Dilantin) decreases cytosol and specific nuclear 3,5,3'-triiodothyronine binding in rat anterior pituitary in vivo and in cultured GC cells. *Endocrinology*. 1984;115:283–290.

69. Solomon DH. Effects of thyrotropin on thyroidal water and electrolytes in the chick. *Endocrinology*. 1961;69:939–957.

70. Starling JR, Hopps BA. Effect of excess iodine on thyroid and liver lysosomal enzymes. *J Surg Res*. 1980;28:57–64.

71. Studer H, Greer MA. A study of the mechanisms involved in the production of iodine-deficiency goiter. *Acta Endocrinol*. 1965;49:610–628.

72. Taurog A. Thyroidal peroxidase–catalyzed iodination of thyroglobulin; inhibition by excess iodide. *Arch Biochem Biophys*. 1970;139:212–220.

73. Taurog A. Thyroid peroxidase and thyroxine biosynthesis. *Recent Prog Horm Res*. 1970;26:189–247.

74. Taurog A. The mechanism of action of thioureylene antithyroid drugs. *Endocrinology*. 1976; 98:1031–1046.

75. Topliss DJ, Kolliniatis E, Barlow JW, Lim C-F, Stockigt JR. Uptake of 3,5,3'-triiodothyronine by cultured rat hepatoma cells in inhibitable by nonbile acid cholephils, diphenylhydantoin, and nonsteroidal antiinflammatory drugs. *Endocrinology*. 1989;124:980–986.

76. Van Heuverswyn B, Leriche A, Van Sande J, Dumont JE, Vassart G. Transcriptional control of thyroglobulin gene expression by cyclic AMP. *FEBS Lett.* 1985;188:192–196.

77. Wartofsky L, Ransil BJ, Ingbar SH. Inhibition by iodine of the release of thyroxine from thyroid glands of patients with thyrotoxicosis. *J Clin Invest.* 1970;49:78–86.

78. Weiss SJ, Philp NJ, Ambesi-Impiombato FS, Grollman EF. Thyrotropin-stimulated iodide transport mediated by adenosine 3',5'-monophosphate and dependent on protein synthesis. *Endocrinology.* 1984;114:1099–1107.

79. Williams JA. Effect of external K^+ concentration on the transmembrane potentials of rabbit thyroid cells. *Am J Physiol.* 1966;211:1171–1174.

80. Williams JA. Effects of TSH on thyroid membrane properties. *Endocrinology.* 1970;86:1154–1158.

81. Wolff J. Transport of iodide and other anions in the thyroid gland. *Physiol Rev.* 1964;44:45–90.

82. Wolff J. Iodine goiter and the pharmacological effects of excess iodide. *Am J Med.* 1969;47:101–122.

83. Wolff J, Halmi NS. Thyroidal iodine transport, V: the role of Na^+-K^+ activated ouabain sensitive adenosine-triphosphate activity. *J Biol Chem.* 1963;238:847–851.

84. Woodbury DM, Woodbury JW. Correlation of micro-electrode potential recordings with histology of rat and guinea pig thyroid glands. *J Physiol (London).* 1963;169:553–567.

85. Yen PM, Darling DS, Chin WW. Basal and thyroid hormone receptor auxiliary protein–enhanced binding of thyroid hormone receptor isoforms to native thyroid hormone response elements. *Endocrinology.* 1991;129:3331–3336.

86. Yen PM, Brubaker JH, Apriletti JW, Baxter JD, Chin WW. Roles of 3,5,3'-triiodothyronine and deoxyribonucleic acid binding on thyroid hormone receptor complex formation. *Endocrinology.* 1994;134:1075–1081.

Endocrine Toxicology, 2nd ed.,
Edited by J. A. Thomas and H. D. Colby
Copyright © 1997 Taylor & Francis

3

Chemically-Induced Changes in the Thyroid

James T. Stevens

Department of Toxicology, Ciba-Geigy Limited, CH-4332 Stein, Switzerland

INTRODUCTION

The follicle cells of the thyroid gland maintain the body economy by regulating the synthesis, storage, and secretion of thyroid hormones necessary for growth, development, and normal body metabolism (39). The regulatory processes of the thyroid gland follicle cells appear to be readily altered by physiologic or chemical means (47). In fact, thyroid disorders are among the most frequently occurring endocrine diseases seen by a physician (11,46). Fortunately, the more serious proliferative lesions of the follicle cells, including tumors, are more prevalent in the thyroid gland of the laboratory rat than that of the human (9,10,28,34,43,50).

Although the mammalian thyroid gland is composed of two embryologically and functionally distinct populations of cells, which produce different classes of hormones (8), the focus of this chapter will be the follicle cells of the thyroid. More details concerning the second type of cells of the thyroid, the C, or parafollicular, cells are provided in Chapter 2 of this volume. In addition, it is essential to understand the basic anatomy, physiology, and biochemistry of the endocrinology of the follicle cells of the thyroid gland before it is possible to appreciate how chemicals can produce their effects on these cells. Although these aspects are discussed in great detail in Chapter 4 of this book, a brief review of the basic economy of the iodothyronines-secreting follicle cells is considered. Potential pathogenic changes in the follicle cells are also discussed.

The primary focus is the response of the follicle cells to an environment altered through chemical injury and chemically induced deficiencies or excesses. Possible mechanisms for these chemically mediated alterations are delineated. Physical processes such as nuclear fallout will not be considered (13, 25).

In the clinical setting, it has been long established that a disturbance in the balance of iodothyronine secretion can result in the production of goiters. Furthermore, it is well known that members of the cabbage family contain iodine-responsive goitrogenic factors (31). Besides the production of goitrogenic effects resulting from iodine deficiencies or phytogoitrogens, discussions will include considerations of synthetic goitrogens (syngoitrogens) and other chemicals that alter the normal homeostasis of the thyroid cells. The clinical significance of the ability of a cadre of chemicals to produce lesions in the follicle cells is often understood, and such lesions are frequently responsive to therapy. On the other hand, the significance of the production of such lesions and tumors in laboratory animals, particularly rodents, is less clear. Species differences are considered to aid in understanding these processes and to help place these findings into proper prospective for human risk assessment.

BASIC ECONOMY OF THYROID FOLLICLE CELLS

The follicle cells that secrete the iodothyronines are responsible for maintaining the basal metabolic rate in tissues essential for their normal function. Although the thyroid gland is not essential for life, malfunction of the follicle cells can result in significant adverse effects on metabolic homeostasis.

Structure and Function

Phylogenetically, the thyroid is the oldest of the endocrine glands. Anderson and Scotti (2) indicate that the follicle cells constitute a basic unit of thyroid tissue–the glandular follicles or acini. This structure, also called a vesicle or alveolus, is unique for an endocrine organ in vertebrates (38). Roughly spherical in shape and lined by a layer of cuboidal epithelial cells, the acini, the alveolus contains a homogenous gelatinous material (colloid) that is primarily thyroglobulin. Thyroglobulin is the stored secretion of acini (6). The luminal borders of the follicles contain many microvilli that are apparently involved in secretion and reabsorption (2). This feature of the thyroid gland, namely, the continuous accumulation and storage of significant amounts of hormonal active substance in the form of colloid, is also a unique feature of the follicle cells of the thyroid (38).

The microscopic structure is subject to considerable variation, depending on diet, nutrition, environment, sex, age, and endocrine status, as well as other factors (51). When the gland is inactive, the colloid is abundant, the follicles are large, and the cells lining them are flat (19). On the other hand, when the gland is active, the acini are small and the cells are cuboidal or columnar, forming many small lacunae for reabsorption.

The follicle is not permanent, as it merely constitutes a transitory phase that alternates between two extremes of the follicle and the interfollicular cell (36). Follicles break up at the apex of disorganization; reorganization results in new follicle formation. A cell is able to produce colloid for a limited period. A period of inactivity to prepare itself for renewal of secretory function is required in conjunction with the interfollicular cell stage, which together initiate a new follicle.

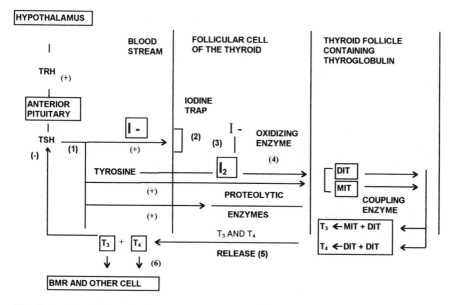

Step 1. Thyrotropin (TSH) Release
Step 2. Iodide Trapping
Step 3. Inhibition of Oxidizing Enzyme
Step 4. Coupling of Tyrosine to Iodine
Step 5. Release of T_3 and T_4
Step 6. Extrathyroidal Effects

Fig. 1. Hormonal and biochemical events involved in the synthesis and secretion of T3 and T4 (Redrawn form (50).

The function of the thyroid follicle cells is regulated by both negative and positive feedback of the anterior pituitary, as well as by a complex series of kinetic interactions (Fig. 1). Each one of these steps represents a possible site of alteration of follicle cell function, both extra- and intrathyroidal. Each of the steps is essential to production of the thyroid hormones. Disruption of these processes can result in imbalances, either directly or indirectly, and in follicle cell pathogenesis.

Follicle Cell Pathogenesis

Thyroid follicle cells are generally cuboidal in appearance under homeostatic hormone balance. When there is an absence of thyrotropin, or thyroid stimulating hormone (TSH), or levels are low, the follicle cells become atrophic, flat, often inactive, and even fibrotic (2). Conversely, an increase in TSH may cause follicle cells to become columnar and undergo both hypertrophy and hyperplasia, with a reduction in thyroglobulin colloid; the mass of the thyroid gland is often greatly increased. Under continuous exposure to TSH stimulation, the gland may undergo hyperplasia with neoplasia, or it may involute with neoplasia. Hemorrhage, cyst formation, fibrosis, and calcification may also occur (39).

Like iodide deficiencies, an excess in dietary iodine may lead to proliferative reactions of follicle cells (8); both conditions result in an excessive TSH secretion in this negative feedback system. Excess iodide inhibits the uptake of iodine by the follicle cells, blocks the peroxidation of I^- to molecular iodine (I_2), interferes with the conversion of diiodotyrosine (DIT) and monoiodotyrosine (MIT), and blocks the release of triiodothyronine (T_3) and thyroxine (T_4), leading to the secretion of TSH (37). In contrast, deficiency of iodide results in a diminished synthesis of iodothyroxine hormones for circulation and in subsequent TSH elevation.

Naturally, substances known as goitrogens have been the focus of studies for a long time (42). These agents alter the iodide-trapping capability of the thyroid and thus the negative feedback on the release of TSH. They are also known to increase the size of the thyroid by proliferation. In humans, this pathogenesis generally stops short of tumor formation (2,9,15,50). In the thyroid follicle cells of rats, however, the proliferative changes lead to an increase in the occurrence of adenomas, as well as follicular cystic hyperplasia and follicular cysts (8–10,50). High iodide intake in rats results in a predisposition to the development of a higher incidence of thyroid adenomas and cystic follicles similar to that resulting from iodide deficiency. Likewise, polychlorinated biphenyls (PCBs), which produce a significant dose-dependent reduction in serum T_4 levels when fed in the diet of rats, result in striking hypertrophy and hyperplasia of the thyroid follicle cells, presumably by enhancing TSH release. These findings are consistent with the thinking that partial destruction of the thyroid, in combination with decreased T_4 production, results in prolonged TSH secretion, which in turn plays a role in tumorigenesis (3).

Thyroid neoplasms, relatively common in most laboratory animals, constitute a spectrum of hyperplastic lesions. However, spontaneous follicle cell adenomas are uncommon in rats (7). Some of these are functional and associated with goitrogenic alterations; others are hyperplastic in the strict morphologic sense and precancerous in their biological behavior (48).

The frequency of thyroid neoplasia is greatest in aged animals, especially those subject to goiters in earlier life (1). These factors often complicate the interpretation of positive oncogenic findings in the follicle cells in the standard rodent bioassays, which are conducted as lifetime experiments, carrying animals into senility.

In a review of experimentally induced thyroid tumors in rats, Van Dyke (55) discussed an increased frequency of tumors in rats in cases where treatment by a variety of agents resulted in TSH stimulation, directly or indirectly. Therefore, tests to evaluate the endocrine status of follicle cells may be useful in connection with lifetime studies to determine the significance of any follicle cell changes manifested. This consideration has been advanced morphologically by Napalkov (38) and mechanistically by Capen (9), Doehler et al. (15), Hill et al. (27), and Paynter et al. (42).

CHEMICALS ALTERING THYROID FOLLICLE CELL HOMEOSTASIS

Thyroid follicle cells respond to prolonged hypersecretion of TSH initially by undergoing hypertrophy and hyperplasia followed by spontaneous neoplasia. Most chemicals that induce changes in these cells act either directly or indirectly on these cells to alter via negative feedback by disrupting the production of T_3 and T_4, by extrathyroidal alteration of peripheral conversion of T_3 and T_4, or by acting directly on the pituitary to stimulate release of TSH. Thus, such patterns of pathogenesis could be anticipated.

Thyrotropin Release

TSH is a hormone released by the anterior pituitary mediated via the thyrotropin-releasing hormone (TRH), a modified tripeptide (pyroglutamylhistidylprolinamide) from the hypothalamus (12). The hypothalamic control by this neurohormone is carried from the median eminence of the hypothalamus to the anterior pituitary via the hypophysial-portal circulation. The TRH binds to the pituicyte membrane on specific receptor sites and causes increased synthesis, as well as secretion, of TSH.

TSH plays a vital role in nearly all the steps of iodothyronine biosynthesis, including stimulation or activation of the iodide trap and activation of proteolytic enzymes that hydrolyze thyroglobulin and make the secretion of the follicle cell hormones possible (see Fig. 1, step 1). Excessive levels of thyroid follicle cell hormones activate a negative feedback effect on TSH release.

It is obvious that agents that alter the release of TRH by the hypothalamus or TSH by the anterior pituitary could significantly affect thyroid follicle cell function. Lybeck et al. (35) demonstrate that methyl parathion exerts an anticholinesterase effect at the hypothalamic–pituitary axis. They suggest that the chemical mediator that liberates TRH from the hypothalamus is acetylcholine; that is, the process is cholinergic in nature. Alternately, Ganong (19) suggests that psychic influences and cold may stimulate release of TRH, whereas warmth and trauma may inhibit TRH release from the hypothalamus.

Iodide Trapping

Follicles actively transport iodide from the blood across the cell into the follicular lumen (see Fig. 1, step 2). An iodide-concentrating mechanism resides in the epithelial membrane of the follicle and can concentrate iodide at levels approximately 30 times higher than found in the plasma (15). The TSH enhances the transport mechanism, whereas it is well known that inorganic ions such as thiocyanate and perchlorate inhibit iodide trapping (39).

In addition, Kuzan and Prahlad (32) have shown that nabam, a dithiocarbamate fungicide that breaks down to ethylene thiourea, inhibits the iodide-trapping mechanism. Likewise, Graham and Hansen (22) show that 500 ppm or more of ethylene thiourea, a degradation product of dithiocarbamate fungicides (eg, zineb and ziram), significantly reduced ^{131}I uptake when administered to rats for a period of 90 days. Goldman et al. (21) obtained a similar response with dichlorodiphenyl-trichloroethane (DDT) after a single dose of 50–200 mg/kg given to rats. Conversely, Florsheim and Velcoff (16) have shown that the herbicide (2,4-dichlorophenoxy)acetic acid enhanced iodide uptake in rats.

Inhibition of Oxidizing Enzyme

Iodide is oxidized to iodine by a peroxidase present in the microvilli membrane (44). Inhibition of peroxidase activity is another mechanism for altering follicle cell function (see Fig. 1, step 3). This process is inhibited by thiouracil and imidazole derivatives (35).

Phytogoitrogens

Goiter formation in humans is due to insufficient iodine intake as a result of (1) deficiency in the soil or water in certain geographical regions, (2) bacterial contamination of water supplies interfering with the availability of iodine, or (3) ingestion of plants containing thiocyanates or thiouracil-like compounds (2). There are numerous naturally goitrogenic substances found in food items ingested by humans. Foods containing these substances include cabbage, brussels sprouts, turnips, and mustard (30), as well as peanuts (49). The pathogenic mechanism for this goitrogenic response may be direct interference with thyroid hormone synthesis or secretion, an increase in thyroid hormone excretion into the bile, or a disruption of the peripheral conversion of T_3 and T_4 (17).

The chemical substance responsible for the goitrogenic activity of turnips is goitrin (L-5-vinyl-2-thiooxazolidone) (27). Goitrin may also be found in the seeds and green parts of other cruciferous plants. In peanuts, the goitrogen is thought to be arachidoside (27).

Syngoitrogens

Since the synthetic goitrogens have been extensively reviewed (14, 42) and their mode of action for altering the thyroid follicle cell and the subsequent pathogenic profile is not dissimilar from the phytogoitrogens, these chemicals will not be considered in great detail. Hill et al. (27) divide the syngoitrogens into three groups by chemical class: thionamides, aromatic amines, and substituted phenols. The primary step in thyroid hormone synthesis that is affected has been described by Capen (9) as an organification defect or as the inhibition of follicle cell peroxidase (see Figure 1, step 3). The syngoitrogens known to alter thyroid hormone synthesis at this level are provided by chemical class in Table 1.

As evident in Table 1, a large number and variety of different zenobiotics can inhibit this important step in thyroid hormone synthesis. Interestingly, Capen (9) points out that there are marked differences between species in the sensitivity of the peroxidase enzyme to inhibition by chemicals. In fact, following a number of long-term studies with sulfonamides, thyroid nodules developed in the more sensitive species (eg, rat, dog, and mouse) but not in those species more resistant to inhibition of peroxidase (eg, monkey, guinea pig, chicken, and human).

Coupling of Tyrosine to Iodine

The amino acid tyrosine, which is transported from the bloodstream, is also needed for the processes of follicle cell hormone synthesis. Iodine is bound to the tyrosine in the endoplasmic reticulum near the apical surface of the follicle cells. These materials are incorporated into the high molecular weight glycoprotein known as

TABLE 1. Syngoitrogens Altering Thyroid Hormone Synthesis by Inhibition of Peroxidase

Class of syngoitrogen	Reference	Syngoitrogen
Thionamides	Barbituric acid	27
	Carbimazole	12
	Ethylene thiourea	22
	Imidazole	50
	Methimazole	12
	Oxazole	27
	Propylthiouracil	33
	Thiouracil	12
	Thiourea	9
	Thiadiazole	27
	Uracil	27
Aromatic amines	Amphenone	9
	Oxydianiline	23
	p-Aminobenzoic acid	9
	p-Aminosalicylic acid	9
	Sulfadiazine	24
	Sulfathiazole	26
	Sulfonamides	42
Substituted phenols	4-Dihydroxybenozoic acid	9
	Hexyresorcinol	27
	Meta-aminophenol	27
	Resorcinol	9
Other	Aminotriazole	53,54
	Antipyrine	9
	Thiamazole	52
	Tricyanoaminopropene	9

thyroglobulin, which is in turn stored as the follicular colloid. Sulfonamide derivatives (39) and propylthiouracil (35) have both been shown to inhibit the coupling of tyrosine to iodine (see Fig. 1, step 4). Thiourea derivatives, such as methimazole, carbimazole, and thiouracil inhibit both incorporation of iodine and coupling of tyrosine to iodine (12).

Release of T_3 and T_4

The metabolic precursors of the thyroid follicle cell hormones are monoiodotyrosine (MIT) and diiodotyrosine (DIT). As the result of coupling enzyme by an ether linkage, MIT and DIT can combine to form 3,5,3'-triiodo-L-thyronine) (T_3), or two DIT molecules can join to form 3,5,3',5'-tetraiodo-L-thyronine (L-thyroxine or T_4). A deiodinase has been observed in the thyroid that can deiodinate MIT and DIT but not the ether-linked T_3 and T_4 (39). This enzyme makes iodine available for the total body pool, as well as for the thyroid.

Generally, the organic forms of iodine are stored in the thyroid as part of thyroglobulin within the acinar wall. This provides for a large storage capacity. Storage of the iodothyronine hormones in thyroglobulin also affords a slow release. Substances that block the synthesis of MIT and DIT, affect the coupling enzyme, or alter the release of iodothyronine hormones from thyroglobulin would also alter the storage process.

Secretion of T_3 and T_4 is initiated by elongation of the microvilli on the follicle cells and by formation of pseudopods in response to TSH production by the anterior pituitary gland (8). The release of the iodothyronines may also be affected (see Fig. 1, step 5).

Kasza et al. (29) showed that repeated exposure to PCBs caused an inhibition of T_3 and T_4 release, as well as striking hypertrophy and hyperplasia of the thyroid follicle cells in rats. Through careful investigative techniques, they determined that the cause of these proliferative changes was interference with the interaction between the colloid droplets and the lysosomal bodies necessary for the release of thyroid hormones. In addition, Ghinea et al. (20) showed that acute exposure to high levels of aminotriazole inhibited the release of T_3 and T_4, whereas the triazine herbicide atrazine stimulated the release of T_3 and T_4 in rats.

Galton and Ingbar (18) demonstrated that in addition to the direct effect of aminotriazole on the thyroid (ie, inhibiting synthesis), this substance also enhances the deiodination of T_4 by the liver, a finding that has been confirmed by Scammell and Fregly (45). It has been shown that PCBs induce hepatic uridine 5'-diphosphate (UDP)-glucuronyl transferase, thereby increasing the excretion of T_4 as a conjugate in the bile (8).

Extrathyroidal Effects

As with all hormonally mediated processes, when the hormone leaves the endocrine organ, there are various mechanisms by which chemicals can alter the hormone in the plasma, at the target site, or both. These mechanisms include a blockade or other type of interference with the synthesis or secretion of one or more hormones, as discussed above. They also include the alteration of protein binding in the plasma, the interference with one or more enzyme systems essential for hormonal transformations or metabolism, and blockade of or competition for receptor sites.

Plasma Protein Binding

Once thyroid hormones are released into the bloodstream, they are bound to T_4-binding proteins, primarily α_1- and α_2-globulins. Normally only about 0.03% of the T_4 in the circulation is free and available for cell membrane penetration, hormone action, metabolism, or elimination (27). The hormones bound to the binding globulin are presumed to be metabolically inactive; bound thyroid hormones are released and subsequently exert their action in the cell. It has been shown, however, that the levels of free thyroid hormones in the plasma may be changed through competitive interactions with certain drugs and xenobiotics (24).

Extrathyroidal protein binding may actually play a remarkable role in determining the level of sensitivity of different species to thyroid pathogenesis (9). Doehler et al. (15) believe that the greater sensitivity of the rodent thyroid to certain pharmaceuticals and other chemicals, as well as to physiologic perturbations, is related to the short half-life of T_4 in the rodent plasma compared with that found in humans; this is associated with the marked species differences in these thyroid hormone–binding proteins.

Enzyme Inducers

In addition to chemicals that affect the availability of thyroid hormones by altering protein binding, there are chemicals that induce hepatic and extrahepatic enzymes. Some of these inducing agents have the potential to enhance the metabolism of T_3 and T_4. An excellent review of this area has been completed by Hill et al. (27).

Oppenheimer et al. (40,41) have shown that treatment of rats with phenobarbital enhances the metabolism of T_4, resulting in a compensatory release of TSH and increased thyroid secretion of new hormone. However, this was not the only effect observed; phenobarbital also increased hepatocellular binding of T_4 and enhanced biliary excretion of the hormone (41). However, these findings suggest that the numerous chemicals in the phenobarbital-type class would have the same capability of altering circulating thyroid hormone levels and inducing thyroid follicle cell pathogenesis.

In addition, this scenario is by no means as simple as enhanced metabolism by phenobarbital-type cytochrome P-450–inducing agents. However, Bastomsky (4) has shown that the so-called cytochrome P-448–inducing agents (eg, 3-methylcholanthrene) induce T_4 UDP-glucuronyl transferase. This again results in a decrease in available, functional T_4 and a compensatory increase in TSH. Indeed, it has been found that the polycyclic aromatic hydrocarbon 2,3,7,8-tetra-chlorodibenzo-p-dioxin (TCDD) is quite capable of altering T_4 metabolism. Bastomsky (5) found that 9 days after the administration of 25 μg/kg to rats T_4 levels were half those found in control rats (5). These findings point to a realm of possibilities where chemicals have the potential to significantly alter the metabolism of thyroid hormones.

HAZARD ASSESSMENT AND RISK EVALUATION

It is clearly possible that a given chemical may affect the follicle cells by any combination of alterations of the pharmacokinetics, thyroid hormone production, or utilization. Agents that indirectly or directly reduce TSH levels do not generally produce proliferative changes in the follicle cell, whereas chemicals that increase TSH levels will effect such changes. It is difficult to relate the proliferative changes seen in bioassays of the laboratory rodent to man, unless such changes can be related to TSH elevation.

The eventual manifestation of pathology in the form of a tumor from long-term exposure to a xenobiotic, at least in most cases, appears to be a secondary or indirect mechanism exhibited by animal models, which are often highly sensitive. In the case of the rodent thyroid tumor, the progression seen for these agents is most commonly the result of compensatory secretion of TSH, leading to an overstimulation of follicle cells. Clearly, such a secondary response would exhibit a no-effect level in most instances, and the substance would be considered to have a threshold below which no remarkable changes in the follicle cells would be exhibited.

In the clinical setting, data regarding human exposure to many of these compounds support the prognosis that the proliferative changes observed do not often proceed beyond hyperplasia. In addition, these differences between humans and the rodent support the view that the hazard and risk concerns arising from long-term rodent bioassays should be kept in proper prospective.

REFERENCES

1. Anderson MP, Capen CC. The endocrine system. In: Benirschke K, Garner FM, Jones TC, eds. *Tumors in Pathology of Laboratory Animals*. New York, NY: Springer-Verlag; 1978;1:424–508.
2. Anderson WAD, Scotti TM. Endocrine glands. In: *Synopsis of Pathology*. 9th ed. St Louis, Mo: CV Mosby; 1976:849–878.
3. Axelrad AA, LeBlond CP. Induction of thyroid tumors in rats by a low iodine diet. *Cancer*. 1955;8:339–367.
4. Bastomsky CH. The biliary excretion of thyroxine and its glucuronic acid conjugate in normal and Gunn rats. *Endocrinology*. 1973;92:35–40.
5. Bastomsky CH. Enhanced thyroxine metabolism and high uptake goiters in rats after a single dose of 2,3,7,8-tetrachlorodibenzo-p-dioxin. *Endocrinology*. 1977;101:292–296.
6. Best CH, Taylor NB. The thyroid gland. In:Best, CH, Taylor, NB, eds. *The Physiological Basis of Medical Practice*, 8th ed. Baltimore, Md: Williams & Wilkins; 1966;1529–1554.
7. Boorman GA. *The Thyroid : Hyperplasia and Neoplasia*. Follicular cell adenomas, thyroid, rat. In: Jones TC, Mohr U, Hunt RD, eds. *Endocrine System*. New York, NY: Springer-Verlag; 1983:177–180.
8. Capen CC. Chemical injury of thyroid: pathologic and mechanistic considerations. In: *Toxicology Forum: 1983 Annual Winter Meeting*. Washington, DC: Bowers Reporting Company; 1983:260–273.

9. Capen CC. Mechanisms of chemical injury of thyroid gland. In: *Prog Clin Bio L Res* 1994:173–191.
10. Capen CC, Martin SL. The effects of xenobiotics on the structure and function of the thyroid follicles and C-cells. *Toxicol Pathol.* 1989;17:266–275.
11. Clark OH, Rollo D, Stroop J, et al. Sensitivity of the thyroid and parathyroid glands to radiation, *J Surg Res.* 1978;24:374–379.
12. Connors JM, Thomas JA. Thyroid and antithyroid drugs. In: Craig CR, Stitzel RE, eds. *Modern Pharmacology.* Boston: Little, Brown; 1982:859–872.
13. Conrad RA, Dobyns BM, Sutow WW. Thyroid neoplasia as a late effect of exposure to radioactive iodine in fallout. *JAMA.* 1970;214:316–324.
14. Cooper DS. Antithyroid drugs. *N Engl J Med.* 1984;311:1353–1362.
15. Doehler KD, Wong CC, von zur Muhlen A. The rat as model for the study of drug effects on thyroid function: consideration of methodological problems. *Pharmacol Ther.* 1979;5:305–318.
16. Florsheim WH, Velcoff SM. Some effects of 2,4-dichlorophenoxyacetic acid on thyroid function in the rat: effects on iodine accumulation. *Endocrinology.* 1962;71:1–6.
17. Furth J. Morphologic changes associated with thyrotropin-secreting pituitary tumors. *Am J Pathol.* 1954;30:421–432.
18. Galton VA, Ingbar SH. Effect of catalase inhibitors on the deiodination of thyroxine. *Endocrinology.* 1964;74:627–634.
19. Ganong WF. The Thyroid Gland, Chapter 18. In: *Review of Medical Physiology* Lange Medical Publications, Los Altos, CA. 1965;248–265.
20. Ghinea E, Simionescu L, Oprescu M. Studies on the action of pesticides upon the endocrines using in vitro human thyroid cells culture and in vivo animal models, I: herbicides aminotriazole (Amitrol) and atrazine.*Rev Roum Med Endocrinol.* 1979;17:185–190.
21. Goldman M, Peaslee M H, Naber SP. The action of DDT on the iodide concentrating mechanism of the thyroid gland in adult male Sprague–Dawley rats. *Am Zool.* 1970;10:301–302.
22. Graham SL, Hansen WH. Effects of short-term administration of ethylene thiourea upon thyroid function of the rat. *Bull Environ Contam Toxicol.* 1972;7:19–25.
23. Hayden DW, Wade GG, Handler AH. Goitrogenic effect of 4,4¥-oxydianiline in rats and mice. *Vet Pathol.* 1978;15:649–662.
24. Haynes RC, Murad F. Thyroid and antithyroid drugs. In: Gilman AG, Goodman LS, Rall TW, Murad F, eds. *The Pharmacological Basis of Therapeutics.* 7th ed. New York, NY: MacMillan; 1985:1389–1411.
25. Hempelmann LH. Risk of thyroid neoplasms after irradiation in childhood. *Science.* 1968;60:159–163.
26. Hill CS, Ibanez ML, Samaan NA, Ahearn MJ, Clark RL. Medullary (solid) carcinoma of the thyroid gland: an analysis of the M.D. Anderson Hospital experience with patients with the tumor, its special features and its histogenesis. *Medicine.* 1973;52:141–171.
27. Hill RN, Erdreich LS, Paynter OE, Roberts PA, Rosenthal SL, Wilkinson CF. Review: thyroid follicular cell carcinogenesis. *Fund Appl Toxicol.* 1989;12:629–697.
28. Kaneko Y, Ohara T, Fujimoto Y. Human medullary carcinoma of the thyroid in tissue culture. *Horm Metab Res.* 1983;15:187–191.
29. Kasza L, Collins WT, Capen CC, Garthoff LH, Friedman L. Comparative toxicity of polychlorinated biphenyl and polybrominated biphenyl in the rat thyroid gland: light and electron microscopic alterations after subacute dietary exposure. *J Environ Pathol Toxicol.* 1978;1:587–599.
30. Kennedy TH, Purves HD. Studies on experimental goitre, I: the effect of Brassica seed diets on rats. *Br J Exp Pathol.* 1941;22:241–247.
31. Kingsbury JM. Phytotoxicology. In: Casarett LJ, Doull J, eds. *Toxicology: The Basic Sciences of Poisons,* New York, NY: MacMillan; 1975:591–604.
32. Kuzan FB, Prahlad KV. The Effect of 1,2,3,4,10,10-hexachloro-1,4,4a,5,8,8a-hexahydroxyendo,exo-5,8-dimethionaphthalene (aldrin) and sodium ethylene-bisdithio-carbomate (nabam) on the chick. *Poultry Science.* 1975;54:1054–1064.
33. Lino ST, Yamada T, Breen MA. Effects of graded doses of propyl thiouracil on biosynthesis of thyroid hormones. *Endocrinology.* 1961;68:582–588.
34. Linsay A, Nichols CW, Chaikoff IL. Naturally occurring thyroid carcinomas in the rat: similarities to human medullary carcinoma. *Arch Pathol.* 1968;86:353–360.
35. Lybeck H, Leppaluoto J, Aito H. The influence of an anticholinesterase, methyl parathion, on the radioiodine uptake of the rat thyroid in vivo and in vitro. *Ann Med Exp Biol Fenn.* 1966;1067(45):76–79.
36. Michaelson SM. Endocrine system. In: Anderson AC, Good LS, eds. *The Beagle as an Experimental Dog.* Ames, Iowa: The Iowa State University Press; 1970:412–452.

37. Nagataki S. Effects of excess quantities of iodide. In: Greep RO, Astwood EB, Greer MA, Solomon DH, Geiger SR, eds. *Handbook of Physiology, Section 7*. Washington, DC: American Physiological Society; 1974;3:329–344.

38. Napalkov NP. Tumours of the thyroid gland. In: Turusov VS, ed. *Pathology in Laboratory Animals, Vol 1, Pt 2: Tumors of the Rat*. Lyon, France: International Agency for Research on Cancer; 1976:239–272.

39. Netter FH. Endocrine system and selected metabolic diseases. In: Forsham PH, ed. *The CIBA Collection of Medical Illustrations*. New York, NY: 1974; 4:41-73.

40. Oppenheimer JH, Bernstein G, Surks MI. Increased thyrxine turnover and thyroidal function after stimulation of hepatocellular binding of thyroxine by phenobarbital. *J Clin Invest*. 1968;47:1399–1406.

41. Oppenheimer JH, Shapiro HC, Schwartz HL, Surks MI. Dissociation between thyroxine metabolism and hormonal action action in phenobarbital-treated rats. *Endocrinology*. 1971;88:115–119.

42. Paynter OE, Brown GJ, Jaeger RB, Gregario CA. Goitrogens and thyroid follicular cell neoplasia: evidence for a threshold process. *Regul Toxicol Pharmacol*. 1988;8:102–119.

43. Raizada RB, Dalta KK, Dikshith TSS. Effect of zineb on male rats. *Bull Environ Contam Toxicol*. 1979;22:208–213.

44. Rosenburg IN. The antithyroid activity of some compounds that inhibit peroxidase. *Science*. 1952;116:503–505.

45. Scammell JG, Fregly MJ. The Effect of 3-amino-1,2,4-triazole on hepatic and renal deiodination of L-thyroxine to 3,5,3'-triiodothyronine. *Toxicol Appl Pharmacol*. 1981;60:45–51.

46. Shank JC. A study of thyroid disease in family practice. *J Fam Pract*. 1976;3:247–252.

47. Simionescu L, Oprescu M, Ghinea E, Ghinea L, Sahleanu V, Dimitriu V. The radioimmunological measurement of thyroglobulin secretion in vitro under the influence of some herbicides. *Rev Roum Mod Endocrinol*. 1977;15:243–248.

48. Squire RA, Goodman DG, Valerio MG, et al. Chapter 12, Tumors In: Benirschke K, Garner FM, Jones TC, eds. *Tumors and Pathology of Laboratory Animals*. New York, NY: Springer-Verlag 1978;2:1052–1283.

49. Srinivasan V, Moudgal NR, Sarma PS. Studies on goitrogenic agents in food, I: goitrogenic action of groundnut. *J Nutr*. 1957;61:87–95.

50. Stevens JT. Effect of chemicals on the thyroid gland. In: Thomas JA, Korach KS, McLachlan JH, eds. *Endocrinology Toxicology*. New York, NY: Raven Press; 1985:135–147.

51. Stockard CR. *The Genetics and Endocrinic Basis for Differences in Form and Behavior*. Philadelphia, Pa: Wistar Institute of Anatomy and Biology; 1941.

52. Stoll R, Faucounau N, Maraud R. Follicular and parafollicular adenomas in the thyroids of rats treated with thiamazole. *Ann Endocrinol (Paris)*. 1978;39:179–189.

53. Taurog A. Thyroid peroxidase and thyroxine biosynthesis. *Recent Prog Horm Res*. 1970;26:189–247.

54. Tsuda H, Takahashi M, Fukushima S, Endo Y. Fine structure and localization of peroxidase activity in aminotriazole goiter.*Nagoya Med J*. 1973;18:183–190.

55. Van Dyke JH. Experimental thyroid tumorigenesis in rats. *Arch Pathol*. 1953;56:613–638.

Endocrine Toxicology, 2nd ed.,
Edited by J. A. Thomas and H. D. Colby
Copyright © 1997 Taylor & Francis

4

Toxicology of the Adrenal Cortex: Role of Metabolic Activation

Howard D. Colby, Yajue Huang, Quinshi Jiang, and Jeffrey M. Voight

*Department of Pharmacology and Toxicology,
Philadelphia College of Pharmacy and Science, Philadelphia, Pennsylvania 19104*

INTRODUCTION

The adrenal cortex is a complex endocrine gland having a variety of physiologic functions. Several types of steroid hormones are secreted by the gland, and control of hormone secretion involves a number of regulatory systems. Perhaps in part because of its complexity, the adrenal cortex is adversely affected by a large number of toxicants. Based on an extensive review of the literature some years ago, Ribelin (92) concluded that chemically induced lesions occurred with greater frequency in the adrenal cortex than in any other endocrine organ. Some of the reasons for this vulnerability of the gland to toxicants will be discussed later.

In this chapter, a brief overview of adrenocortical physiology is presented before any consideration of toxicology. To understand the functional consequences of toxicant interactions with any target organ requires some appreciation of the underlying physiologic processes. This is particularly relevant for a multifunctional organ like the adrenal cortex. The discussion of adrenal toxicology will include some general aspects, such as the types of chemicals causing adrenocortical lesions and the factors affecting toxicity. However, the focus of this chapter is on adrenal xenobiotic metabolism and its role in toxicity. In particular, recent work on some of the cytochrome P-450 isozymes that are involved in adrenal bioactivation reactions is described. For other aspects of adrenocortical toxicology, the reader is referred to several recent review articles (13,38,106).

ADRENOCORTICAL PHYSIOLOGY (11)

The steroid hormones that are secreted by the adrenal cortex (Table 1) have far-reaching physiologic effects throughout the body. As a result, the actions of toxicants on the adrenal cortex may cause a wide variety of functional changes. The glucocorticoids, typified by cortisol, have important roles in the regulation

TABLE 1. *Types and Functions of the Major Steroids Secreted by the Adrenal Cortex.*

Secretory product	Type of hormone	Function
Cortisol	Glucocorticoid	Regulation of intermediary metabolism
Aldosterone	Mineralocorticoid	Electrolyte balance
DHEA[a] and DHEA-sulphate	Androgen	Sexual development in females

[a]DHEA, dehydroepiandrosterone.

of intermediary metabolism, particularly carbohydrate and lipid metabolism. Other actions of glucocorticoids include their involvement in adaptation to stress and modulation of behavior. Stress is a potent stimulus for cortisol secretion and is not well tolerated by individuals with inadequate adrenocortical function. However, the specific role(s) of glucocorticoids in the response to stress has yet to be resolved. Similarly, although it has long been recognized that disorders of the adrenal cortex are associated with behavioral abnormalities, the mechanism(s) are still not fully understood.

Mineralocorticoids are the other major class of steroid hormones produced exclusively by the adrenal cortex. The physiologically most important mineralocorticoid is aldosterone whose actions are concerned primarily with electrolyte balance and blood pressure homeostasis. Aldosterone interacts with receptors in the distal tubular cells of the kidney, effecting an increase in the renal reabsorption of sodium ions, as well as increases in potassium and hydrogen ion excretion. One of the consequences of mineralocorticoid actions is an increase in plasma sodium concentrations, with the resulting osmotic effect promoting expansion of the extracellular fluid volume. Thus, disorders of aldosterone secretion are usually characterized by blood pressure abnormalities and/or electrolyte imbalances.

The adrenal cortex secretes large amounts of androgenic hormones, but adrenal androgens are far less potent than their testicular counterpart, testosterone. Otherwise, adrenal and gonadal androgens have similar effects. The quantitatively most important adrenal androgen is dehydroepiandrosterone (DHEA), which is secreted as both the free steroid and sulfated conjugate (see Table 1). The physiologic significance of adrenal androgens in males is uncertain, but as the major source of androgens in females, they are of importance in normal sexual maturation. The adrenal cortex also produces small amounts of estrogens that, except in some adrenal disorders, are believed to be of little functional significance.

The relative amounts of different hormones produced by cells of the adrenal cortex varies among the different anatomic zones of the gland. This relationship between anatomic location and steroidogenic function is known as the functional zonation of the adrenal cortex (67). The outermost zone of the cortex, lying directly beneath the capsule of the gland, is the *zona glomerulosa* (Table 2). This zone is the sole site of aldosterone production within the gland; it does not produce glucocorticoids or androgens. The latter steroids are produced by the cells of the middle and inner zones of the gland, the *zona fasciculata* and *zona reticularis,* respectively. There appear to be some functional differences between these

TABLE 2. *Functional Zonation of the Adrenal Cortex.*

Zone	Hormone(s) secreted
Zona glomerulosa	Aldosterone
Zona fasciculata	Cortisol, DHEA[a]
Zona reticularis	Cortisol, DHEA[a]

[a]DHEA, dehydroepiandrosterone.

two zones, but the physiologic significance has yet to be clearly defined. It is important to be aware of the functional zonation that exists in the adrenal cortex when considering the impact of toxicants on the gland. Some adrenal toxicants have highly localized sites of action, and any resulting functional changes would therefore depend on the hormones produced by the affected zone.

The functional zonation of the adrenal cortex is a consequence of zonal differences in the expression of the enzymes required for steroid hormone production. All steroid hormones are synthesized by the enzymatic modification of the precursor molecule, cholesterol (Fig. 1). The adrenal cortex stores large amounts of cholesterol, mostly as cholesterol esters, in organelles known as lipid droplets. Much of the cholesterol stored in the adrenal is obtained by the receptor-mediated uptake of plasma lipoproteins, although some de novo synthesis also occurs within adrenal cells. As needed, adrenal cholesterol esters are hydrolyzed enzymatically to provide free cholesterol as substrate for steroidogenesis.

The conversion of cholesterol to adrenal steroid hormones is dominated by a series of site-specific hydroxylation reactions on the steroid nucleus (see Fig. 1). Each of these reactions is catalyzed by a specific cytochrome P-450 isozyme (36). As discussed later, cytochromes P-450 are also of importance in adrenal toxicology as sources of reactive oxygen species and in the bioactivation of protoxicants. Some of the steroidogenic P-450 isozymes are located within mitochondrial membranes in adrenal cells, and others are associated with the endoplasmic reticulum. As a result, there is an intracellular migration of the steroid substrate between subcellular compartments in the course of steroid hormone synthesis. The factors controlling this migration have yet to be clearly resolved, although a role for transport or carrier proteins has been postulated. Once produced, steroid hormones are not stored in appreciable quantities; their lipophilicity allows for rapid diffusion across cell membranes and entry into the blood. Thus, synthesis and secretion are inseparable processes, and steroid hormone output is controlled by regulation of steroidogenesis.

The first step in the steroidogenic pathway, cholesterol side-chain cleavage (see Fig. 1), is the rate-limiting reaction, and therefore it is not surprising that it is the site of action of most regulatory factors. The mitochondrial P-450 isozyme (P-450scc) that catalyzes this reaction is essential for the production of all steroid hormones and accordingly is expressed in all steroidogenic organs. However, other P-450–dependent steroid hydroxylases are differentially expressed in different organs, resulting in a unique profile of hormone synthesis that is characteristic of

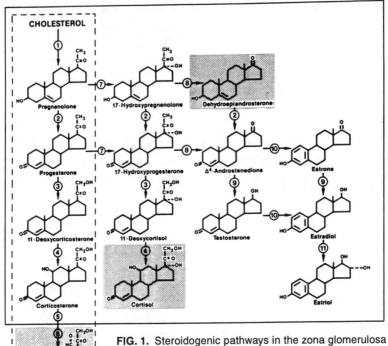

FIG. 1. Steroidogenic pathways in the zona glomerulosa (within broken lines) and zona fasciculata–zona reticularis (within solid lines) of the human adrenal cortex. The major secretory products are shaded. Enzymes: *1*, Cholesterol side-chain cleavage; *2*, 3β-hydroxysteroid dehydrogenase–isomerase; *3*, 21-hydroxylase; *4*, 11β-hydroxylase; *5*, 18-hydroxylase; *6*, 18-hydroxysteroid dehydrogenase; *7*, 17α-hydroxylase; *8*, C17–20-lyase; *9*, 17-hydroxysteroid dehydrogenase; *10*, aromatase; *11*, 16α-hydroxylase. (From ref. 11, with permission.)

each. For example, since the 11β-hydroxylase (P-450c11b) and 21-hydroxylase (P-450c21) are expressed only in the adrenal cortex, mineralocorticoid and glucocorticoid syntheses are limited to this organ. Similarly, the functional zonation within the adrenal cortex is the result of enzymatic differences between the zona glomerulosa and the inner zones of the gland. The 17α-hydroxylase (P-450c17), an enzyme required for both cortisol and DHEA synthesis, is not expressed in the cells of the zona glomerulosa; however, all of the enzymes needed for aldosterone production are expressed there. On the other hand, the cells of the zona fasciculata and zona reticularis express the P-450c17, but not the P-450 isozyme (P-450c11b2) that catalyzes the final step in aldosterone biosynthesis. Consequently, only the zona glomerulosa synthesizes aldosterone, and production of cortisol and DHEA is limited to the zona fasciculata and zona reticularis.

Owing to the different functions and sites of synthesis of the various types of adrenal hormones, more than one regulatory mechanism might be expected. In

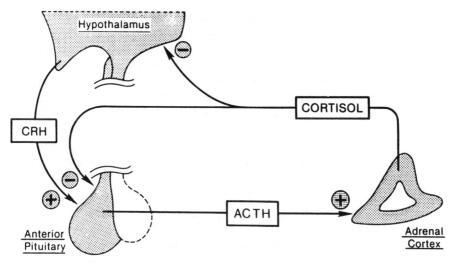

FIG. 2. Regulation of cortisol secretion by the hypothalamic–pituitary axis (+, stimulation; -, inhibition). (From ref. 11, with permission.)

fact, there are several multicomponent regulatory systems that participate in the overall control of adrenal steroidogenesis. As a result, there are many potential target sites for toxicants that could cause disruption of adrenocortical function. Cortisol secretion is regulated principally by a negative feedback loop that includes the anterior pituitary gland and hypothalamus (Fig. 2). Blood cortisol concentrations are the regulated component of the feedback system, and adrenocorticotropic hormone (ACTH) is the direct modulator of cortisol secretion by the cells of the zona fasciculata and zona reticularis. ACTH interacts with membrane receptors in its target cells, activating adenylyl cyclase and increasing cyclic adenosine monophosphate (cAMP) production. The cAMP is believed to mediate both the acute effects of ACTH on cortisol secretion and its longer-term effects on growth of the inner zones of the adrenal cortex. The rapid stimulation of cortisol output by ACTH results from an increase in the transport of cholesterol to the mitochondrial P-450scc (79), thereby increasing enzyme activity and steroid synthesis. Among the chronic actions of ACTH is the maintenance of adrenal steroidogenic enzymes by cAMP-mediated enhancement of gene expression (79,98).

Secretion of aldosterone by the cells of the zona glomerulosa may also be stimulated by ACTH, but this effect is of minor physiologic significance. Blood pressure and plasma electrolytes (potassium, sodium) are the major factors involved in the regulation of aldosterone secretion (11). The regulatory effects of blood pressure and plasma sodium concentrations on aldosterone production are mediated by the renin–angiotensin system. Angiotensin II is the component of the system that interacts with membrane receptors in zona glomerulosa cells to promote aldosterone secretion. Plasma potassium concentrations, acting independently of the renin–angiotensin system, also influence aldosterone secretion in a feedback relationship that further ensures electrolyte homeostasis.

The regulation of adrenal androgen production remains an area of some controversy. Secretion of adrenal androgens generally parallels glucocorticoid output by the gland, suggesting a major role for ACTH in the regulation of both (74,88). However, there are a number of circumstances characterized by a dissociation between cortisol and androgen secretion. One of the clearest examples occurs late in life when adrenal androgen secretion declines markedly while there is little change in cortisol output. Several mechanisms have been proposed to account for this dissociation. However, none can adequately account for the divergence of adrenal cortisol and androgen secretion under the variety of physiologic and pathologic circumstances that have been reported (74,88), indicating the need for further investigation.

ADRENOCORTICAL TOXICOLOGY

Adrenal Vulnerability to Toxicants

As noted by Ribelin (92), the incidence of chemical-induced lesions in the adrenal cortex exceeds that for any other endocrine gland. This conclusion was based on literature reports on the appearance of morphologic changes in adrenal cells after exposure to numerous substances. It is not known to what extent these structural alterations are necessarily accompanied by changes in adrenocortical function. Similarly, there are many reports in the literature of chemical-induced changes in adrenal function with no indication of whether there are associated morphologic lesions. For relatively few adrenal toxicants has the relationship between structural and functional alterations been thoroughly investigated.

If designation as an adrenal toxicant includes those chemicals that cause changes in either the structure or the function of the gland, there are a large number of compounds in the group. Many of these substances have been identified and discussed in earlier reviews (13,38,92,106). The reader is referred to these articles for a comprehensive overview of chemicals causing adrenal toxicity. Some of the more widely recognized or recently described adrenal toxicants are included in Table 3. The nature of the compounds listed in the table ranges from drugs to environmental carcinogens. As noted by Ribelin (92), the diversity of substances that adversely affect the adrenal cortex makes it impossible to classify them in any simple chemical scheme. In addition, mechanisms of action remain largely unresolved. Investigations on the effects of most adrenal toxicants have not progressed beyond the descriptive stage. Although investigations in recent years have been more mechanism-based than before, progress has been slow.

Additional research is also needed on the factors affecting the actions of adrenal toxicants. The results of some studies indicate that a variety of physiologic and pharmacologic factors can influence adrenal toxicity. For example, the effects of some toxicants are highly species-dependent, making it difficult to extrapolate the results of animal studies to humans. It has also been found that age, gender,

TABLE 3. *Compounds Causing Structural and/or Functional Changes in the Adrenal Cortex.*

Compound	Reference
Acrylonitrile	107
Carbon tetrachloride (CCl4)	10
Chloramphenicol	72
Chlordecone (Kepone)	28
Chloroform	44
Chlorphentermine	40
Cyclosporine-A	73
Cyproterone acetate	87
o,p'-DDD (Mitotane)	39
7,12-Dimethylbenz[a]anthracene (DMBA)	52
α-(1,4-Dioxido-3methylquin-oxalin-2-yl)- N-Methylnitrone (DMNM)	119
Doxorubicin (Adriamycin)	23
Etomidate	90
Gossypol	35
Ketoconazole	29
Melengestrol acetate	93
Metals	
Cadmium	85
Copper	112
Tin-protoporphyrin	70
3-Methylsulfonyl-DDE	56
Nicotine	4
Nifurtimox	24
PD132301-2	113
Phenytoin	42
Polychlorinated biphenyls (PCBs)	54
Mifepristone (RU 486)	2
Spironolactone	62
Suramin	3
Tamoxifen	68
2,3,7,8-Tetrachlorodibonzo-p-dioxin (TCDD)	25
Δ9-Tetrahydrocannabinol	117
Toxaphene	81
Triaryl phosphates	65

hormonal environment, and other variables can influence the severity of adrenal toxicity caused by some chemicals. In most cases, the mechanisms responsible for this physiologic modulation of toxicity have not been determined. Because of the large number of substances that have the potential to affect the adrenal cortex adversely, it is important to understand the factors that predispose to adrenal toxicity in order to minimize risk whenever possible.

It is not known with certainty why the adrenal cortex is more susceptible to chemical-induced toxicities than other endocrine organs. However, there are a number of factors that probably contribute to the relatively high incidence (Table 4).

TABLE 4. *Factors Contributing to Toxicity of the Adrenal Cortex.*

High lipid content
Abundant blood supply
P-450–related formation of active oxygen species
Potential for lipid peroxidation
Metabolism (bioactivation) of xenobiotics

Accumulation of Xenobiotics by the Adrenal Cortex

The adrenal cortex has an excellent blood supply, facilitating the delivery of toxic substances to the gland. When expressed per gram of tissue, blood flow to the adrenal is as great as that to any other organ in the body. Accumulation of foreign compounds within the adrenal cortex may be further enhanced by its lipophilic nature. Most xenobiotics that enter the body must be lipid-soluble in order to cross cell membranes and be absorbed. Such substances tend to be retained and accumulate in organs that have a high lipid content, including the adrenal cortex. Thus, potentially toxic substances may reach higher concentrations in the adrenal cortex than in many other organs.

The nature of the blood supply to the adrenal cortex may also contribute to the zonal patterns of toxicity caused by some substances. As noted by Ribelin (92), many adrenal toxicants cause lesions that are highly localized to specific regions of the cortex. Cortical cells are perfused by a capillary system that drains from the outer to the inner region of the gland before uniting in a plexus at the corticomedullary border (46,114). Thus, the blood reaching the inner regions of the cortex first perfuses the cells in the outer portions of the gland. As a result, removal by cortical cells of substances delivered to the adrenal in the blood would tend to establish concentration gradients across the gland with outer zone cells exposed to the highest levels. By contrast, metabolic products of either endogenous or exogenous substances that are released by adrenal cells would probably accumulate at higher concentrations in the inner regions of the cortex. A differential distribution of either toxicants or protective substances within the adrenal could establish regions of high and low vulnerability, resulting in zone-specific toxicities.

Cytochromes P-450 and Peroxidative Damage

The abundance of cytochromes P-450 throughout the adrenal cortex may be a major factor in the frequency of chemical-induced toxicities. The continuous production of steroid hormones by the gland requires the ongoing activities of many P-450–dependent steroid hydroxylases. The mechanism of action of these enzymes may contribute to the risk of local toxicities. Oxygen activation is an obligatory step in the catalytic cycle of all P-450 enzymes (50,51). As a result, reactive forms of oxygen such as the superoxide anion are produced and may escape from the active site of the enzyme to cause oxidative damage. In addition, it has been proposed that some hydroxylated steroid metabolites (pseudosubstrates) bind to steroidogenic P-450 isozymes but cannot be further metabolized, causing an increase in the release of oxygen radicals (47). If this hypothesis is correct, accumulation of pseudosubstrates in certain regions of the adrenal cortex could selectively increase the potential for toxicity at such sites.

The formation of reactive oxygen species may be particularly problematic for the adrenal cortex because of the potential for peroxidation of membrane lipids. Adrenocortical membranes have high concentrations of polyunsaturated fatty acids (Table 5), the substrates for lipid peroxidation. Very high rates of lipid peroxidation have been demonstrated in adrenal mitochondrial and microsomal preparations *in vitro* (100–102), and adrenal glands *in vivo* contain large amounts of lipofuscin, believed to be indicative of peroxidative damage (48). It is known that lipid peroxidation can adversely affect cellular membrane integrity, thereby compromising a variety of important functions (50,51,95). Included among the consequences of lipid peroxidation is degradation of cytochromes P-450 (22,66,110). It has been demonstrated that initiation of lipid peroxidation in adrenocortical mitochondria or microsomes effects declines in steroid hydroxylase activities as a result of P-450 inactivation (9,53,58,116). Thus, exposure of the adrenal to substances that promote lipid peroxidation may diminish the capacity for steroid hormone production.

Perhaps because of its vulnerability to lipid peroxidation or other oxidative damage, the adrenal cortex contains very high concentrations of several antioxidants (50,51), most notably α-tocopherol (α-T) and ascorbic acid (Table 6). The adrenal content of α-T, a fat-soluble vitamin localized principally in membranes, is higher than that of any other tissue (30). However, very little definitive information is available on the mechanisms responsible for this localization or the functional significance of adrenal antioxidants. Several investigators have

TABLE 5. *Free Fatty Acid Concentrations in Guinea Pig Adrenocortical Microsomes.*

C:DB[a]	Fatty acid concentration (μg/g equivalent tissue)
14:0	0.6 ± 0.1 (1)
16:0	16.3 ± 2.1 (22)
16:1	1.1 ± 0.2 (1)
18:0	10.8 ± 0.9 (14)
18:1	23.8 ± 2.0 (32)
18:2	6.3 ± 0.9 (8)
18:3	0.9 ± 0.2 (1)
20:4	15.3 ± 0.5 (20)

Values are expressed as the mean ± SE of eight experiments; numbers in parentheses indicate the percentage of the total fatty acid concentration
[a]C, number of carbon atoms; DB, number of double bonds in fatty acid chain.
(From ref. 100, with permission.)

TABLE 6. *Cytosolic Ascorbic Acid and Microsomal α-Tocopherol Concentrations in Guinea Pig Adrenal Cortex and Liver.*[a]

Tissue	Ascorbic acid (mg/g tissue)	α-Tocopherol (μg/g tissue)
Adrenal	1.4 ± 0.2	57 ± 7
Liver	0.3 ± 0.1	6 ± 1

[a]Values are expressed as means ± SE of 6–7 experiments.
(From ref. 100, with permission.)

demonstrated that adrenocortical function is compromised and lipid peroxidation is high in α-T–deficient animals (59,5), but relatively little is known about the mechanisms responsible for the functional changes. The results of some studies suggest that adrenal antioxidants may be important for protecting P-450 enzymes from oxidant species produced as by-products of steroidogenesis (49–51). α-T is a potent inhibitor of lipid peroxidation (69,84), and its effects on steroidogenesis may be the result of its modulating peroxidative damage to P-450 isozymes or its modifying the lipid environment of these membrane-bound enzymes. Staats and co-workers have found that within the guinea pig adrenal cortex, there are large regional differences in α-T concentrations that are inversely related to lipid peroxidation activity in the different zones of the gland (101,102). The mechanisms responsible for the differential distribution of α-T within the adrenal cortex have yet to be resolved.

Ascorbic acid (AA) is another antioxidant that is found in higher concentrations in the adrenal cortex than in any other organ (45). AA can exert both prooxidant and antioxidant effects, but at the concentrations normally found in the adrenal, AA would be expected to act as an antioxidant (50,51). However, we have reported that the antioxidant activity of AA in the adrenal cortex, as in other organs, is highly dependent on the accompanying concentrations of α-T (99). It was first proposed by Tappel (108) that AA and α-T synergistically interact as part of an electron transport system that terminates free radical chains. According to this hypothesis, the tocopheroxyl radical formed in the course of free-radical scavenging, is reduced back to α-T by AA, thereby enhancing the antioxidant effectiveness of each α-T molecule. Thus, the role of AA within the adrenal cortex may be intimately associated with the actions of α-T and, in fact, may serve principally to preserve adequate α-T levels in the gland.

The high concentrations of α-T and AA found in the adrenal would suggest that the gland is well protected from oxidative damage. However, the adequacy of antioxidant protection can be meaningfully assessed only in relation to the level of oxidative stress to which the gland is exposed. The latter, of course, is not readily quantifiable, but the ongoing activities of steroidogenic P-450 isozymes might be expected to generate high levels of free radicals. In addition, the differential distribution of antioxidants such as α-T within the adrenal cortex may result in some regions of the gland being more vulnerable to oxidative injury than others.

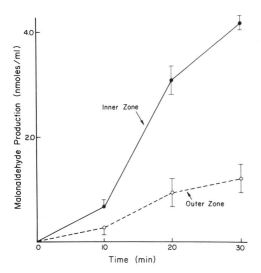

FIG. 3. Time-courses of Fe^{2+}-induced lipid peroxidation (malonaldehyde production) in adrenal inner (zona reticularis) and outer (zona fasciculata and zona glomerulosa) zone mitochondrial preparations. (From ref. 100, with permission.)

For example, it has been demonstrated that in the guinea pig adrenal cortex, the zona reticularis has far lower concentrations of α-T than does the rest of the gland and consequently is subject to higher levels of lipid peroxidation (Fig. 3) (100–102). A more complete understanding of the physiology and pathophysiology of the adrenal cortex will probably be necessary before the adequacy of its antioxidant protection can be determined.

Bioactivation of Xenobiotics

It has long been recognized that the metabolism of xenobiotics in the body may result in the formation of products that have greater or less biologic activity than the parent compound (41). The production of active metabolites from inactive precursors is known as bioactivation. In some cases, highly reactive metabolites or intermediates are produced, resulting in toxicity (41). The enzymes most often implicated in such bioactivation reactions are cytochromes P-450 and many protoxicants are activated only by specific P-450 isozymes. Thus, the organ-specific distribution of certain P-450 isozymes that catalyze bioactivation accounts for the site-selective actions of some toxicants.

Until recently, the role of bioactivation in adrenal toxicity received relatively little attention, in part because adrenal P-450 isozymes were thought to participate exclusively in steroidogenesis. However, it is now recognized that a wide variety of xenobiotics are metabolized by adrenocortical enzymes (12,13,38,57). Among the substrates for adrenal P-450 isozymes are toxicants that are known to require activation for the expression of their toxicity. The toxic agents for which adrenal activation has been clearly implicated include carbon tetrachloride (10), 7,12-dimethylbenz[a]anthracene (86), o,p'-DDD (39), spironolactone (96), chloroform, and 1-aminobenzotriazole (118). It is possible that other adrenal toxicants also undergo metabolic activation, but for most this possibility has not been investigated.

The adrenal enzymes responsible for xenobiotic metabolism include both steroidogenic and nonsteroidogenic P-450 isozymes. Among the former, bioactivation of protoxicants has been found to be catalyzed by the P-450c11 (39), the P-450c21 (43), and the P-450c17 isozymes (62). However, the vast majority of adrenal xenobiotic metabolizing and bioactivation reactions appear to be catalyzed by nonsteroidogenic P-450 isozymes that have yet to be completely characterized (6,8,86). The remainder of this chapter will focus on P-450c17 and P-4502D16 as examples of steroidogenic and nonsteroidogenic P-450 isozymes that are involved in adrenal xenobiotic metabolism. The studies described will serve to illustrate some of the experimental approaches used to establish the functional significance of these enzymes in the metabolism of xenobiotics. They may also be indicative of studies to be done with other less well-characterized isozymes.

P-450c17 (17α-Hydroxylase)

The P-450c17 is a microsomal isozyme that has an essential role in the biosynthesis of glucocorticoids, androgens, and estrogens (11). This enzyme catalyzes two sequential reactions in the steroidogenic pathway, 17α-hydroxylation and cleavage of the C17–20 bond (C17—20-lyase; see Fig. 1). Purification and reconstitution experiments (37, 61), as well as cloning and expression studies (120), have established that both reactions are catalyzed by the same protein. However, the two activities are separable by site-directed mutagenesis-induced changes of as little as a single amino acid (60).

Recently, other steroid-metabolizing reactions have also been attributed to the P-450c17 (75,105). Meadus and co-workers (75) found that purified P-450c17 from porcine testis or adrenal glands or from bovine adrenals, when reconstituted with cytochrome b_5, catalyzed the conversion of pregnenolone to 5,16-androstadien-3β-ol (andien-β synthase). In the absence of cytochrome b, activity was not demonstrable. These studies confirmed some of the earlier observations of Nakajin et al. (82). In addition, Swart et al. (105) reported that COS 1 cells transfected with a full-length human P-450c17 cDNA converted progesterone to both 17α-hydroxyprogesterone and 16α-hydroxyprogesterone, indicating that the protein had 16α-hydroxylase as well as 17α-hydroxylase activity. Antibodies raised against porcine P-450c17 inhibited equally the 17α-hydroxylation and 16α-hydroxylation of progesterone by human fetal adrenal microsomes, providing further evidence that P-450c17 has 16α-hydroxylase activity. Thus, the P-450c17 appears to be multifunctional with respect to steroid metabolism.

The results of several studies indicate that P-450c17 also has xenobiotic-metabolizing activities. Suhara and co-workers (103) found that a purified P-450c17 from pig testis catalyzed a variety of reactions with different xenobiotic

TABLE 7. *Steroid and Xenobiotic-metabolizing Activities in Guinea Pig Adrenal Microsomes and in Reconstituted Systems with P-450c17 and P-450c21.*

Reaction	Adrenal microsomes (nmol/min per mg prot)	Reconstituted system (nmol/min per nmol cytochrome P-450)	
		P-450c17	P-450c21
21-Hydroxylation	6.1 ± 0.6	<0.1	18.1 ± 0.3
17α-Hydroxylation	7.7 ± 0.7	5.8 ± 0.6	<0.1
Benzo[a]pyrene hydroxylation	0.52 ± 0.02	1.48 ± 0.07	<0.01
2-Nitropropane denitrification	7.6 ± 0.3	25.9 ± 1.2	4.8 ± 1.1
Aminopyrine N-demethylation	6.0 ± 0.2	5.0 ± 0.1	1.4 ± 0.3
7-Ethoxycoumarin dealkylation	<0.01	<0.01	<0.01

(From ref. 80, with permission.)

substrates. Among the enzymatic activities of the reconstituted enzyme preparation were N-demethylation (aminopyrine, benzphetamine), O-dealkylation (7-ethoxy-coumarin, p-nitroanisol), denitration (1-nitropropane, 2-nitropropane), and hydroxylation (acetanilide, benzo[a]pyrene). Inhibition of P-450c17-catalyzed xenobiotic metabolism by a number of structurally unrelated steroids further demonstrated that many different compounds could interact with the enzyme.

Mochizuki et al. (80) reported that a purified P-450c17 from guinea pig adrenal glands, when reconstituted with NADPH–P-450 reductase and lipid, had xenobiotic-metabolizing activities, as well as 17α-hydroxylase activity. The reconstituted enzyme preparation catalyzed benzo[a]pyrene hydroxylation, aminopyrine N-demethylation, and 2-nitropropane denitrification (Table 7), in confirmation of the findings by Suhara et al. (103). However, the adrenal P-450c17, unlike the testicular enzyme (103), had no detectable 7-ethoxycoumarin deethylase activity (see Table 7). Mochizuki and co-workers (80) also found that a reconstituted P-450c21 from bovine adrenals exhibited little or no activity with the same xenobiotic substrates.

The benzo[a]pyrene hydroxylase activity of the reconstituted 17α-hydroxylase from guinea pig adrenals was completely inhibited by antibody raised against the P-450c17 (Fig. 4) but was unaffected by anti–P-450c21 IgG (80). In contrast, studies with guinea pig adrenal microsomes, which catalyze high rates of benzo[a]pyrene hydroxylation (17), revealed that anti–P-450c17 IgG decreased activity by a maximum of approximately 30% (Fig. 5). The same antibody completely inhibited microsomal 17α-hydroxylation but had no effect on 21-hydroxylation. The results indicate that P-450c17 has xenobiotic-metabolizing activity but may not account for all of the benzo[a]pyrene hydroxylase activity in guinea pig adrenal microsomes. Since the guinea pig P-450c17 has recently been cloned and sequenced by Tremblay and co-workers (109) and by us (Fig. 6), it will be of interest to determine if the expressed protein catalyzes the same enzymatic reactions as the purified preparation of Mochizuki et al. (80). It will also be possible

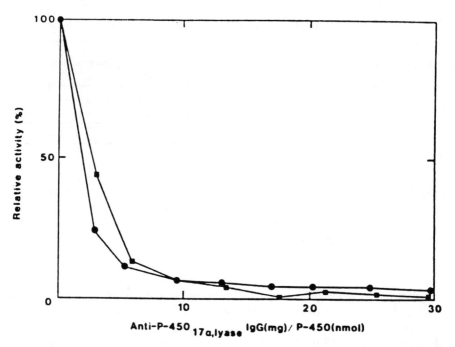

FIG. 4. Effects of anti–P-450c17 (17α,lyase) IgG on 17α-hydroxylase and benzo[a]pyrene hydroxylase activities of a reconstituted 17α-hydroxylase system. ●, benzo[a]pyrene hydroxylase; ■, 17α-hydroxylase. (From ref. 80, with permission.)

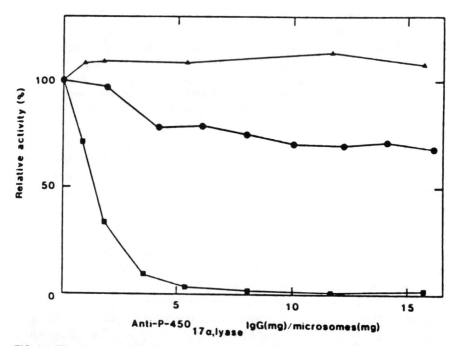

FIG. 5. Effects of anti–P-450c17 (17α,lyase) IgG on steroid and benzo[a]pyrene hydroxylase activities of guinea pig adrenal microsomes. ▲, 21-hydroxylase; ●, benzo[a]pyrene hydroxylase; ■, 17α-hydroxylase. (From ref. 80, with permission.)

to determine if differences in the amino acid sequences of P-450c17 from various species (Fig. 7) influence the xenobiotic-metabolizing activities of each enzyme.

One of the well-studied adrenal toxicants that appears to be activated by the P-450c17 is the diuretic agent, spironolactone. Spironolactone is used clinically in the treatment of congestive heart failure and other edematous states (94). The

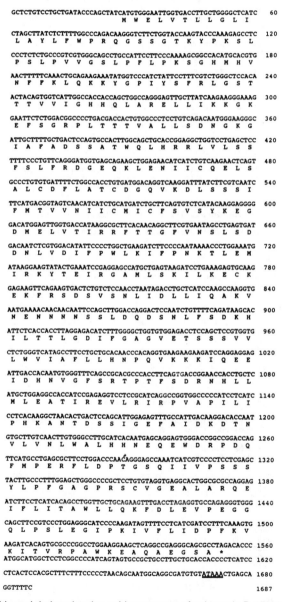

FIG. 6. Nucleotide and deduced amino acid sequences of guinea pig P-450c17 cDNA. The coding region stops at the position indicated by the asterisk. The one-letter amino acid code is used in the second position of each codon. The polyadenylation signal is underlined.

drug competitively binds to renal mineralocorticoid receptors, thereby promoting sodium excretion and potassium retention. In recent years, spironolactone has also been used effectively in the treatment of hirsutism as a result of its anti-androgenic activity (31).

```
GPI     MWELVTLLGLILAYLFWPRQGSSGTKYPKSLPSLPVVGSLPFLPKSGHMH      50
RAT     MWELVGLLLLILAYFFWVKSKTPGAKLPRSLPSLPLVGSLPFLPRRGHMH      50
HUM     MWELVALFLLTLAYLFWPKRRCPRAKYPKSLLSLPLVGSLPFLPRHGHMH      50
BOV     MWLLLAVFLLTLAYLFWPKTKHSGAKYPRSLPSLPLVGSLPFLPRRGQQH      50
        ** *.... *.***.**  .    . .* *.** ***.********. *. *

GPI     VNFFKLQKKYGPIYSFRLGSTTTVVIGHHQLARELLIKKGKEFSGRPLTT     100
RAT     VNFFKLQEKYGPIYSLRLGTTTTVIIGHYQLAREVLIKKGKEFSGRPQMV     100
HUM     NNFFKLQKKYGPIYSVRMGTKTTVIVGHHQLAKEVLIKKGKDFSGRPQMA     100
BOV     KNFFKLQEKYGPIYSFRLGSKTTVMIGHHQLAREVLLKKGKEFSGRPKVA     100
        ****** ****** *.*.***..**.***.*.*.**** **** .

GPI     TVALLSDNGKGIAFADSSATWQLHRRLVLSSFSLFRDGEQKLENIICQEL     150
RAT     TQSLLSDQGKGVAFADAGSSWHLHRKLVFSTFSLFKDG-QKLEKLICQEA     149
HUM     TLDIASKNRKGIAFADSGAHWQLHRRLAMATFALFKDGDQKLEKIICQEI     150·
BOV     TLDILSDNQKGIAFAGHGAHWQLHRKLALNAFALFKDGNLKLEKIINQEA     150
        * .. *,. **.***. .. *.***.*,....*.**.** ***..* **

GPI     SALCDFLATCDGQVKDLSSSIFMTVVNIICMICFSVSYKEGDMELVTIRR     200
RAT     KSLCDMMLAHDKESIDLSTPIFMSVTNIICAICFNISYEKNDPKLTAIKT     199
HUM     STLCDMLATHNGQSIDISFPVFVAVTNVISLICFNTSYKNGDPELNVIQN     200
BOV     NVLCDFLATQHGEAIDLSEPLSLAVTNIISFICFNFSFKNEDPALKAIQN     200
        . ***... .. *.* ....*.*.*. ***. *.*.  . .*.

GPI     FTTGFVNSLSDDNLVDIFPWLKIFPNKTLEMIRKYTEIRGAMLSKILKEC     250
RAT     FTEGIVDATGDRNLVDIFPWLTIFPNKGLEVIKGYAKVRNEVLTGIFEKC     249
HUM     YNEGIIDNLSKDSLVDLVPWLKIFPNKTLEKLKSHVKIRNDLLNKILENY     250
BOV     VNDGILEVLSKEVLLDIFPVLKIFPSKAMEKMKGCVQTRNELLNEILEKC     250
        ..*...  .. *.*. * *.***.*,.* ...  ...*,..*. *,....

GPI     KEKFRSDSVSNLIDLLIQAKVNENNNNSSLDQDSNLFSDKHILTTLGDIF     300
RAT     REKFDSQSISSLTDILIQAKMNSDNNNSCEGRDPDVFSDRHILATVGDIF     299
HUM     KEKFRSDSITNMLDTLMQAKMNSDNNNAGPDQDSELLSDNHILTTIGDIF     300
BOV     QENFSSDSITNLLHILIQAKVNADNNNAGPDQDSKLLSNRHMLATIGDIF     300
        .*.* *.*.... . *.***.*..*.*,  ..*....*..*.*.*.****

GPI     GAGVETSSSVVLWVIAFLLHNPQVKKKIQEEIDHNVGFSRTPTFSDRNHL     350
RAT     GAGIETTTTVLKWILAFLVHNPEVKKKIQKEIDQYVGFSRTPTFNDRSHL     349
HUM     GAGVETTTSVVKWTLAFLLHNPQVKKKLYEEIDQNVGFSRTPTISDRNRL     350
BOV     GAGVETTTSVIKWIVAYLLHHPSLKKKRIQDDIDQIIGFNRTPTISDRNRL     350
        ***.**...*. *..*.*.* .**.. ..**. .**.****..**..*

GPI     LMLEATIREVLRIRPVAPILIPHKANTDSSIGEFAIDKDTNVLVNLWALH     400
RAT     LMLEATIREVLRIRPVAPMLIPHKANVDSSIGEFTVPKDTHVVVNLWALH     399
HUM     LLLEATIREVLRLRPVAPMLIPHKANLDSSIGEFAVDKGTEVIINLWALH     400
BOV     VLLEATIREVLRIRPVAPTLIPHKAVIDSSIGDLTIDKGTDVVVNLWALH     400
        ..*********.***** ****** *****.... *.*.*..*****

GPI     HNEQEWDRPDQFMPERFLDPTGSQIIVPSSSYLPFGAGPRSCVGEALARQ     450
RAT     HDENEWDQPDQFMPERFLDPTGSHLITPTQSYLPFGAGPRSCIGEALARQ     449
HUM     HNEKEWHQPDQFMPERFLNPAGTQLISPSVSYLPFGAGPRSCIGEILARQ     450
BOV     HSEKEWQHPDLFMPERFLDPTGTQLISPSLSYLPFGAGPRSCVGEMLARQ     450
        *.*.**..** ******.*..  .* *.*.************.** ****

GPI     EIFLITAWLLQKFDLEVPEGGQLPSLEGIPKIVFLIDPFKVKITVRPAWK     500
RAT     ELFVFTALLLQRFDLDVSDDKQLPRLEGDPKVVFLIDPFKVKITVRQAWM     499
HUM     ELFLIMAWLLQRFDLEVPDDGQLPSLEGIPKVVFLIDSFKVKIKVRQAWR     500
BOV     ELFLFMSRLLQRFNLEIPDDGKLPSLEGHASLVLQIKPFKVKIEVRQAWK     500
        *.*..*.*.*...... **.*** ...*. *,.*****,**.**.

GPI     EAQAEGSA-     508
RAT     DAQAEVST-     507
HUM     EAQAEGST-     508
BOV     EAQAEGSTP     509
        .**** *.
```

FIG. 7. Alignment of the amino acid sequences of P-450c17 from guinea pig (GPI), rat, human (HUM), and bovine (BOV). The asterisks indicate amino acids that are identical in all sequences; the dots indicate amino acids that are similar in all sequences. The numbers indicate amino acid positions. Hyphens represent gaps introduced to optimize sequence alignment.

Among the side effects of spironolactone is inhibition of steroidogenesis in the adrenal cortex and testis. Administration of the drug to guinea pigs or dogs decreases adrenal cortisol production, apparently as the result of declines in the activities of several steroid hydroxylases that are required for hormone synthesis (32,34,76–78). A number of clinical investigations similarly indicated the potential for inhibition of adrenocortical function in humans by spironolactone. Changes in cortisol, aldosterone, and adrenal androgen secretion were observed in patients receiving the drug (1,104,111).

Studies on the mechanism of action of spironolactone on adrenocortical function revealed a decline in microsomal P-450 concentrations after administration of the drug to experimental animals (32,34,78). In vitro experiments similarly indicated that spironolactone effected the degradation of cytochromes P-450 in adrenal microsomes, suggesting, in addition, that metabolic activation of the drug was required for this effect (34,76,77). Incubation of adrenal microsomes with spironolactone plus NADPH caused a decline in P-450 concentrations, but in the absence of NADPH spironolactone had no effect on cytochromes P-450 (Table 8). Accompanying the decline in P-450 caused by spironolactone in vitro was a decrease in the P-450–catalyzed 17α-hydroxylase activity. The NADPH requirement for P-450 inactivation by spironolactone, as well as its prevention by monooxygenase inhibitors (76,77), suggested that a microsomal P-450 isozyme was responsible for activation of the drug.

Experiments that were designed to characterize the activation pathway for spironolactone-mediated P-450 degradation revealed that at least two enzymatic steps were required (96). When guinea pig adrenal microsomes were incubated with spironolactone in the absence of NADPH, the drug was converted to its deacetylated metabolite, 7α-thiospirolactone (7α-thio-SL), as the only metabolite (Fig. 8). By contrast, in the presence of NADPH, when degradation of P-450 occurred, very little 7α-thio-SL was recovered from the adrenal incubations, suggesting that it was further metabolized by NADPH-dependent enzymes. Incubation of adrenal

TABLE 8. *Effects of Preincubating Adrenal Microsomes with Spironolactone and/or NADPH on 17α-Hydroxylase Activity and on Cytochrome P-450 Concentrations.*

	Preincubation Conditions			
	Controls	Spironolactone	NADPH	Spironolactone+ NADPH
17α-Hydroxylation (nmol/min x mg protein)	12.2 ± 1.1	11.5 ± 1.4	11.9 ± 1.3	7.1 ± 1.0[a]
Cytochrome P-450 (nmol/mg protein)	1.8 ± 0.2	1.8 ± 0.3	1.7 ± 0.2	1.2 ± 0.2[a]

[a]$P<0.05$ vs. control value.
(From ref. 96, with permission.)

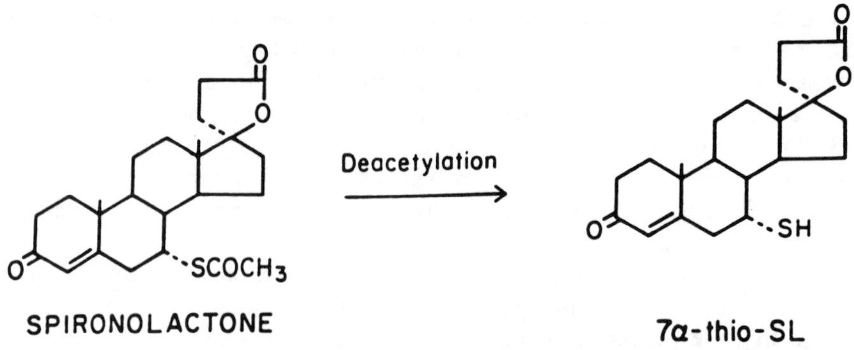

FIG. 8. Chemical structures of spironolactone and its deacetylated metabolite 7α-thio-SL.

microsomes with 7α-thio-SL as the substrate confirmed that its metabolism was stimulated by NADPH (96) and that there was an accompanying loss of cytochrome P-450 (Table 9). Since 7α-thio-SL was far more potent than spironolactone in catalyzing the degradation of adrenal microsomal P-450, it appeared that the metabolite might mediate the actions of the parent drug. This hypothesis was confirmed by experiments with dimethyl *p*-nitrophenyl phosphate (DPNP), an esterase inhibitor that blocks the conversion of spironolactone to 7α-thio-SL. In the presence of DPNP, the SL-mediated degradation of P-450 in adrenal microsomes was prevented, whereas that mediated by 7α-thio-SL was unaffected (Table 10). The results established that 7α-thio-SL was an obligatory intermediate in the actions of spironolactone on adrenal P-450 but that further metabolism of the intermediate was required for toxicity. It has been proposed that 7α-thio-SL is oxidized to a highly reactive sulfenic acid derivative, but definitive identification of the toxic metabolite has yet to be established.

Although the identity of the active metabolite of spironolactone remains uncertain, there is an abundance of evidence that implicates the P-450c17 in its

TABLE 9. *Effects of Incubation of Adrenal Microsomes with 7α-Thio-SL[a] and/or an NADPH-generating System on P-450 Content and on 17α-Hydroxylase and 21-Hydroxylase Activities.*

Incubation conditions	P-450 (%)	17α-Hydroxylase (%)	21-Hydroxylase (%)
Control	103 ± 6	97 ± 4	89 ± 4
NADPH	95 ± 9	103 ± 2	95 ± 4
7α-Thio-SL	105 ± 3	104 ± 12	92 ± 9
NADPH + 7α-Thio-SL	57 ± 3[b]	47 ± 5[b]	92 ± 13

[a]7α-Thio-SL, 7α-thiospirolactone.
[b]$P<0.05$ vs. corresponding control.
(From ref. 96, with permission.)

TABLE 10. *Effects of the Esterase Inhibitor DPNP on Spironolactone- and 7α-Thio-SL–mediated Destruction of Cytochrome P-450 in Adrenal Microsomes.*[a]

Preincubation conditions	Cytochrome P-450 concentration (% of control)
NADPH	100
NADPH + DPNP (100 μM)	95.2 ± 1.9
NADPH + spironolactone (100 μM)	74.5 ± 2.3[b]
NADPH + spironolactone + DPNP	92.8 ± 1.8
NADPH + 7α-thio-SL (100 μM)	47.0 ± 1.2[b]
NAPDH + 7α-thio-SL + DPNP	46.8 ± 1.5[b]

[a]DPNP, dimethyl *p*-nitrophenyl phosphate; 7α-thio-SL, 7α-thiospirolactone.
[b]$P<0.05$ vs. NADPH alone.
(From ref. 96, with permission.)

formation. Early investigations demonstrated that spironolactone caused P-450 degradation only in organs that had 17α-hydroxylase activity, such as the adrenal cortex and testes (76–78). Similarly, in those species such as rats and mice that lack expression of the P-450c17 in adrenal glands, spironolactone administration did not affect adrenal P-450 concentrations. In vitro studies also demonstrated a relationship between 17α-hydroxylase activity and the extent of P-450 degradation in adrenal microsomes (97). Steroid substrates for the 17α-hydroxylase competitively blocked the spironolactone-mediated loss of P-450, but 17α-hydroxylated compounds, which are not substrates, had no effect. Observations such as these, in combination with studies demonstrating that spironolactone caused a decline in 17α-hydroxylase activity, led Menard and co-workers (76,77) to propose that spironolactone was a suicide substrate for the P-450c17. The kinetics of P-450 degradation by spironolactone were also consistent with a mechanism-based inhibition (76,77).

Direct evidence for involvement of the P-450c17 in the activation of spironolactone by adrenal microsomes was provided by Kossor et al. (62). These investigators utilized a purified and reconstituted 17α-hydroxylase preparation consisting of P-450c17, NADPH–P-450 reductase, cytochrome b_5, and dilauroylphosphatidylcholine, to investigate the activation of spironolactone and its deacetylated metabolite, 7α-thio-SL. They found that incubation of the reconstituted system with 7α-thio-SL in the presence of NADPH resulted in the degradation of the P-450c17 and complete loss of 17α-hydroxylase activity (Table 11). In contrast, spironolactone, when incubated under the same conditions, had no effect. These data demonstrate that 7α-thio-SL is activated directly by the purified 17α-hydroxylase, causing inactivation of the P-450c17. They also confirm that spironolactone must first be converted to 7α-thio-SL before activation by the enzyme can occur. The latter conclusion was further supported by spectral studies suggesting that 7α-thio-SL, but not spironolactone, was a substrate for the purified P-450c17 (62).

TABLE 11. *Effects of Preincubation of a Reconstituted 17α-Hydroxylase/lyase Preparation with 7α-Thio-SL, Spironolactone, or Progesterone and an NADPH-generating System on P-450c17 Concentrations and 17α-Hydroxylase Activities.*[a]

Preincubation conditions	P-450c17 (% of control)	17α-Hydroxylation (nmol/min x nmol P-450)
NADPH + progesterone	82 ± 5	16.3 ± 0.6
NADPH + spironolactone	64 ± 5	13.9 ± 0.1
NADPH + 7α-thio-SL	<1[b]	<1[b]

[a]7α-thio-SL, 7α-thiospirolactone.
[b]Below detectable levels in all experiments.
(From ref. 62, with permission.)

Investigations with guinea pig adrenal microsomes provided further evidence for the involvement of P-450c17 in spironolactone activation (62). The effects of anti–P-450c17 IgG on 7α-thio-SL–mediated P-450 degradation were studied. When adrenal microsomes were preincubated with the P-450c17 antibody, there was a greater than 90% decline in 17α-hydroxylase activity

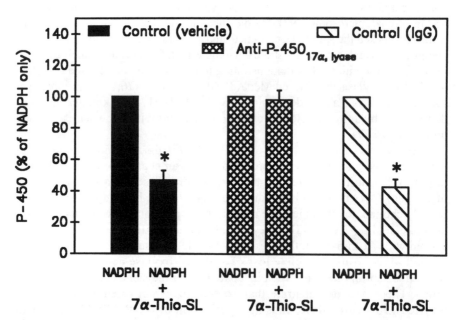

FIG. 9. Effects of anti–P-450c17 (17α,lyase) and control IgG on the 7α-thio-SL–mediated degradation of P-450 in adrenal microsomes. Microsomal suspensions were preincubated with or without anti–P-450c17 IgG or control IgG and then incubated with an NADPH-generating system in the presence or absence of 7α-thio-SL. *P<0.05 vs. corresponding NADPH-only value. (From ref. 62, with permission.)

but no change in the rate of 21-hydroxylation. As a result of the preincubation with the antibody, the subsequent degradation of microsomal P-450 by spironolactone or by 7α-thio-SL (Fig. 9) was completely blocked. The results of these investigations demonstrate that the 17α-hydroxylase is responsible for the activation of spironolactone, resulting in the degradation of P-450c17 and inhibition of steroidogenesis. Further investigation will be necessary to determine if any of the other xenobiotics metabolized by the P-450c17 is also converted to a toxic metabolite.

Cytochrome P-4502D16

It has been known for many years that most of the xenobiotic-metabolizing activity in adrenal glands cannot be attributed to steroidogenic P-450 isozymes. However, definitive characterization of the specific enzymes involved is only just beginning to occur. The guinea pig has been commonly employed in studies on adrenal xenobiotic metabolism, probably because of the high levels and diversity of enzymatic reactions catalyzed (14,63). In addition, the large size of the adrenal glands in guinea pigs, compared with other laboratory animals, provides a relative abundance of tissue for investigation.

Early studies provided indirect evidence that xenobiotic metabolism in the guinea pig adrenal was catalyzed by different P-450 isozymes than those involved in steroidogenesis. For example, a number of physiologic variables were found to have different effects on adrenal steroid and xenobiotic metabolism. As guinea pigs age, adrenal microsomal metabolism of xenobiotics such as ethylmorphine and benzo[a]pyrene increases substantially (Fig. 10). By contrast, neither 17α-hydroxylase nor 21-hydroxylase activity is affected by the age of the animal (16,33,89). In sexually mature guinea pigs, adrenal xenobiotic-metabolizing activities are considerably greater in males than in females, but there are no gender differences in adrenal P-450–catalyzed steroid metabolism (89). In addition, strain differences in adrenal xenobiotic metabolism in guinea pigs have been noted with no apparent influence on steroidogenic enzymes (21). In inbred Strain 13 and Strain 2 guinea pigs, the rates of adrenal xenobiotic metabolism are far greater and less variable than in outbred animals (Fig. 11), but 17α- and 21-hydroxylase activities are not strain-dependent (21). As discussed below, these inbred strains have been very useful for characterization of the P-450 isozymes that catalyze adrenal xenobiotic metabolism.

Like other regulatory influences, ACTH has divergent effects on adrenal xenobiotic and steroid metabolism (17,19,71). It is well established that ACTH increases the synthesis of adrenal steroidogenic P-450 isozymes by cAMP-mediated enhancement of gene expression (98,79). As a result, enzyme activities and steroid synthesis are enhanced by ACTH treatment. However, ACTH administration to guinea pigs decreases the rates of adrenal xenobiotic metabolism and lowers microsomal P-450 concentrations (Fig. 12). Colby et al. (17,18) also noted that ACTH treatment decreased the apparent binding of xenobiotic

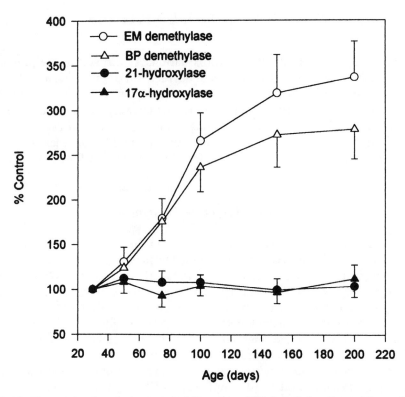

FIG. 10. Changes in adrenal microsomal ethylmorphine (EM) demethylase, benzo[a]yrene (BP) hydroxylase, 21-hydroxylase, and 17α-hydroxylase activities with aging in guinea pigs.

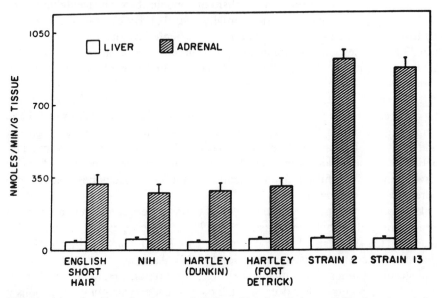

FIG. 11. Adrenal and hepatic microsomal ethylmorphine demethylase activities in various strains of guinea pigs. (From ref. 21, with permission.)

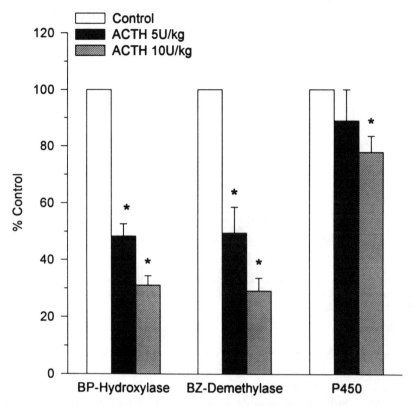

FIG. 12. Effects of ACTH administration to guinea pigs for 7 days on adrenal microsomal benzo[a]pyrene (BP) hydroxylase and benzphetamine (BZ) *N*-demethylase activities and cytochrome P-450 concentrations. *P<0.05 vs. corresponding control values.

substrates to adrenal cytochromes P-450 without affecting steroid binding. These observations suggested that ACTH effected a selective down-regulation of adrenal xenobiotic-metabolizing P-450 isozymes, but the mechanism(s) involved were not determined.

An important advance in the characterization of the P-450 isozymes responsible for adrenal xenobiotic metabolism in guinea pigs was the demonstration by Martin and Black (71) that enzyme activities were highly localized to the innermost zone (zona reticularis) of the cortex. These investigators described a microdissection technique for separating the guinea pig adrenal into an inner zone, consisting principally of zona reticularis, and an outer zone, comprising the zona fasciculata and zona glomerulosa. They found that ethylmorphine demethylase activity was far greater in inner-zone than in outer-zone microsomal preparations. Subsequently, it was reported that other xenobiotics such as benzo[a]pyrene (Fig. 13), benzphetamine, ethoxycoumarin, and chlorinated biphenyls were also metabolized far more rapidly by inner- than by outer-zone microsomes (10,27). It is possible that the low activities in the outer-zone preparations represent con-

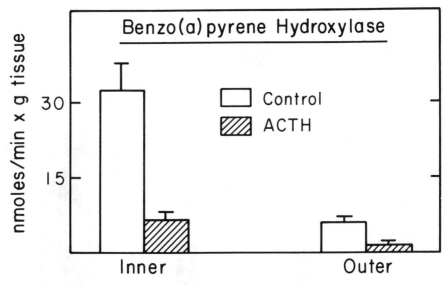

FIG. 13. Benzo[a]pyrene hydroxylase activities in adrenal inner (zona reticularis) and outer (zona fasciculata plus zona glomerulosa) zone microsomes from control and ACTH-treated (10 IU/day x 7 days) guinea pigs.

tamination by inner-zone tissue. In contrast to xenobiotic metabolism, steroids are rapidly metabolized by both inner- and outer-zone microsomes (26).

The localization of xenobiotic metabolism to the zona reticularis of the guinea pig adrenal cortex provides an explanation for the zone-specific actions of some adrenal toxicants. For example, it has been recognized for several decades that carbon tetrachloride (CCl_4) causes adrenocortical necrosis in humans and experimental animals (115). In guinea pigs, the adrenal necrosis caused by CCl_4 is limited to the zona reticularis, with no apparent toxicity to the outer zones (10). Since cytochrome P-450–catalyzed bioactivation is required for the toxicity of CCl_4 (15,91), it was proposed that conversion of CCl_4 to its reactive metabolite, probably the trichloromethyl radical, occurred only in the zona reticularis. Experimental support for this hypothesis was provided by Brogan and co-workers (10), who demonstrated that CCl_4 was activated in vitro by adrenal inner-zone, but not outer-zone, microsomes. These investigators found that incubation of inner-zone microsomes with CCl_4 plus NADPH initiated lipid peroxidation and catalyzed the covalent binding of CCl_4-derived radioactivity to microsomal protein (Fig. 14). In the absence of NADPH, CCl_4 had no effect, indicating that the activation was catalyzed by NADPH-dependent, inner-zone microsomal enzymes.

It was subsequently demonstrated that adrenal activation of CCl_4 was not catalyzed by either of the microsomal steroid hydroxylases, but by an unidentified P-450 isozyme (20). When adrenal microsomes were preincubated with anti–P-450c17 or anti–P-450c21 IgG to inhibit 17α-hydroxylase or 21-hydroxylase activity, there was no effect on microsomal activation of CCl_4, as measured by

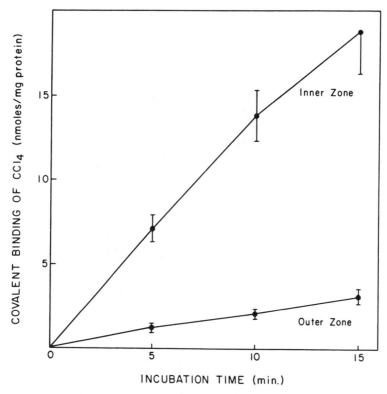

FIG. 14. Covalent binding of radioactivity to microsomal protein following the incubation of guinea pig adrenal inner- and outer-zone microsomes with $^{14}CCl_4$ and NADPH. (From ref. 10, with permission.)

initiation of lipid peroxidation (Fig. 15) or covalent binding to protein. However, preincubation with 1-aminobenzotriazole, a suicide substrate for adrenal xenobiotic-metabolizing P-450 isozymes (118), blocked the activation of CCl_4 by adrenal microsomes (see Fig. 15). Collectively, these results demonstrated that the metabolic activation of CCl_4 is catalyzed by a nonsteroidogenic microsomal P-450 isozyme that is localized to the inner zone (zona reticularis) of the adrenal cortex. Using similar experimental approaches, we have recently found that chloroform, another adrenal toxicant that causes necrosis of the zona reticularis (44), is probably activated by the same isozyme.

Identification of the enzyme(s) responsible for xenobiotic metabolism in the guinea pig adrenal was advanced by the findings of Black and co-workers (7,8) that inner-zone microsomes contained a unique protein, having the characteristics of a P-450 isozyme, that was not present in the outer zone. As estimated by SDS-polyacrylamide gel electrophoresis, its molecular weight was 52 kDa and it was found to be immunoreactive with anti–P-4501A1/1A2 antibody. Despite the immunoreactivity, it seemed unlikely that the adrenal isozyme was

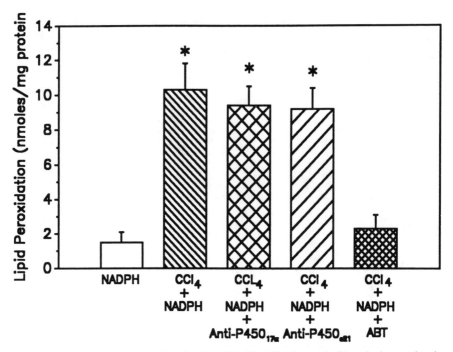

FIG. 15. Effects of anti–P-450c17 and anti–P-450c21 antibodies and of 1-aminobenzotriazole (ABT) on CCl_4-initiated lipid peroxidation in guinea pig adrenal microsomes. $P<0.05$ vs. NADPH group. (From ref. 20, with permission.)

the same as hepatic P-4501A1 or P-4501A2, since, for example, potent inducers of the hepatic isozymes had no effect on adrenal xenobiotic metabolism. Prior investigations had also demonstrated that hepatic and adrenal xenobiotic metabolism in guinea pigs was independently regulated by a number of physiologic factors (21,89), suggesting that different enzymes were involved. In addition, we found that the patterns of metabolism of some xenobiotic substrates, such as benzo[a]pyrene, are different for adrenal and hepatic microsomes (Fig. 16), indicating catalysis by different P-450 isozymes (17).

The adrenal microsomal 52-kDa protein described by Black et al. (7,8) has been found to be highly correlated with xenobiotic metabolism in the guinea pig adrenal cortex. In addition to its inner-zone localization, concentration of the protein increases with aging, coinciding with increases in the rates of adrenal xenobiotic metabolism. ACTH treatment decreases microsomal content of the protein and simultaneously decreases adrenal xenobiotic-metabolizing activities. A close correspondence between changes in adrenal xenobiotic metabolism and in concentrations of the protein as effected by other physiologic variables has also been described (6–8). Collectively, these observations provide strong indirect evidence for the involvement of the 52-kDa protein in adrenal xenobiotic metabolism.

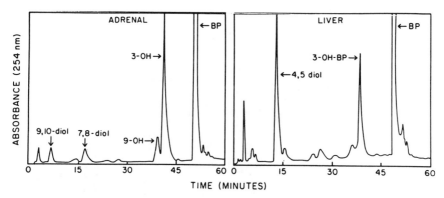

FIG. 16. Metabolism of benzo[a]pyrene (BP) by guinea pig adrenal and hepatic microsomal preparations. *3-OH*, 3-hydroxy-BP; *9,10-diol*, BP-9,10-dihydrodiol; *7,8-diol*, BP-7,8-dihydrodiol; *4,5-diol*, BP-4,5-dihydrodiol. (ref. 17 with permission.)

In order to fully characterize this protein and definitively determine its role in adrenal xenobiotic metabolism, we began a series of microsequencing and molecular cloning studies. Initially, SDS-PAGE conditions were established for optimal separation of this protein from the two major adrenal microsomal steroidogenic P-450 isozymes, P-450c17 and P-450c21 (Fig. 17). Perhaps because of the modified conditions, the protein of interest had an apparent molecular weight of 50 kDa rather than the 52 kDa reported previously (7,8). Identification of the appropriate protein band was established by its inner-zone localization and immunoreactivity with polyclonal antibody to P-4501A1/1A2 as described by Black et al. (8). After transferring the microsomal proteins from gels to PVDF membranes, the band of interest was cut out for microsequencing analysis.

N-terminal microsequencing of the isolated protein revealed the identities of the first 38 amino acids. The sequence obtained was highly homologous with P-4502D subfamily members in a variety of species. The homology with dog P-4502D15, for example, was approximately 84%. Because of the high homology of the protein with P-4502D isozymes, we used a full-length cDNA for human P-4502D6 as a probe to screen a guinea pig adrenal cDNA library. A number of positive clones were obtained, including several that were longer than 1500 base pairs. Nucleotide sequencing identified a full-length clone having an open reading frame that encodes a 500-amino-acid protein (Fig. 18). The deduced amino acid sequence included 38 amino acids that were identical to those obtained by N-terminal microsequencing.

The amino acid sequence encoded by the full-length clone is approximately 70% homologous with other P-4502D isozymes (55) and is therefore a member of the same subfamily. In accordance with the recommended nomenclature (83), this new isozyme has been designated P-4502D16 (CYP2D16). To confirm that

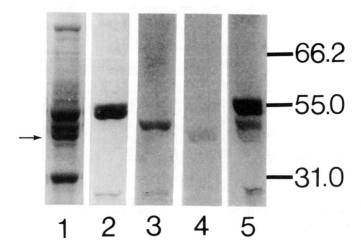

FIG. 17. Electrophoretic and Western blot analyses of guinea pig adrenal microsomes. Lanes are labeled as follows: *1*, Coomassie-stained gel; *2*, anti–P-450c17 immunoblot; *3*, anti–P-450c21 immunoblot; *4*, anti–P-4501A1/1A2 immunoblot; *5*, combined anti–P-450c17, anti–P-450c21, and anti–P-4501A1/1A2 immunoblot. The band used for microsequencing is indicated by the arrow. (From ref. 55, with permission.)

this isozyme is expressed in the guinea pig adrenal gland, RNA was prepared from adrenal inner- and outer-zone tissue, and Northern analysis was done using our full-length P-4502D16 cDNA as the probe. A strong signal was obtained with the inner-zone RNA and a much weaker one with the outer-zone preparation (55).

The high level of expression of P-4502D16 in the inner zone of the guinea pig adrenal cortex and its apparent immunoreactivity with anti–P-4501A1/1A2 antibodies suggest that this is the P-450 isozyme found by Black and co-workers (7,8) to be associated with xenobiotic metabolism. Some of the catalytic capabilities reported for other P-4502D subfamily members overlap with those of adrenal microsomal preparations (64). Others, including benzo[a]pyrene hydroxylation, have not been attributed to P-4502D isozymes but are catalyzed by adrenal microsomes. Thus, the extent to which P-4502D16 accounts for overall xenobiotic metabolism in the guinea pig adrenal cortex remains to be determined. This issue should soon be resolved by expression of the isozyme and assessment of its enzymatic capabilities. It seems likely that P-4502D16 will be found to have a major role in the xenobiotic-metabolizing capabilities of the guinea pig adrenal cortex.

CONCLUSION

It has been proposed that adrenal activation of xenobiotics contributes to the frequency of chemical-induced lesions in the gland. Although this phenomenon has been clearly demonstrated for a number of adrenal toxicants, the overall

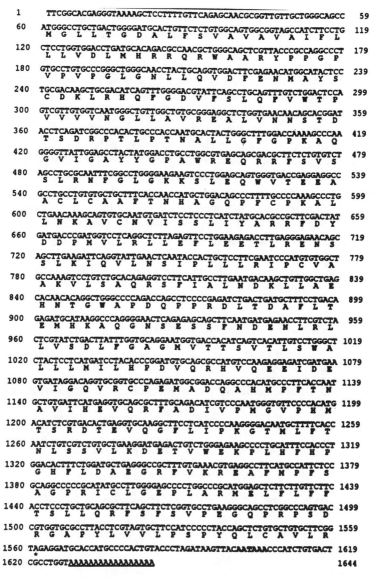

```
1     TTCGGCACGAGGGTAAAAGCTCCTTTTGTTCAGAGCAACGCGGTTGTTGCTGGGCAGCC      59

60    ATGGGCCTGCTGACTGGGGATGCACTGTTCTCTGTGGCAGTGGCGGTAGCCATCTTCCTG     119
      M  G  L  L  T  G  D  A  L  F  S  V  A  V  A  V  A  I  F  L

120   CTCCTGGTGGACCTGATGCACAGACGCCAACGCTGGGCAGCTCGTTACCCGCCAGGCCCT     179
      L  L  V  D  L  M  H  R  R  Q  R  W  A  A  R  Y  P  P  G  P

180   GTGCCTGTGCCCGGGCTGGGCAACCTACTGCAGGTGGACTTCGAGAACATGGCATACTCC     239
      V  P  V  P  G  L  G  N  L  L  Q  V  D  F  E  N  M  A  Y  S

240   TGCGACAAGCTGCGACATCAGTTTGGGGACGTATTCAGCCTGCAGTTTGTCTGGACTCCA     299
      C  D  K  L  R  H  Q  F  G  D  V  F  S  L  Q  F  V  W  T  P

300   GTCGTTGTGGTCAATGGGCTGTTGGCTGTGCGGGAGGCTCTGGTGAACAACAGCACGGAT     359
      V  V  V  V  N  G  L  L  A  V  R  E  A  L  V  N  N  S  T  D

360   ACCTCAGATCGGCCCACACTGCCCACCAATGCACTACTGGGCTTTGGACCAAAAGCCCAA     419
      T  S  D  R  P  T  L  P  T  N  A  L  L  G  F  G  P  K  A  Q

420   GGGGTTATTGGAGCCTACTATGGACCTGCCTGGCGTGAGCAGCGACGCTTCTCTGTGTCT     479
      G  V  I  G  A  Y  Y  G  P  A  W  R  E  Q  R  R  F  S  V  S

480   AGCCTGCGCAATTTCGGCCTGGGGAAGAAGTCCCTGGAGCAGTGGGTGACCGAGGAGGCC     539
      S  L  R  N  F  G  L  G  K  K  S  L  E  Q  W  V  T  E  E  A

540   GCCTGCCTGTGTGCTGCTTTCACCAACCATGCTGGACAGCCCTTTTGCCCCAAAGCCCTG     599
      A  C  L  C  A  A  F  T  N  H  A  G  Q  P  F  C  P  K  A  L

600   CTGAACAAAGCAGTGTGCAATGTGATCTCCTCCCTCATCTATGCACGCCGCTTCGACTAT     659
      L  N  K  A  V  C  N  V  I  S  S  L  I  Y  A  R  R  F  D  Y

660   GATGACCCGATGGTCCTCAGGCTCTTAGAGTTCCTGGAAGAGACCTTGAGGGAGAACAGC     719
      D  D  P  M  V  L  R  L  L  E  F  L  E  E  T  L  R  E  N  S

720   AGCTTGAAGATTCAGGTATTGAACTCAATACCACTGCTCCTTCGAATCCCATGTGTGGCT     779
      S  L  K  I  Q  V  L  N  S  I  P  L  L  L  R  I  P  C  V  A

780   GCCAAAGTCCTGTCTGCACAGAGGTCCTTCATTGCCTTGAATGACAAGCTGTTGGCTGAG     839
      A  K  V  L  S  A  Q  R  S  F  I  A  L  N  D  K  L  L  A  E

840   CACAACACAGGCTGGGCCCCAGACCAGCCTCCCGAGATCTGACTGATGCTTTCCTGACA     899
      H  N  T  G  W  A  P  D  Q  P  P  R  D  L  T  D  A  F  L  T

900   GAGATGCATAAGGCCCAGGGGAACTCAGAGAGCAGCTTCAATGATGAGAACCTTCGTCTA     959
      E  M  H  K  A  Q  G  N  S  E  S  S  F  N  D  E  N  L  R  L

960   CTCGTATCTGACTTATTTGGTGCAGGAATGGTGACCACATCAGTCACATTGTCCTGGGCT    1019
      L  V  S  D  L  F  G  A  G  M  V  T  T  S  V  T  L  S  W  A

1020  CTACTCCTCATGATCCTACACCCGGATGTGCAGCGCCATGTCCAAGAGGAGATCGATGAA    1079
      L  L  L  M  I  L  H  P  D  V  Q  R  H  V  Q  E  E  I  D  E

1080  GTGATAGGACAGGTGCGGTGCCCAGAGATGGCGGACCAGGCCCACATGCCCTTCACCAAT    1139
      V  I  G  Q  V  R  C  P  E  M  A  D  Q  A  H  M  P  F  T  N

1140  GCTGTGATTCATGAGGTGCAGCGCTTTGCAGACATCGTCCCAATGGGTGTTCCCCACATG    1199
      A  V  I  H  E  V  Q  R  F  A  D  I  V  P  M  G  V  P  H  M

1200  ACATCTCGTGACACTGAGGTGCAAGGCTTCCTCATCCCCAAGGGGACAATGCTTTTCACC    1259
      T  S  R  D  T  E  V  Q  G  F  L  I  P  K  G  T  M  L  F  T

1260  AATCTGTCGTCTGTGCTGAAGGATGAGACTGTCTGGGAGAAGCCCCTGCATTTCCACCCT    1319
      N  L  S  S  V  L  K  D  E  T  V  W  E  K  P  L  H  F  H  P

1320  GGACACTTTCTGGATGCTGAGGGCCGCTTTGTGAAACGTGAGGCCTTCATGCCATTCTCC    1379
      G  H  F  L  D  A  E  G  R  F  V  K  R  E  A  F  M  P  F  S

1380  GCAGGCCCCCGCATATGCCTTGGGGAGCCCCTGGCCCGCATGGAGCTCTTCTTGTTCTTC    1439
      A  G  P  R  I  C  L  G  E  P  L  A  R  M  E  L  F  L  F  F

1440  ACCTCCCTGCTGCAGCGCTTCAGCTTCTCGGTGCCTGAAGGGCAGCCTCGGCCCAGTGAC    1499
      T  S  L  L  Q  R  F  S  F  S  V  P  E  G  Q  P  R  P  S  D

1500  CGTGGTGCGCCTTACCTCGTAGTGCTTCCATCCCCCTACCAGCTCTGTGCTGTGCTTCGG    1559
      R  G  A  P  Y  L  V  V  L  P  S  P  Y  Q  L  C  A  V  L  R

1560  TAGAGGATGCACCATGCCCCACTGTACCCTAGATAAGTTACAATAAACCCATCTGTGACT    1619
         *

1620  CGCCTGGTAAAAAAAAAAAAAAAAAAAA                                   1644
```

FIG. 18. Nucleotide and deduced amino acid sequences of guinea pig adrenal P-4502D16. The coding region stops at the position indicated by the asterisk. The one-letter amino acid code is used in the second position of each codon. The polyadenylation signal is bolded and the poly-A tail is underlined. (From ref. 55, with permission.)

significance remains to be determined. The limited distribution of certain activating enzymes is known to account for the organ-specific toxicities of some chemicals; it also seems to provide an explanation for the zone-specific lesions caused by some adrenal toxicants. Similarly, the effects of various physiologic factors on adrenal vulnerability to some toxicants may be mediated by modulation of activation processes. Differences in adrenal metabolism of xenobiotics also account for the species-specific toxicities of some chemicals.

Until recently, studies on the enzymes involved in adrenal activation reactions were largely descriptive in nature. However, reports on the purification and cloning of some adrenal xenobiotic-metabolizing P-450 isozymes now offer the opportunity for in-depth functional and molecular characterization of these enzymes. Future investigations will likely provide important data on the catalytic capabilities of as well as on the regulatory mechanisms for the nonsteroidogenic adrenal cytochromes P-450. Such information should contribute to more complete understanding of the role of these enzymes in adrenal toxicology. In addition, it will be of interest to determine if these xenobiotic-metabolizing P-450 isozymes also have an as yet unknown physiologic function, perhaps related to adrenal steroid metabolism.

REFERENCES

1. Abshagen V, Sporl S, Schoneshofer M, Oelkers W. Increased plasma 11-deoxycorticosterone during spironolactone medication. *J Clin Endocrinol Metab*. 1977;44:1190–1197.
2. Albertson BD, Hill RB, Sprague KA, Wood KE, Nieman LK, Loriaux DL. Effect of the antiglucocorticoid RU 486 on adrenal steroidogenic enzyme activity and steroidogenesis. *Eur J Endocrinol*. 1994;130:195–200.
3. Ashby H, DiMattina M, Linehan WM, Robertson CN, Queenan JT, Albertson BD. The inhibition of human adrenal steroidogenic enzyme activities by suramin. *J Clin Endocrinol Metab*. 1989;68:505–508.
4. Barbieri RL, York CM, Cherry ML Ryan, KJ. The effects of nicotine, cotinine and anabasine on rat adrenal 11β-hydroxylase and 21-hydroxylase. *J Steroid Biochem*. 1987;28:25–28.
5. Barnes MM, Lees D, Smith AJ. In: DeDuve C, Hayaishi, O, eds. *Tocopherol, Oxygen, and Biomembranes*. Amsterdam, The Netherlands: Elsevier; 1978:221–240.
6. Black VH. Immunodetectable cytochromes P-450I, II, and III in guinea pig adrenal-hormone responsiveness and relationship to capacity for xenobiotic metabolism. *Endocrinology*. 1990;127:1153–1159.
7. Black VH, Barilla JR, Martin KO. Effects of age, adrenocorticotropin, and dexamethasone on a male-specific cytochrome P-450 localized in the inner zone of the guinea pig adrenal. *Endocrinology*. 1989;124:2494–2498.
8. Black VH, Barilla JR, Russo JJ, Martin KO. A cytochrome P-450 immunochemically related to P-450c,d (P-450I) localized to smooth microsomes and inner zone of the guinea pig adrenal. *Endocrinology*. 1989;124:2480–2493.
9. Brogan WC, Miles PR, Colby HD. Effects of lipid peroxidation on adrenal microsomal monooxygenases. *Biochim Biophys Acta*. 1983;758:114–120.
10. Brogan WC, Eacho PI, Hinton DE, Colby HD. Effects of carbon tetrachloride on adrenocortical structure and function in guinea pigs. *Toxicol Appl Pharmacol*. 1984;75:118–127.
11. Colby HD. The adrenal cortex. In: Hedge GA, Colby HD, Goodman RL, eds. *Clinical Endocrine Physiology*. Philadelphia, Pa: WB Saunders; 1987:127–159.
12. Colby HD. Adrenal gland toxicity: chemically induced dysfunction. *J Am Coll Toxicol*. 1988;7:45–69.
13. Colby HD, Longhurst PA. Toxicology of the adrenal gland. In: Atterwill CK, Flack JD, eds. *Endocrine Toxicology*. Cambridge, UK: Cambridge University Press; 1992:243–284.
14. Colby HD, Rumbaugh RC. Adrenal drug metabolism. In: Gram TE, ed. *Extrahepatic Metabolism of Drugs and Other Foreign Compounds*. Jamaica, NY: Spectrum Publications; 1980:239–266.

15. Colby HD, Brogan WC, Miles PR. Carbon tetrachloride–induced changes in adrenal microsomal mixed function oxidases and lipid peroxidation. *Toxicol Appl Pharmacol*. 1981;60:492–499.
16. Colby HD, Rumbaugh RC, Stitzel RE. Changes in adrenal microsomal cytochrome(s) P-450 with aging in the guinea pig. *Endocrinology*. 1980;107:1359–1363.
17. Colby HD, Johnson PB, Pope MR, Zulkoski JS. Metabolism of benzo(a)pyrene by guinea pig adrenal and hepatic microsomes. *Biochem Pharmacol*. 1982;5:639–646.
18. Colby HD, Johnson PB, Zulkoski JS, Pope MR. Differential effects of adrenocorticotropic hormone on adrenal microsomal xenobiotic and steroid metabolism in guinea pigs. *Drug Metab Dispos*. 1982;10:326–329.
19. Colby HD, Levitt M, Pope MR, Johnson PB. Differential effects of adrenocorticotropic hormone on steroid hydroxylase activities in the inner and outer zones of the guinea pig adrenal cortex. *J Steroid Biochem Mol Biol*. 1992;42:329–335.
20. Colby HD, Purcell H, Kominami S, Takemori S, Kossor DC. Adrenal activation of carbon tetrachloride: role of microsomal P-450 isozymes. *Toxicology*. 1994;94:31–40.
21. Colby HD, Rumbaugh RC, Marquess ML, Johnson PB, Pope MR, Stitzel RE. Strain differences in adrenal xenobiotic metabolism in guinea pigs. *Drug Metab Dispos*. 1979;7:270–273.
22. Cross CE, Halliwell B, Borish ET, *et al*. Oxygen radicals and human disease. *Ann Intern Med*. 1987;107:526–545.
23. Cuellar A, Escamilla E, Ramirez J, Chavez E. Adriamycin as an inhibitor of 11β-hydroxylase activity in adrenal cortex mitochondria. *Arch Biochem Biophys*. 1984;235:538–543.
24. DeCastro CR, DeToranzo EGD, Carbone M, Castro JA. Ultrastructural effects of nifurtimox on rat adrenal cortex related to reductive biotransformation. *Exp Mol Pathol*. 1990;52:98–108.
25. DiBartolomeis MJ, Moore RW, Peterson RE, Christian BJ, Jefcoate CR. Altered regulation of adrenal steroidogenesis in 2,3,7,8-tetrachlorodibenzo-*p*-dioxin–treated rats. *Biochem Pharmacol*. 1987;36:59–67.
26. Eacho PI, Colby HD. Differences in microsomal steroid metabolism between the inner and outer zones of the guinea pig adrenal cortex. *Endocrinology*. 1985;116:536–541.
27. Eacho PI, O'Donnell JP, Colby HD. Metabolism of 4-chlorobiphenyl by guinea pig adrenocortical and hepatic microsomes. *Biochem Pharmacol*. 1984;33:3627–3632.
28. Eroschenko VP, Wilson WO. Cellular changes in the gonads, livers and adrenal glands of Japanese quail as affected by the insecticide Kepone. *Toxicol Appl Pharmacol*. 1975;31:491–504.
29. Feldman D. Ketoconazole and other imidazole derivatives as inhibitors of steroidogenesis. *Endocrinol Rev*. 1986;7:409–420.
30. Gallo-Torres HE. Vitamin E transport and metabolism. In: Machlin LJ, ed. *Vitamin E: A Comprehensive Treatise*. New York, NY: Marcel Dekker; 1980:193–267.
31. Givens JR. Treatment of hirsutism with spironolactone. *Fertil Steril*. 1985;43:841–843.
32. Greiner JW, Kramer RE, Jarrell J, Colby HD. Mechanism of action of spironolactone on adrenocortical function in guinea pigs. *J Pharmacol Exp Ther*. 1976;198:709–715.
33. Greiner JW, Kramer RE, Rumbaugh RC, Colby HD. Differential control of adrenal drug and steroid metabolism in the guinea pig. *Life Sci*. 1977;20:1017–1026.
34. Greiner JW, Rumbaugh RC, Kramer RE, Colby HD. Relation of canrenone to the actions of spironolactone on adrenal cytochrome P-450–dependent enzymes. *Endocrinology*. 1978;103:1313–1320.
35. Gu Y, Lin YC. Suppression of adrenocorticotropic hormone (ACTH)–induced corticosterone secretion in cultured rat adrenocortical cells by gossypol and gossypolone. *Res Commun Chem Pathol Pharmacol*. 1991;72:27–38.
36. Hall PF. Cytochromes P-450 and the regulation of steroid synthesis. *Steroids*. 1986;48:131–196.
37. Hall PF. Cytochrome P-450 C_{21scc}: One enzyme with two actions: hydroxylase and lyase. *J Steroid Biochem Mol Biol*. 1991;40:527–532.
38. Hallberg E. Metabolism and toxicity of xenobiotics in the adrenal cortex, with particular reference to 7,12-dimethylbenz(a)anthracene. *J Biochem Toxicol*. 1990;5:71–90.
39. Hart MM, Reagan RL, Adamson RH. The effect of isomers of DDD on the ACTH-induced steroid output, histology and ultrastructure of the dog adrenal cortex. *Toxicol Appl Pharmacol*. 1973;24:101–113.
40. Hartmann F, Jentzen F. Effect of chlorphentermine on hormone content and function of the adrenal cortex in rats. *Horm Metab Res*. 1979;11:158–160.
41. Hinson JA, Pumford NR, Nelson SD. The role of metabolic activation in drug toxicity. *Drug Metab Rev*. 1994;26:395–412.
42. Hirai M, Ichikawa M. Changes in serum glucocorticoid levels and thymic atrophy induced by phenytoin administration in mice. *Toxicol Lett*. 1991;56:1–6.
43. Hiwatashi A, Ichikawa Y. Purification and reconstitution of the steroid 21-hydroxylase system (cytochrome P-450–linked mixed function oxidase system) of bovine adrenocortical microsomes. *Biochim*

Biophys Acta. 1981;664:33–48.

44. Hoerr N. The cells of the suprarenal cortex in the guinea pig. Their reaction to injury and their replacement. *Am J Anat.* 1931;48:139–197.

45. Hornig D. Distribution of ascorbic acid, metabolites and analogues in man and animals. *Ann N Y Acad Sci.* 1975;258:103–118.

46. Hornsby PJ . The regulation of adrenocortical function by control of growth and structure. In: Anderson DC, Winter JSD, eds. *Adrenal Cortex.* London, UK: Butterworth; 1985:1–31.

47. Hornsby PJ. Cytochrome P-450/pseudosubstrate interactions and the role of antioxidants in the adrenal cortex. *Endocrine Res.* 1986;12:469–494.

48. Hornsby PJ. Physiological and pathological effects of steroids on the function of the adrenal cortex. *J Steroid Biochem.* 1987;27:1161–1171.

49. Hornsby PJ. Steroid and xenobiotic effects on the adrenal cortex: Mediation by oxidative and other mechanisms. *Free Radical Biol Med.* 1989;6:103–115.

50. Hornsby PJ, Crivello JF. The role of lipid peroxidation and biological antioxidants in the function of the adrenal cortex, part 1: a background review. *Mol Cell Endocrinol.* 1983;30:1–20.

51. Hornsby PJ, Crivello JF. The role of lipid peroxidation and biological antioxidants in the function of the adrenal cortex, part 2. *Mol Cell Endocrinol.* 1983;30:123–147.

52. Huggins C, Morii S. Selective adrenal necrosis and apoplexy induced by 7,12-dimethylbenz(a)anthracene. *J Exp Med.* 1961; 114:741–760.

53. Imataka H, Suzuki K, Tamaoki B. Effect of Fe^{2+}-induced lipid peroxidation upon microsomal steroidogenic enzyme activities of porcine adrenal cortex. *Biochem Biophys Res Commun.* 1985;128:657–663.

54. Inao S. Adrenocortical insufficiency induced in rats by prolonged feeding of Kanechlor (chlorobiphenyl). *Kumamoto Med J.* 1970; 23:27–31.

55. Jiang Q, Voigt JM, Colby HD . Molecular cloning and sequencing of a guinea pig cytochrome P-4502D (CYP2D16): high level expression in adrenal microsomes. *Biochem Biophys Res Commun.* 1995; 209: 1149–1156

56. Jönsson C-J, Lund B-O. In vitro bioactivation of the environmental pollutant 3-methylsulphonyl-2,2-bis(4-chlorophenyl)-1,1-dichloroethene in the human adrenal gland. *Toxicol Lett.* 1994;71:69–175.

57. Juchau MR, Pedersen MG. Drug biotransformation reactions in the human fetal adrenal gland. *Life Sci.* 1973;12:193–204.

58. Kitabchi AE. Inhibition of steroid C-21 hydroxylase by ascorbate: alterations of microsomal lipids in beef adrenal cortex. *Steroids.* 1967;10:567–576.

59. Kitabchi AE. Hormonal status in vitamin E deficiency. In: Machlin LJ, ed. *Vitamin E: A Comprehensive Treatise.* New York, NY: Marcel Dekker; 1980:348–371.

60. Kitamura M, Buczko E, Dufau ML. Dissociation of hydroxylase and lyase activities by site-directed mutagenesis of the rat P-45017α. *Mol Endocrinol.* 1991;5:1373–1380.

61. Kominami S, Shinzawa K, Takemori S. Purification and some properties of cytochrome P-450 specific for steroid 17α-hydroxylation and C17-20 bond cleavage from guinea pig adrenal microsomes. *Biochem Biophys Res Commun.* 1982;109:916–921.

62. Kossor DC, Kominami S, Takemori S, Colby HD. Role of the steroid 17α-hydroxylase in spironolactone-mediated destruction of adrenal cytochrome P-450. *Mol Pharmacol.* 1991;40:321–325.

63. Kupfer D, Orrenius S. Characteristics of guinea pig liver and adrenal monooxygenase systems. *Mol Pharmacol.* 1970;6:221–230.

64. Larrey D, Distlerath LM, Dannon GA, Wilkinson GR, Guengerich FP. Purification and characterization of the rat liver microsomal cytochrome P-450 involved in the 4-hydroxylation of debrisoquine, a prototype for genetic variation in oxidative drug metabolism. *Biochemistry.* 1984;23:2787–2795.

65. Latendresse JR, Azhar S, Brooks CL, Capen CC. Pathogenesis of cholesteryl lipidosis of adrenocortical and ovarian interstitial cells in F344 rats caused by tricresyl phosphate and butylated triphenyl phosphate. *Toxicol Appl Pharmacol.* 1993;122:281–289.

66. Logani MK, Davies RE. Lipid oxidation: biological effects and antioxidants–a review. *Lipids.* 1980;15:485–495.

67. Long JA. Zonation of the mammalian adrenal cortex. In: Geiger SR, exec ed. *Handbook of Physiology: A Critical Comprehensive Presentation of Physiologic Knowledge and Concepts.* Baltimore, Md: Williams & Wilkins; 1975:6:13–24.

68. Lullman H, Lullman-Rauch R. Tamoxifen-induced generalized lipidosis in rats subchronically treated with high doses. *Toxicol Appl Pharmacol.* 1981;61:138–146.

69. Machlin LJ, Bendich A. Free radical tissue damage: protective role of antioxidant nutrients. *FASEB J* 1987;1:441–445.

70. Maines MD, Trakshel. Tin-protoporphyrin: a potent inhibitor of hemoprotein-dependent steroidogenesis in rat adrenals and testes. *J Pharmacol Exp Ther.* 1992;260:909–916.

71. Martin KO, Black VH. Effects of age and adrenocorticotropin on microsomal enzymes in guinea pig adrenal inner and outer cortices. *Endocrinology*. 1983;112:573–579.

72. Mazzocchi G, Nussdorfer GG. Effects of chloramphenicol on the long term trophic action of ACTH on rat adrenocortical cells: a combined stereological and enzymological study. *J Anat*. 1985;140: 607–612.

73. Mazzocchi G, Markowoska A, Andreis PG, *et al.* Effects of Cyclosporine-A on Steroid Secretio of dispersed rat adrenocortical cells. *Exp Toxicol Pathol*. 1993;45:481–488.

74. McKenna TJ, Cunningham SK. The control of adrenal androgen secretion. *J Endocrol*. 1991;192:1–3.

75. Meadus WJ, Mason JI, Squires EJ. Cytochrome P-450c17 from porcine and bovine adrenal catalyzes the formation of 5,16-androstadien-3β-ol from pregnenolone in the presence of cytochrome b_5. *J Steroid Biochem Mol Biol*. 1993;46:565–572.

76. Menard RH, Guenthner TM, Kon H, Gillette JR. Studies on the destruction of adrenal and testicular cytochrome P-450 by spironolactone. *J Biol Chem*. 1979;254:1726–1733.

77. Menard RH, Guenthner TM, Taburet AM, et al. Specificity of the in vitro destruction of adrenal and hepatic microsomal steroid hydroxylases by thiosteroids. *Mol Pharmacol*. 1979;16:997–1010.

78. Menard RH, Martin HF, Stripp B, Gillette JR, Bartter FC. Spironolactone and cytochrome P-450: impairment of steroid hydroxylation in the adrenal cortex. *Life Sci*. 1975;15:1639–1648.

79. Miller WR. Molecular biology of steroid hormone synthesis. *Endocrinol Rev*. 1988;9:295–318.

80. Mochizuki H, Kominami S, Takemori S. Examination of differences between benzo(a)pyrene and steroid hydroxylases in guinea pig adrenal microsomes. *Biochim Biophys Acta*. 1988;964:83–89.

81. Mohammed A, Hallberg E, Rydstrom J, Slanina P. Toxaphene: accumulation in the adrenal cortex and effect on ACTH-stimulated corticosteroid synthesis in the rat. *Toxicol Lett*. 1985;24:137–143.

82. Nakajin S, Takahasi M, Shinoda M, Hall PF. Cytochrome b_5 promotes the synthesis of delta-16 C19 steroids by homogenous cytochrome P-450 C21 sidechain cleavage from pig testis. *Biochem Biophys Res Commun*. 1985;132:708–713.

83. Nelson DR, Kamataki T, Waxman DJ, et al. The P-450 superfamily: update on new sequences, gene mapping, accession numbers, early trivial names of enzymes, and nomenclature. *DNA Cell Biol*. 1993;22:1–51.

84. Niki E. Antioxidants in relation to lipid peroxidation. *Chem Physics Lipids*. 1987;44:227–53.

85. Nishiyama S, Nakamura K. Effect of cadmium on plasma aldosterone and serum corticosterone concentrations in male rats. *Toxicol Appl Pharmacol*. 1984;76:420–425.

86. Otto S, Marcus C, Pidgeon C, Jefcoate C. A novel adrenocorticotropin-inducible cytochrome P-450 from rat adrenal microsomes catalyzes polycyclic aromatic hydrocarbon metabolism. *Endocrinology*. 1991;129:970–982.

87. Panesar NS, Herries DG, Stitch SR. Effects of cyproterone and cyproterone acetate on the adrenal gland in the rat: studies in vivo and in vitro. *J Endocrinol*. 1979;80:229–238.

88. Parker LN. Adrenarche. *Endocrinol Metab Clin North Am*. 1991;20:71–83.

89. Pitrolo DA, Rumbaugh RC, Colby HD. Maturational changes in adrenal xenobiotic metabolism in male and female guinea pigs. *Drug Metab Dispos*. 1979;7:52–56.

90. Preziosi P, Vacca M. Adrenocortical suppression and other endocrine effects of etomidate. *Life Sci*. 1988;42:477–489.

91. Recknagel RO, Glende EA, Dolak JA, Waller RL. Mechanisms of carbon tetrachloride toxicity. *Pharmacol Ther*. 1989;43:139–154.

92. Ribelin WE. The effects of drugs and chemicals upon the structure of the adrenal gland. *Fundam Appl Toxicol*. 1984;4:105–119.

93. Robertson WR, Lambert A, Mitchell R, Kendle K, Petrow V. The effect of some antiprostatic steroids upon cortisol production by guinea pig adrenal cells stimulated by ACTH. *Biochem Pharmacol*. 1989; 38:3669–3671.

94. Saunders FJ, Alberti RL. *Aldactone (Spironolactone): A Comprehensive Review*. New York, NY: Searle, Inc; 1978.

95. Sevanian A, Hochstein P. Mechanisms and consequences of lipid peroxidation in biological systems. *Annu Rev Nutr*. 1985;5:365–390.

96. Sherry JH, Flowers L, O'Donnell JP, LaCagnin LB, Colby HD. Metabolism of spironolactone by adrenocortical and hepatic microsomes: relationship to cytochrome P-450 destruction. *J Pharmacol Exp Ther*. 1986;236:675–683.

97. Sherry JH, Johnson PB, Levitt M, Bergstrom J, Colby HD. Regional differences in adrenal activation of spironolactone: relationship to steroid 17α-hydroxylase activity. *Drug Metab Dispos*. 1989;17:709–710.

98. Simpson ER, Waterman MR. Regulation of the synthesis of steroidogenic enzymes in adrenal cortical cells by ACTH. *Annu Rev Physiol*. 1988;5:427–440.

99. Staats DA, Colby HD. Modulation of the effects of ascorbic acid on lipid peroxidation by tocopherol in adrenocortical mitochondria. *J Steroid Biochem*. 1989;32:609–611.

100. Staats DA, Lohr D, Colby HD. Relationship between mitochondrial lipid peroxidation and alpha-tocopherol levels in guinea pig adrenal cortex. *Biochim Biophys Acta.* 1988;961:279–284.
101. Staats DA, Lohr D, Colby HD. Effects of tocopherol depletion on the regional differences in adrenal microsomal lipid peroxidation and steroid metabolism. *Endocrinology.* 1988;123:975–980.
102. Staats DA, Lohr D, Colby HD. αTocopherol depletion eliminates the regional differences in adrenal mitochondrial lipid peroxidation. *Mol Cell Endocrinol.* 1989;62:189–195.
103. Suhara K, Fujimura Y, Shiroo M, Katagiri M. Multiple catalytic properties of the purified and reconstituted cytochrome P-450 (P-450$_{sccII}$) system of pig testis microsomes. *J Biol Chem.* 1984;259:8729–8736.
104. Sundsfjord JA, Marton P, Jorgensen H, Aakvaag A. Reduced aldosterone secretion during spironolactone treatment in primary aldosteronism: report of a case. *J Clin Endocrinol Metab.* 1974;39:734–739.
105. Swart P, Swart AC, Waterman MR, Estabrook RW, Mason JI. Progesterone 16α-hydroxylase activity is catalyzed by human cytochrome P-450 17α-hydroxylase. *J Clin Endocrinol Metab.* 1993;77:98–102.
106. Szabo S, Lippe IT. Adrenal gland: Chemically induced structural and functional changes in the cortex. *Toxicol Pathol.* 1989; 17:317–329.
107. Szabo S, Hütter I, Kovacs K, Horvath E, Szabo D, Horner HC. Pathogenesis of experimental adrenal hemorrhagic necrosis ("apoplexy"). Ultrastructural, biochemical, neuropharmacologic, and blood coagulation studies with acrylonitrile in the rat. *Lab Invest.* 1980;42:533–546.
108. Tappel AL. Will antioxidant nutrients slow aging processes? *Geriatrics.* 1968;23:97–105.
109. Tremblay Y, Fleury A, Beadoin C, Vallèe M, Bèlanger A. Molecular cloning and expression of guinea pig cytochrome P-450c17 cDNA (steroid 17α-hydroxylase/17,20 lyase): tissue distribution, regulation, and substrate specificity of the expressed enzyme. *DNA Cell Biol.* 1994;13:1199–1212.
110. Tribble DL, Aw TY, Jones DP. The pathophysiological significance of lipid peroxidation in oxidative cell injury. *Hepatology.* 1987;7:377–386.
111. Tuck ML, Sowers JR, Fittingoff DB, et al. Plasma corticosteroid concentrations during spironolactone administration: evidence for adrenal biosynthetic blockade in man. *J Clin Endocrinol Metab.* 1981;52:1057–1061.
112. Veltman JC, Maines MD. Regulatory effect of copper on rat adrenal cytochrome P-450 and steroid metabolism. *Biochem Pharmacol.* 1986;35:2903–2909.
113. Vernetti LA, MacDonald JR, Wolfgang GHI, Dominick MA, Pegg DG. ATP depletion is associated with cytotoxicity of a novel lipid regulator in guinea pig adrenocortical cells. *Toxicol Appl Pharmacol.* 1993;118:30–38.
114. Vinson GP, Kenyon CJ. Steroidogenesis in the zones of the mammalian adrenal cortex. In: Chester Jones I, Henderson IW, eds. *General, Comparative, and Clinical Endocrinology of the Adrenal Cortex.* New York, NY: Academic Press, 1978;2:201–264.
115. von Oettingen WF. In: *The Halogenated Aliphatic, Olefinic, Cyclic, Aromatic, and Aliphatic-aromatic Hydrocarbons Including the Halogenated Insecticides: Their Toxicity and Potential Dangers.* Washington, DC: Public Health Service Publications; 1955.
116. Wang HP, Kimura T. Ferrous ion-mediated cytochrome P-450 degradation and lipid peroxidation in adrenal cortex mitochondria. *Biochim Biophys Acta.* 1976;423:374–381.
117. Warner W, Harris LS, Carchman RA. Inhibition of corticosteroidogenesis by delta-9-tetrahydrocannabinol. *Endocrinology.* 1977;101:1815–1820.
118. Xu D, Voigt JM, Mico BA, Kominami S, Takemori S, Colby HD. Inhibition of adrenal cytochromes P-450 by 1-aminobenzotriazole in vitro. *Biochem Pharmacol.* 1994;48:1421–1426.
119. Yarrington JT, Loudy DE, Sprinkle DJ, Gibson JP, Wright CL, Johnston JO. Degeneration of the rat and canine adrenal cortex caused by α-(1,4-dioxido-3-methylquinoxalin-2-yl)-*N*-methylnitrone (DMNM). *Fundam Appl Toxicol.* 1985;5:370–381.
120. Zuber MX, Simpson ER, Waterman MR. Expression of bovine 17α-hydroxylase cytochrome P-450 cDNA in nonsteroidogenic (COS 1) cells. *Science.* 1986;234:1258–1261.

Endocrine Toxicology, 2nd ed.,
Edited by J. A. Thomas and H. D. Colby
Copyright © 1997 Taylor & Francis

5

Chemically-Induced Lesions
in the Adrenal Cortex

Sandor Szabo and Zsuzsa Sandor

*Departments of Pathology and Pharmacology, University of California at Irvine, and
Veterans Affairs Medical Center, Long Beach, California 90822*

The most well-known causes of cell and tissue injury are hypoxia, chemical and physical factors, biologic (eg, infectious, immunologic) agents, and genetic determinants. Among these etiologic agents, chemicals represent the most common agents affecting endocrine glands; in decreasing frequency these include the adrenals, testis, ovary, and other glands (22). This may be the reason that systematic structure-activity studies have been performed only with adrenocorticolytic chemicals (25,28,31). Our purpose here is to review the patterns of cell and tissue injury in the endocrine glands starting with etiology and progressing through pathogenesis and structural (ie, morphologic) and functional (eg, pathophysiologic) changes.

A variety of chemicals produce adrenal necrosis in experimental animals. Mechanical blockade of adrenal vessels results in a similar pattern of focal necrosis, originating in the inner cortical layers (7). The correlation between structural and functional adrenal changes caused by chemicals and ischemia has been reviewed (25). New data indicate a relationship between the chemical structure of a drug and its toxicity for the adrenal cortex (5); for example, a good correlation exists between the number of sulfhydryl groups and the adrenocorticolytic effect of the molecule. There has also been a structure-activity study involving adrenocorticolytic chemicals, some of which induce duodenal ulcer (28).

In our review, we will provide some data on the most important drugs causing adrenocortical lesions. The most rapidly acting adrenolytic chemical is acrylonitrile, which induces adrenal apoplexy in about 2 hours. Cysteamine, pyrazole and thioguanine, the most extensively studied adrenocorticolytic agents, cause adrenocortical necrosis in 2–5 days. Other compounds such as 7,12-dimethylbenz[a]anthracene (DMBA) and hexadimethrine bromide will also be reviewed.

ACRYLONITRILE

Acrylonitrile (CH_2=$CHCN$, vinyl cyanide) is one of the most important components used in the manufacture of plastics, fibers and synthetic rubber. Vinyl cyanide is otherwise the unsaturated homologue of the duodenal ulcerogen propionitrile. Acute and chronic toxic effects of the chemical, proved by animal experiments and learned from accidental human poisonings, involve mainly the adrenal glands, stomach, duodenum, brain, and lungs (11,25,29,32,33).

The acute adrenocorticolytic effect of acrylonitrile was described in 1971 (26). The first really detailed pathogenetic and morphologic studies were published in 1976 and 1980 (27,33). In the majority of experiments, acrylonitrile was injected intravenously in a dose of 5 mg or 15 mg/100 g body weight. The smaller dose caused mild adrenocortical damage and no mortality, whereas the larger dose induced hemorrhagic adrenal necrosis and 100% mortality within 2 hours (33). Acrylonitrile is the fastest-acting adrenocorticolytic agent because one large intravenous dose in rats causes adrenal hemorrhage and necrosis in 90–120 minutes in 100% of cases.

Morphologic Changes

Extensive ultrastructural, histochemical, and light-microscopic studies have been performed with only a few adrenocorticolytic agents, with acrylonitrile

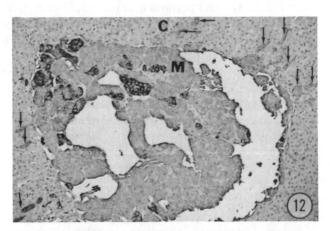

FIG. 1. Special stain to demonstrate medullary catecholamines, light brown-black adrenaline and dark brown-black noradrenaline secretory granules in the medulla of the adrenal of a rat given acrylonitrile (60 minutes). Note the sharp demarcation of cortex (C) and medulla (M). However, several cortical capillaries are also filled with silver-positive materials *(arrows)*, probably originating from the medulla. (Grimelius stain, ×95.) (Reproduced with permission from Szabo S, Hüttner I, Kovacs K, Horvath E, Szabo D, Horne HC, *Lab Invest* 1980; 42:533-546.)

probably the most widely investigated. Electron microscopic time-course studies with acrylonitrile injected intravenously in rats revealed an early endothelial injury in the adrenal cortex. This coincided with mild congestion and focal labeling of blood vessels with the vascular tracer colloidal carbon in the adrenals of rats killed 30 minutes after injection of acrylonitrile; these changes were especially notable at the corticomedullary junction. Occasional blackened vessels were seen even in the zona fasciculata. The carbon deposition was more prominent and extensive (eg, even in subcapsular areas) at 60 minutes than at 30 minutes. Fragments of silver-positive (dark brown, black) granular tissue in the lumen of capillaries mostly in the inner cortex were visible with Grimelius' stain for argyrophil granules, less often in the subcapsular regions (Fig.1). Focal deposition in the medullary vessels and less frequently along the wall of cortical capillaries was seen with fibrin stain. These fibrin thrombi caused only narrowing; complete occlusion of the lumen was not seen. The congestion was more advanced at 60 minutes than 30 minutes, and eosinophilic amorphous (plasma-like) material filled up the place of very rare cell drop-outs. Severe congestion and focal hemorrhages were observed in the zona reticularis and, in a few cases only, in the zona glomerulosa. The bleeding first appeared usually in the inner cortex and less frequently in the middle of the zona fasciculata or outer cortex (Fig. 2). Black deposits were seen around the bleeding site in the adrenals of animals injected with carbon. Fibrin deposition was more prominent than at earlier time intervals, and more suboocclusive thrombi were detected.

Macroscopically, the adrenals from acrylonitrile-injected rats had focally or uniformly red capsular surface. Microscopically, they showed small or extensive

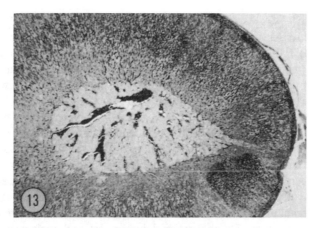

FIG. 2. Extensive hemorrhagic necrosis (developed in 120 minutes) involving the outer layers of cortex in the adrenal of a rat which received acrylonitrile. (Luna's stain for hemoglobin, ×25.) (reproduced with permission from Szabo S, Hüttner I, Kovacs K, Horvath E, Szabo D, Horner HC. *Lab Invest* 1980; 42:533-546.)

blood lakes involving the cortex and often extending into the subcapsular space.

Experiments with rats ingesting 0.002%, 0.01%, 0.05, or 0.2% of acrylonitrile in drinking water for 7, 21, or 60 days revealed a biphasic, dose- and time-dependent effect on the adrenal gland (32). Namely, initial atrophy was followed by normalization of weight or slight but statistically significant enlargement. Despite these macroscopic and microscopic changes in the adrenals, the cortex remained hypofunctional (see below).

Functional Alterations

Acrylonitrile is a very reactive chemical that interacts with body constituents (24,25) and undergoes metabolic transformations. It rapidly depletes reduced glutathione in several organs (29,37). In this brief biochemical and functional overview, emphasis is placed on neuroendocrine alterations.

After injection of equimolar amounts of acrylonitrile and its saturated analog propionitrile (which does not exert any adrenocorticolytic effect), catecholamine levels in the adrenal and brain were measured in rats. Acrylonitrile steadily increased the concentration of dopamine in the adrenals (+25%, +49%, and +52% at 15, 30, and 60 minutes, respectively, after the injection) but not in the brain. The levels of noradrenaline after a transient rise in the adrenals (+38% at 15 minutes) showed a tendency to decrease, especially in the brain (eg,–32% at 60 minutes). Minor and transient elevation of dopamine in the adrenals (eg, +25% at 30 minutes) was caused only by the saturated and duodenal ulcerogen analog propionitrile. The rapid development (ie, within hours) of often hemorrhagic necrosis of the adrenal cortex is usually not accompanied by an immediate decrease in the circulating level of corticoids, which have a relatively long biologic half-life (ie, hours, days).

Acrylonitrile was also administered to rats in drinking water (0.01–0.2%) or gavage for 3 weeks and resulted in dose-dependent decrease in circulating corticoids (Fig. 3). Pair-feeding with the highest concentration of acrylonitrile (0.2%) also diminished the plasma levels of both corticoids, indicating that the stressor effect and/or decreased food intake were also responsible for the low circulating levels of steroids.

The adrenal weight was reduced in 7- and 21-day experiments, but it was increased in the 60-day studies (32). Dose-dependent adrenal atrophy was observed when the rats were ingesting up to 0.2% acrylonitrile. However, 0.05% and 0.2% acrylonitrile in drinking water caused decreased food and water intake accompanied by decreased body weight. To avoid this complication of treatment, rats were given equivalent amounts of acrylonitrile by intragastric gavage. This resulted in adrenal enlargement, but circulating corticoid levels were diminished, indicating a syndrome of hypofunctional, hyperplastic adrenals or increased corticoid turnover (32).

Plasma corticosterone was more sensitive than aldosterone to acrylonitrile, and the nitrile was more active when given by daily gavage than when ingested

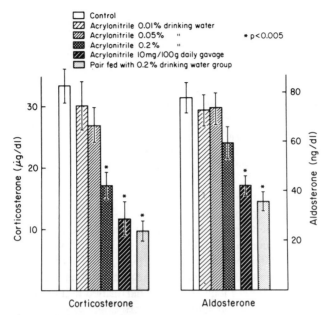

FIG. 3. Effect of acrylonitrile ingestion for 3 weeks on plasma corticosterone and aldosterone levels in the rat. (reproduced with permission from Szabo S, Gallagher GI, Silver EH, Maull EA, Horner HC, Komanicky P, *et al. J Appl Toxicol* 1984; 4:131–140.)

spontaneously through drinking water (32). The level of plasma corticosterone decreased in 7-day experiment only when acrylonitrile was administered by gavage, whereas the in 21-day experiment the chemical depressed corticosterone and aldosterone levels after either spontaneous ingestion or gavage. Age was also an important contributing factor, since young rats were more susceptible to acrylonitrile than adult rats, as reflected by depression of plasma corticosterone and aldosterone levels (32).

The mechanism of chronic action of acrylonitrile on the adrenals and on circulating corticoids is poorly understood. In the absence of ultrastructural changes in the adrenocortical parenchymal cells in rats after chronic acrylonitrile ingestion, a major interference with the synthesis of steroids by the nitrile is difficult to reconcile, although subtle biochemical alterations (eg, inhibition of enzymes in corticoid synthesis) may take place. The compensatory enlargement (eg, following unilateral adrenalectomy) was not impaired by chronic ingestion of acrylonitrile. The elevation of plasma corticosterone level induced by ACTH, on the other hand, was significantly less prominent in acrylonitrile-treated rats than in controls (Table 1). Namely, ACTH caused a marked elevation in plasma corticosterone concentrations, but the increases were significantly attenuated by either 0.01% or 0.05% acrylonitrile in drinking water. Acrylonitrile-induced enhancement of corticosterone clearance from plasma might be a very likely

TABLE 1. *Influence of Chronic Acrylonitrile Ingestion in Drinking Water on Adrenocortical Response to ACTH in Rats.*

Group	Treatment	Plasma corticosterone (µg/dL)
1	None	17.3 ± 4.3
2	ACTH	63.8 ± 2.7^a
3	Acrylonitrile (0.01%) + ACTH	$54.0 \pm 2.9^{a(b)}$
4	Acrylonitrile (0.05%) + ACTH	$49.2 \pm 4.7^{b(b)}$

[a]$P<0.005$ compared with group 1.
[b]$P<0.05$ compared with group 1; (), compared with group 2.
(From ref. 32, with permission.)

explanation for these results, similar to that described in cadmium-treated rats (20). The resulting low levels of circulating steroids may thus trigger, through negative feedback, an enhanced ACTH release, leading to adrenal enlargement, as we have found in our 60-day experiments, especially with acrylonitrile (32). Alternatively, acrylonitrile may decrease the adrenal sensitivity of ACTH.

Recently, in vitro experiments were also performed to investigate the possible direct or indirect effect of acrylonitrile on steroidogenesis (32,35). Isolated zona fasciculata and zona glomerulosa cells were incubated with acrylonitrile to test the hypothesis that acrylonitrile might inhibit the basal and ACTH-stimulated corticosterone and aldosterone production. No evidence for any damaging effect of acrylonitrile in vitro was found either by light microscopy or electron microscopy. No effect of the chemical on adrenocortical steroidogenesis was seen, not even when the adrenocortical cells were incubated in the presence of acrylonitrile and liver microsomes containing drug-metabolizing enzymes. In addition, acrylonitrile did not interfere with the ACTH-stimulated corticosterone production.

The decreased plasma levels of corticosterone in rats chronically ingesting acrylonitrile might thus be explained by increased turnover of corticosterone from the plasma. The increased release of ACTH to compensate for enhanced corticoid turnover might then explain the enlargement of adrenal glands in animals with low circulating levels of corticosterone.

Toxicologic and Clinical Implications

Acrylonitrile is among the 50 most extensively synthesized chemicals in the United States, and its annual production is increasing. Because of its large production and extensive use, the chemical has occupational relevance, especially since case reports of acute and chronic exposure have been published (4,14,18,20,35,37). Its carcinogenic effect has been investigated in both epidemiologic and animal studies (4,14,18,20).

Animal toxicity studies provided insight into the mechanisms of action of acrylonitrile and related saturated and unsaturated nitriles (25,28). These structure-activity studies revealed that the adrenocorticolytic potency of alkyl nitriles is associated with a 2–3 carbon nucleus bearing one or two nucleophilic radicals (eg, – SH, – CN). Branching and unsaturation of the carbon nucleus increased the adrenocorticolytic potency (25,28). The subsequent biochemical, functional and morphologic studies provided a good animal model to investigate the pathogenesis of adrenal apoplexy in the Waterhouse–Friderichsen syndrome (27). The very early alterations in catecholamine secretion, the retrograde embolization of medullary tissue into cortical capillaries, and the primary endothelial lesions *preceding* the parenchymal cortical cell damage could have been discovered only in animal models (24,27,29,32,33). This pathogenetic sequence, nevertheless, was confirmed in most of these elements in human autopsy and surgical pathology material (31).

Although acrylonitrile (Fig. 4.) and the related nitriles are relatively toxic, the structure-activity studies should help to design adrenocorticolytic agents with acceptable safety to produce selective functional or structural inactivation of adrenal cortex for therapeutic purposes.

CYSTEAMINE AND PYRAZOLE

Cysteamine, a naturally occurring derivative of cysteine, is used for the treatment of cystinosis; it is also an antidote and free radical scavenger that protects against radiation damage. Pyrazole is a cyclic drug (1,2-diazole) and experimentally used as a gastroprotective agent (6). In large doses, it causes thyroid necrosis (30), while its derivative, 4-methylpyrazole, is a potent inhibitor of alcohol dehydrogenase.

Morphologic Changes

The structural lesions caused by cysteamine and pyrazole in the adrenals are qualitatively similar to those produced by acrylonitrile. The difference is in the speed of development of structural alterations, since both chemicals act more slowly than acrylonitrile. Nevertheless, cysteamine is faster: Microscopically and grossly, visible hemorrhagic necrosis is seen in rats within 24–48 hours after cysteamine administration. The same changes are seen following pyrazole administration within 3–5 days (1).

In the medulla, signs of degranulation and cellular damage were shown by ultrastructural studies at 8 hours after treatment with cysteamine (17). Localized congestion and cellular debris were seen in medullary capillaries and in the lumina of blood vessels of the zona reticularis and zona fasciculata. Areas of focal necrosis were noted in the corticomedullary region by 12 hours after cysteamine administration. Medullary cell debris was seen in many of the vessels of the corticomedullary junction and extended from this region up into the capillaries of the zona fasciculata. Parenchymal cells of the cortex appeared normal, although the number of necrotic cells increased slightly.

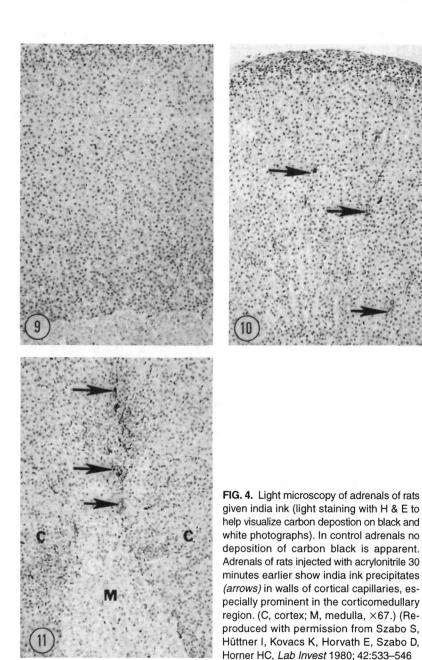

FIG. 4. Light microscopy of adrenals of rats given india ink (light staining with H & E to help visualize carbon depostion on black and white photographs). In control adrenals no deposition of carbon black is apparent. Adrenals of rats injected with acrylonitrile 30 minutes earlier show india ink precipitates *(arrows)* in walls of cortical capillaries, especially prominent in the corticomedullary region. (C, cortex; M, medulla, ×67.) (Reproduced with permission from Szabo S, Hüttner I, Kovacs K, Horvath E, Szabo D, Horner HC, *Lab Invest* 1980; 42:533–546

There were no additional changes by 20–24 hours after treatment with cysteamine in the medullary cells. Congestion was reduced, although medullary cell debris could still be seen in the zona reticularis, along with leakage of red blood cells and platelets into the perivascular space. A breakdown in the structural integrity of this region was widespread, and the zona fasciculata and glomerulosa showed signs of severe congestion. Endothelial cells in all layers showed blabbing, and many were ruptured and necrotic. Polymorphonuclear leukocytes and mononuclear cells were also noted inside and outside the capillaries (17).

Special histochemical studies revealed aggregates of argyrophil granules, shown by Grimelius' stain and light microscopy, in the capillaries of the medulla and corticomedullary junction of the adrenals 2 and 4 hours after the administration of cysteamine. Large fragments of silver-positive medullary tissue were seen at 6 hours and later in the capillaries of otherwise normal looking cortex. Severe congestion and mild edema in the medulla and at the corticomedullary area were prominent at these early time intervals. Focal hemorrhages in the cortex and a few cells with pyknotic nuclei as a sign of single cell necrosis were seen after 12 hours. By 24 hours after cysteamine administration, massive hemorrhage and necrosis of parenchymal cells were common in the swollen adrenal cortex. Multifocal and nonocclusive deposits of fibrin in medullary and corticomedullary vessels were observed by special stains (17).

Based on ultrastructural, histochemical, and light-microscopic studies, two forms of adrenocortical lesions induced by cysteamine or pyrazole may be distinguished. In the first of these forms, frequently focal and later extensive hemorrhage developed where parenchymal cells, showing no histologic abnormalities, were surrounded by a large number of extravasated red blood cells. This type of injury may lead to ischemia and necrosis. The second form of adrencortical lesion, rarer than the first, is marked by single cell necrosis or apoptosis ("dropout" cells), which may be the only form of cortical injury, involving part or most of the cortex. This may or may not be associated with hemorrhage (17,31).

Functional Alterations

Biochemical and functional studies have been performed with cysteamine and pyrazole as well. Adrenal concentration of dopamine rose rapidly and significantly after cysteamine administration. The concentration of noradrenaline was elevated but returned to control levels in 4 hours after cysteamine injection, compared with the longer-lasting effect on dopamine for 24 hours. The hemorrhagic adrenocortical necrosis caused by cysteamine was also markedly reduced by medullectomy, phenoxybenzamine, and labetalol, suggesting an etiologic or pathogenetic role for catecholamines and α-adrenergic receptors in adrenal damage (Table 2). In this regard, the possible role of catecholamines in the mechanism of action of cysteamine is similar to the mode of action of the rapidly acting adrenocorticolytic acrylonitrile and that of pyrazole, which causes cortical necrosis in

TABLE 2. *Reduction of Chemically Induced Adrenocortical Necrosis by Medullectomy and Adrenergic Antagonists in the Rat.*[a]

Pretreatment	Treatment		
	Acrylonitrile	Cysteamine	Pyrazole
Sham medullectomy	76	85	107
Medullectomy	6[b]	5[b]	14[b]
Phenoxybenzamine	41[b]	50[b]	–
Propranolol	65[c]	95	–

[a]Results are expressed as percentage reduction from that seen in untreated controls.
[b]$P<0.05$.
[c]$P<0.01$.
(From ref. 31, with permission.)

3–5 days (ie, more slowly than cysteamine). Catecholamines, thus, might be one of the common mediators or modulators of both these drugs in chemically induced adrenocortical necrosis and in "spontaneous" adrenal necrosis occurring during hypotension or very severe stress (56,57). Further studies are needed to clarify the role of catecholamines in this type of cell and tissue injury.

Plasma corticosterone levels were significantly elevated in 15, 30 and 60 minutes after administration of a single low dose of cysteamine insufficient to produce adrenocortical necrosis (18). In 2 hours, the hormone concentration returned to normal and did not change at 3 and 6 hours (at the end of that experiment). This transient elevation of glucocorticoid secretion might thus be a nonspecific stressor effect. The influence of large doses and prolonged administration of cysteamine on adrenocortical function have not been investigated.

Toxicologic and Clinical Implications

Cysteamine and its derivatives were also part of the initial structure-activity studies with adrenocorticolytic chemicals. Cysteamine is less toxic than acrylonitrile and hence may be a better candidate to develop potent, nontoxic and specific adrenocortical drugs than the nitrile compounds. The adrenocorticolytic effect of cysteamine may be a part of the clinical toxicologic profile, especially of lethargy, noted in patients treated with high doses of this thiol drug to counteract the hepatotoxic effect of acetaminophen.

Pyrazole is a potent gastroprotective agent in animal models, although it is relatively toxic (6). Its derivative, 4-methylpryrazole, has been used in humans to inhibit alcohol dehydrogenase (10). Unfortunately, the adrenocorticolytic potency of this derivative has not been tested. Nevertheless, pyrazole derivatives might represent yet another chemically distinct group of compounds that can be developed for human pharmacologic use.

One of the most useful outcomes of studies concerning the adrenal effects of cysteamine and pyrazole is that animal models were established in which the progression of adrenocorticolytic lesions was slower than that found with the very rapidly acting acrylonitrile. Hence, new pathogenetic factors such as the two pathways of cell and tissue injury in the adrenal cortex were elucidated: (1) primary endothelial damage followed by secondary destruction of parenchymal cells; and (2) primary single and multiple cell "drop-out" in the cortex when early cellular damage in the cortical tissue proper is followed by secondary vascular injury, extravasation of erythrocytes, and hemorrhage. Furthermore, since pyrazole, unlike cysteamine, also causes thyroid necrosis (30), the use of pyrazole provides the so far only available, chemically induced Schmidt's syndrome, allowing parallel (ie, in the same animal model) investigation of the pathogenesis of adrenocortical and thyroid lesions.

Investigation of cysteamine and pyrazole in animal models provided qualitatively novel and quantitatively substantial new information about mechanisms of cell and tissue injury in the adrenal *and* thyroid glands; thus, each is not only "yet another" adrenocorticolytic agent. The two structurally different chemicals, with their participation in structure-activity studies (1,3,4), also represent model chemicals to design selective and potent adrenocorticolytic drugs with minimal side effects and systemic toxicity.

7,12-DIMETHYLBENZ[A]ANTHRACENE (DMBA)

DMBA produces mammary tumors in experimental animals. The adrenocorticolytic action of this carcinogen was discovered during carcinogenic studies (9), providing thus one of the first animal models of slowly progressing adrenal necrosis.

Morphologic Changes

A single 50-mg dose of DMBA dissolved in 2 mL oil, taken by mouth, is sufficient to trigger the adrenocorticolytic process. One day after administration of DMBA, electron microscopy showed marked focal alterations in the capillaries of the adrenal cortex (8). The continuity of the capillary endothelium was almost completely destroyed, and the basement membrane disappeared or was blurred. Cortical cells in the areas with intact capillaries did not show any remarkable changes, while some of the parenchymal cells surrounding the impaired capillaries demonstrated severe alterations. Rarely, "giant" mitochondria with partly tubular and tubulovesicular structures were also seen.

Numerous capillaries demonstrated gaps with fenestrations interrupted, and the remaining parts of the endothelium were often edematous, containing vacuoles with disorganized organelles 48 hours after the administration of DMBA. In some of the capillaries, only remnants of the endothelium could be recognized, and the basement membrane was also blurred. Platelet thrombi were often seen. Some of the parenchymal cells surrounding the ruptured capillaries essentially demonstrated the same necrotic lesions described above. Later, 72 hours after DMBA administration, if no hemorrhage occurred in the zona reticularis, neither the alterations in the capillaries nor those in the parenchymal cells became more severe.

Huggins and Morii (9) assumed that the necrosis developing in the inner layers of the adrenal cortex after oral administration of DMBA was caused primarily by a cytotoxic action. They observed that the DMBA-induced adrenal necrosis did not develop in infantile or hypophysectomized rats, whereas ACTH promoted the development of necrosis. The administration of 11β-hydroxylase inhibitors such as metyrapone also prevented the necrosis induced by DMBA.

Early vascular changes in the adrenal cortex of rats given DMBA were shown by Horvath et al. (8). They demonstrated severe circulatory disturbances leading to ischemic changes in the adrenals followed by extensive hemorrhage and necrosis. Namely, 24 hours after oral administration of DMBA, when no substantial histologic alterations were present, except perhaps in the inner layers of the adrenal cortex, marked capillary damage was detected and became more pronounced on the next day. Platelet thrombi occasionally caused complete occlusion of the damaged capillaries. The primary changes apparently involved opening of the endothelial gaps, rupture of the fenestrae, edematous swelling of the endothelium, and its partial or complete destruction. Severe alterations in the parenchymal cells with injury to the cell membrane, destruction of the organelles, and necrosis were observed only in the areas of the ruptured capillaries.

It cannot be excluded that ACTH release induced by DMBA is involved in the pathogenesis of the capillary lesions. The prevailing suggestion is that DMBA-induced necrosis of the adrenal cortex is due to ischemia caused primarily by injury to the capillary endothelium.

Toxicologic and Clinical Implications

DMBA has not been widely used as an adrenocorticolytic drug because of its carcinogenic effect. Nevertheless, the two time-course and ultrastructural studies (8,9) represent the first pathogenetic investigation aimed at understanding the mechanism of adrenal necrosis.

THIOGUANINE

In contrast to the single-dose administration of other adrenocorticolytic agents, multiple injections of thioguanine are needed to produce hemorrhagic necrosis of the adrenal cortex in rats. After daily divided dosing, electron microscopic studies using the diffusion tracer horseradish peroxidase revealed that endothelial damage preceded the hemorrhagic necrosis of parenchymal cells (34). Prior to studies with thioguanine, similar inferences were made only with regard to DMBA.

After one dose (8 mg/100 g) of thioguanine, there were no gross abnormalities in the adrenal glands of rats. Given two injections of thioguanine, rats showed congested adrenals with focal light-brown and red areas indicating true apoplexy. These changes were more prominent and extensive in animals receiving three doses.

Morphologic Changes

After one injection of thioguanine, light microscopy revealed cellular swelling and congestion in the inner cortical layers similar to those occurring during stress. Two injections of thioguanine caused focal necrosis and hemorrhages in the outer part of the zona fasciculata. After three doses, these changes were more pronounced, showing massive bleeding and necrosis in the outer part of the adrenal cortex. No abnormalities were seen in the medulla, and no thrombosis of the adrenal veins was found.

The adrenal glands were hemorrhagic in 100% of rats given thioguanine for 4 or 5 days, while mortality was 80%. No evidence of necrosis was seen in hypophysectomized animal treated with thioguanine. The mortality in this group was 100%, but the survival time was not significantly shorter than in unoperated and thioguanine-injected rats.

Electron microscopy showed that the cortical capillaries sustained the earliest damage, eg, discontinuity of endothelial cells and rupture of capillary basement membrane with escape of platelets and erythrocytes into the intercellular space of zona fasciculata. In rats injected with horseradish peroxidase, early endothelial damage was especially prominent, and accumulation of platelets was seen later. The adrenocortical cells showed swelling of mitochondria and vesiculation of endoplasmic reticulum.

Functional Alterations

Although no functional studies (ie, measurement of blood levels of corticoids) have been performed with thioguanine, studies with hypophysectomized animals indicate that a fully functional adrenal cortex is necessary for thioguanine-induced adrenal apoplexy (34). Thioguanine is similar to acrylonitrile, which cannot induce adrenocortical necrosis in hypophysectomized rats or in animals treated with the 11β-hydroxylase inhibitor metyrapone or the -adrenergic antagonist phenoxybenzamine (33).

Toxicologic and Clinical Implications

Thioguanine is an antimetabolite used in the treatment of human leukemias. Since it is used in patients, thioguanine is an especially good candidate for "medical adrenalectomy" (ie, pharmacologic inactivation of the adrenal cortex) as an adjunct therapy for breast cancer.

Animal experiments indicate that thioguanine may first affect the endothelial lining of capillaries in the zona fasciculata, resulting in platelet aggregation. Parenchymal cell injury is manifested by mitochondrial swelling and dilation of the endoplasmic reticulum. The pattern of parenchymal changes correspond to ischemic injury that might be due to a direct toxic effect of thioguanine on the cells or to vasospasm resulting in ischemia and damage of the endothelial cells. The localization of early lesions at the level of the endothelium may suggest a secondary, ischemic nature of parenchymal cell damage.

Thioguanine-induced adrenocortical necrosis is clearly pituitary-dependent since it is prevented by hypophysectomy. Pituitary ablation also protects against the adrenal necrosis caused by diphtheria toxin, DMBA, acrylonitrile, or thioacetamide.

HEXADIMETHRINE BROMIDE

Hexadimethrine bromide induces necrosis of the zones of adrenal cortex (3), in addition to its effect on the pituitary gland of the rat. This drug causes two different lesions in the cortex: (1) toxic damage to the zona glomerulosa and (2) ischemic necrosis of the zonae fasciculata and reticularis, produced only by large doses.

Morphologic Changes

In about 6 hours after administration of hexadimethrine bromide, the first changes appeared in the zona glomerulosa of rats' adrenal cortex. Most of the cells showed a distinct vacuolation of cytoplasm under light microscopy (3). At 24 hours, many of the parenchymal cells appeared to have disappeared completely, leaving only a network of stroma. At 48 hours, only a loose meshwork and occasional large foamy cells were seen. During the next few days, the zones would become condensed to a very thin band, which at many points disappeared completely.

The basic lesions in the inner zones (fasciculata and reticularis) were infarct and wedge-shaped patches of cortex with narrow ends toward the medulla. The patches varied in size and number; sometimes only one or two were present, whereas in other adrenals they became confluent and replaced almost the entire deep cortex. In the typical lesion, the outer edge of the infarct extended to about 70–100 μm from the capsule, and only a thin layer of surviving zona fasciculata separated the infarcted area from the damaged zona glomerulosa.

In very severe cortical lesions, the medullary circulation may also be impaired, resulting in a small medullary infarct beneath the necrotic cortex. The first evidence of circulatory arrest was seen in about 6 hours. At 24 hours, the lesions developed into an ordinary infarct, with a central dead area and peripheral transitional zone showing lysis and disappearance of cells. At 48 hours, the nuclei in the central dead area showed little further change, but those in the peripheral zone were fading and the columns were beginning to break up. In 4 days, the nuclei in the central cells completely disappeared, and the cytoplasm became very pale.

Toxicologic and Clinical Implications

Hexadimethrine bromide causes two kinds of lesions in the adrenal gland of the rat: (1) a toxic necrosis of the entire zona glomerulosa and (2) a patchy infarct of the zona fasciculata and zona reticularis, produced by large doses of the drug.

OTHER ADRENOCORTICOLYTIC AGENTS

A few other chemicals have also been found to induce adrenal necrosis, as documented in brief case reports or short morphologic descriptions. Systematic pathogenetic studies have not been performed with most of these agents, and we give only a brief description here.

Basic polyglutaminic acid derivatives injected intravenously in rats produced adrenal apoplexy often accompanied by hemorrhagic lesions in the liver and in the lung (14). Extensive hemorrhages in the adrenal cortex, mainly in the zona fasciculata, with early signs of necrosis were found at histologic examination of the adrenals. The incidence of hemorrhagic lesions in the adrenals, liver, and lung showed a positive correlation with the viscosity of these basic polyglutaminic acid derivatives. The adrenal lesions and mortality were reduced only by pretreatment with spironolactone, and not by the other microsomal enzyme inducer pregnenolone-16α-carbonitrile (PCN), the glucocorticoid triamcinolone, or hypophysectomy (14).

Certain chemicals produce only nonhemorrhagic lesions in the adrenal cortex. Among these, derivatives of dichlorodiphenyltrichloroethane (DDT) are the best known, but their effect was demonstrated mainly in dogs (23). In rats, aniline caused marked adrenal enlargement, excessive accumulation of lipid droplets and cholesterol crystals, degeneration of mitochondria, hypertrophy of smooth endoplasmic reticulum, dilation of Golgi complex, and slight increase in the number of lysosomes (12). These changes were especially prominent in the inner cortical layers and often led to cell necrosis. Spironolactone (23), vinblastine (13), and mevinolin (16) cause ultrastructural alterations in the adrenal cortex affecting mainly the endoplasmic reticulum, mitochondria, microtubules, and smooth endoplasmic reticulum plus peroxisomes. Although some of these changes are irreversible, they rarely lead to cell death in the adrenal cortex.

SUMMARY

This chapter provides an overview of morphologic and functional lesions in the adrenal cortex produced by chemicals (mostly drugs of therapeutic or diagnostic value). The biochemical mechanisms of pathogenesis are also emphasized whenever studies were available for analysis. The clinical and occupational relevance, whenever appropriate, is emphasized as well as the availability of animal models to elicit the pathogenesis of chemically induced endocrine lesions.

REFERENCES

1. Adrenal hemorrhage, apoplexy, and infarction. *Lancet.* 1976;2:295. Editorial
2. Alford WC Jr, Meador CK, Mihalevich J, *et al.* Acute adrenal insufficiency following cardiac surgical procedures. *J Thorac Cardiovasc Surg.* 1979;78:489–493.
3. Carroll R, Kovács K, Tapp E, Lipool MB. Experimental hexadimethrine necrosis of zona glomerulosa and inner layers of adrenal cortex. *Lancet.* 1964;2:921–924.32.
4. Gallagher GT, Maull EA, Kovács K, Szabo S. Neoplasms in rats ingesting acrylonitrile for two years. *J Am Coll Toxicol.* 1988;7:603–615.
5. Giampaolo C, Gray AT, Olshen RA, Szabo S. Predicting chemically induced duodenal ulcer and adrenal necrosis with classification trees. *Proc Natl Acad Sci U S A.* 1991;88:6298–6302.
6. Hauser H, Szabo S. Extremely long protection by pyrazole derivatives against ethanol-induced gastric mucosal injury. *FASEB J.* 1988;2:A1052.
7. Horváth E, Kovács K. Effect of temporary ischemia on the fine structure of the rat adrenal cortex. *Pathol Eur.* 1973;8:43–60.
8. Horváh E, Kovcs K, Szabo D. An electron-microscopic study of the adrenocortical lesion induced by 7,12-dimethylbenzanthracene in rats. *J Pathol.* 1969;97:277–282.
9. Huggins C, Morii S. Selective adrenal necrosis and apoplexy induced by 7,12-dimethylbenz[a]anthracene. *J Exp Med.* 1961;114:741–760.
10. Jacobsen D, Sebastioan CS, Blomstrand R, McMartin KE. 4-Methylpyrazole: a controlled study of safety in healthy human subjects after single, ascending doses. *Alcohol Clin Exp Res.* 1988;12:516
11. Jaeger RJ, Cote IL, Silver EM, Szabo S. Effect of hypoxia on the acute toxicity of acrylonitrile. *Res Commun Chem Path Pharm.* 1982;36:345–248.
12. Kovács K, Blascheck JA, Yeghiayan E, Hatakeyama S, Gardell C. Adrenocortical lipid hyperplasia induced in rats by aniline: a histologic and electron microscopy study. *Am J Pathol.* 1971;62:17–29.
13. Kovács K, Horváth E, Szabo S, *et al.* Effect of vinblastine on the fine structure of the rat adrenal cortex. *Horm Metab Res.* 1975;7:365–366.
14. Lazar G, Szabo S, Husztik E. The experimental production of hemorrhagic lesions in the rat adrenal, liver and lung by basic polyglutamic acid derivatives. *Res Exp Med.* 1972;159:58–64.
15. Maltoni C, Ciliberti A, DiMaio V. Carcinogenicity bioassays on rats of acrylonitrile administered by inhalation and by ingestion. *Med Lav.* 1977;69:401
16. Mazzocchi G, Rebuffat P, Belloni AS, Gottardo G, Meneghelli V, Nussdorfer GG. Effects of mevinolin, an inhibitor of cholesterol synthesis, on the morphological and functional responses of rat adrenal zona fasciculata to a prolonged treatment with 4-aminopyrazol-pyrimidine. *Anat Rec.* 1988;221:700–706.
17. McComb DJ, Kovács K, Horner HC, *et al.* Cysteamine-induced adrenocortical necrosis in rats. *Exp Mol Pathol.* 1981;35:422–434.
18. Narasaki Y, Yabana T. On the mechanism of duodenal ulcer formation after administration of cysteamine in rat. *Sapporo Med J.* 1979;47:415–428.
19. *NIOSH Criteria for a Recommended Standard. Occupational Exposure to Nitriles.* Atlanta, Ga: Centers for Disease Control; 1978:1–155. US Dept of Health, Education, and Welfare publication.
20. Nishiyama S, Takata T. Effects of cadmium on the level of serum corticosterone and adrenocortical function in male rats. *Res Commun Chem Pathol Pharm.* 1982;37:65–79.
21. Occupational exposure to acrylonitrile (vinyl cyanide). Proposed standard and notice of hearing. *Federal Register* 1978;2586–2621.
22. Ribelin WE. The effects of drugs and chemicals upon the structure of the adrenal gland. *Fundam Appl Toxicol.* 1984;4:105–119.
23. Riddel RH, ed. *Pathology of Drug-Induced and Toxic Diseases.* New York, NY: Churchill Livingstone; 1982.
24. Silver EH, Szabo S, Cahill, Jaeger RJ. Time-course studies of the distribution of [1-14C] acrylonitrile in rats after intravenous administration. *J Appl Toxicol.* 1987;7:303–306.
25. Szabo S, Lippe IT. Adrenal gland: chemically induced structural and functional changes in the cortex. *Toxicol Pathol.* 1989;17:317–329.
26. Szabo S, Selye H. Adrenal apoplexy and necrosis produced by acrylonitrile. *Endokrinologie.* 1971;57:405–408.
27. Szabo S, Reynolds ES, Kovács K. Animal model of human disease: Waterhouse–Friderichsen syndrome; animal model: acrylonitrile-induced adrenal apoplexy. *Am J Pathol.* 1976;82:653–656.

28. Szabo S, Reynolds ES, Unger SH. Structure-activity relations between alkyl nucleophilic chemicals causing duodenal ulcer and adrenocortical necrosis. *J Pharmacol Exp Ther*. 1982;223:68–76.
29. Szabo S, Bailey KA, Boor PJ, Jaeger RJ. Acrylonitrile and tissue glutathione: differential effect of acute and chronic interactions. *Biochem Biophys Res Commun*. 1977;79:32–37.
30. Szabo S, Horváth E, Kovács K, Larsen PR. Pyrazole-induced thyroid necrosis. A distinct organ lesion. *Science*. 1978;199:1209–1210.
31. Szabo S, McComb DJ, Kovacs K, Hüttner I. Adrenocortical hemorrhagic necrosis: the role of catecholamines and retrograde medullary-cell embolism. *Arch Pathol Lab Med*. 1981;105:536–539.
32. Szabo S, Gallagher GT, Silver EH, et al. Subacute and chronic action of acrylonitrile on adrenals and gastrointestinal tract: biochemical, functional and ultrastructural studies in the rat. *J Appl Toxicol*. 1984;4:131–140.
33. Szabo S, Hütner I, Kovács K, Horváth E, Szabo D, Horner HC. Pathogenesis of experimental adrenal hemorrhagic necrosis ("apoplexy"). Ultrastructural, biochemical, neuropharmacologic and blood coagulation studies with acrylonitrile in the rat. *Lab Invest*. 1980;42:533–546
34. Szabo S, Kovács K, Horváth E, Szabo D, Hüttner I, Garg BD. Thioguanine induced adrenocortical necrosis and its prevention by hypophysectomy in rats. *Exp Mol Pathol*. 1977;26:155–168.
35. Szalay KS, Szabo D, Szeberenyi S, Toth IE, Szabo S. Lack of direct effect of acrylonitrile on corticoid production of isolated zona fasciculata and zona glomerulosa cells. *J Mol Cell Toxicol*. 1987;1:163–169.
36. Tambura CH. Chemical hepatitis: pathogenesis, detection and management. *Med Clin North Am*. 1979;63:545.
37. Vaino H, Makinen A. Styrene and acrylonitrile induced depression of hepatic non-protein sulfhydryl content in various rodent species. *Res Commun Chem Pathol Pharm*. 1977;17:115–124.
38. Zeller H, Hofmann HT, Thiess AM, Hey W. Zur Toxizat der Nitrile. *Zentralbl Arbeitsmed Arbeitsschutz*. 1969;19:225.

Endocrine Toxicology, 2nd ed.,
Edited by J. A. Thomas and H. D. Colby
Copyright © 1997 Taylor & Francis

6

Steroid Receptors

Nasir Bashirelahi, B. Koffman, and *Robert J. Sydiskis

*Departments of Oral and Craniofacial Biological Sciences and *Biochemistry
University of Maryland Dental School, Baltimore, Maryland 21201*

STEROID RECEPTOR LOCALIZATION AND MECHANISM OF ACTION

There are three classes of steroid hormones: adrenal steroids (cortisol, aldosterone), sex steroids (progesterone, estrogen, and testosterone), and vitamin D_3 (100,137). These hormones have a chemical structure similar to that of cholesterol and in most cases are derived from cholesterol (137).

Classical Steroid Hormone Actions

Steroid hormones enter most cells by diffusion (93,307,353) and bind to macromolecules or hormone receptors in the target cells with high affinity, with the equilibrium dissociation constant (K_d) typically 10^{-10}–10^{-8} mol/L (18,125,198,227).

Without steroid hormones, the steroid receptors exist associated with several proteins in a nontransformed state unable to bind DNA. The nontransformed androgen, progesterone, glucocorticoid, and estrogen receptors were shown to be associated with the 90-kd heat shock protein (hsp90) (181,363), and also with a protein of 56–59 kd. A 70-kd protein has been shown in the nontransformed progesterone- and glucocorticoid-receptor complexes, but not in other steroid-receptor complexes (213,355,330).

Steroid hormone receptors are large proteins whose location remains controversial (126,386). Localization of unoccupied steroid hormone receptors was initially thought to be cytoplasmic (178). In 1984, Welshons et al. (394) used enucleation studies and King and Greene (198) used immunocytochemical studies with antibodies specific for estrogen receptor to conclude that estrogen receptor in the presence or absence of steroid hormone is located in the nucleus. Unoccupied receptors for estrogen, progesterone, vitamin D, and androgen are localized to the nucleus.

Similar enucleation studies were done to localize the glucocorticoid receptor and progesterone receptor to the nucleus in the presence or absence of steroid hormone (393). However, immunocytochemical studies concluded that unoccupied glucocorticoid receptor is located in the cytoplasm, while occupied glucocorticoid receptor is located in the nucleus (111,399). Gorski et al. (126) contend that there is light staining in the nuclei, even in the absence of hormone, in the photographs of the study by Fuxe et al. (111), and cite Brink et al. (48), who showed that fixation procedures are critical for maintaining immunocytochemical activity of unoccupied glucocorticoid receptor; Brink and co-workers also concluded that unoccupied glucocorticoid receptor is nuclear.

Webster et al. (386) countered the arguments of Gorski et al. (126) that unoccupied glucocorticoid receptor is nuclear by citing two other studies. In one study, enucleation of rat hepatoma cells localized unoccupied glucocorticoid receptor to the cytoplasts (cytoplasm) (267), while in the other study localization of the glucocorticoid receptor varied: The L-cell cell line had unoccupied glucocorticoid receptor in the cytoplasm and nucleus, while GH_3 cells had unoccupied glucocorticoid receptor solely in the nucleus (223). Webster et al. (386) concluded that the unoccupied glucocorticoid receptor resides in the cytoplasm and translocates to the nucleus on hormone binding and possibly shuttles back and forth (386).

Since then, Rossini and Malaguti (324), using cross-linking methods, found untransformed glucocorticoid receptor in cytoplasm and nuclei of HTC cells in a ratio of approximately 2:1. Using the same procedures, they found untransformed glucocorticoid receptor in the cytoplasm and nuclei of HeLa S_3 (85.4% and 14.6%, respectively) and MCF-7 cells (75.2% and 24.8%, respectively) (325). The nuclear fraction of unoccupied glucocorticoid receptor was relatively consistent in nanomolar concentrations, while the cytosolic concentration varied as much as 50-fold in the three cell types. The matter of unoccupied glucocorticoid receptor localization remains controversial.

Binding of steroid to cytosolic receptor results in dissociation of the receptor-protein complex (nontransformed state) to reveal the DNA-binding domain of the receptor (formation of an activated or transformed steroid-receptor complex), which now has affinity for certain nuclear binding sites. Receptor-steroid complexes may bind to DNA, nuclear matrix, and nuclear membranes (60,217).

Although previously thought to occur in the cytoplasm, transformation may also occur in the nucleus (87,350). Receptor-steroid complexes then dimerize, bind to DNA, and participate in transcription (60). Steroid hormone receptors, retinoic acid receptors, and vitamin D receptors interact with DNA using a zinc-finger motif (297). The first zinc finger recognizes a specific target DNA sequence (30,86,130), while a second zinc finger orients the receptor for DNA binding (30), stabilizes the DNA-protein interaction (30,130), contains a site directly involved in transcription activation (336), and provides a dimerization interface (244).

The resulting biological events that occur because of the interaction of receptor-steroid complexes with genetic material include mRNA transcription, processing, and translation into protein. After interaction with genetic material, the receptor is recycled into unoccupied receptor and the steroid is eliminated from the cell.

Proto-oncogenes such as c-*myc*, c-*fos*, c-*jun*, and c-*myb* play a role in growth in normal cells, and their levels are altered by several factors, including steroid hormones and polylpeptide growth factors. They have come to be known as immediate early genes, and their gene products are transcription factors that influence the expression of late genes (343).

Nonclassical Steroid Hormone Actions

Evidence has accumulated that steroid hormones exert their effects by nonclassical actions (46), such as via steroid membrane receptors that primarily bind to progesterone or one of its derivatives. There is evidence that steroid hormones can have rapid effects that are not mediated by genomic or nuclear steroid receptors in oocytes (26), hepatocytes (331), and neurons (251,404).

Recent studies argue for the existence of a surface plasma progesterone receptor in spermatazoa able to induce an increase in Ca^{2+} influx and acrosomal reaction (40,271). This subject is reviewed by Revelli et al. (318), who also propose several possible mechanisms of action.

Alphaxalone (3$\propto$-hydroxy-5$\propto$-pregnane-11,20-dione) is a major constituent of Althesin, used clinically for induction of anesthesia (64). The β-hydroxy isomer of this compound is inactive, suggesting the possibility that it works via a receptor. Electrophysiologic and radioligand binding methods were used to investigate the interaction of alphaxalone (147). An allosteric neurosteroid site was found to exist on the inhibitory $GABA_A$ neurotransmitter receptor distinct from sites recognized by benzodiazepines and barbiturates. Of the naturally occurring steroids, allopregnanolone (3$\propto$-hydroxy-5$\propto$-pregnan-20-one), a progesterone derivative, is one of the most potent and markedly enhances responses to $GABA_A$ receptor agonists (412). Neuroactive steroids are steroids with actions at the membranes of excitable cells (22,79,113,147,252,299).

Some neurosteroids also modulate excitatory events mediated by glutamate. Pregnenolone sulfate potentiates *N*-methyl-D-aspartate (NMDA)–mediated responses when measured by electrophysiologic recording techniques (404) or determination of NMDA-induced increases in intracellular calcium concentration (172).

Other potential nonclassical mechanisms of steroid hormones include alteration of cell membrane fluidity by steroid hormone and activation of steroids by other factors, such as dopamine or epidermal growth factor. In addition, there is also the possibility that steroid hormone intercalates directly with DNA and acts as a transcription factor without involvement of steroid hormone receptor. These possibilities are reviewed in detail by Brann et al. (46).

Plasma Steroid–Binding Proteins (323)

Besides albumin, two plasma proteins (glycoproteins) bind steroids. Cortisol and progesterone are the ligands for corticosteroid-binding globulin (CBG, transcortin), and testosterone, dihydrotestosterone (DHT), and estradiol are the ligands for sex hormone–binding globulin (SHBG; testosterone-binding globulin, TeBG; or steroid-binding protein).

The gene for CBG is located on chromosome 14 (14q31-q32.1). CBG has over 30% homology with the serine protease inhibitor superfamily and is considered a member of this protein family. The gene for SHBG is located on chromosome 17 (17p12-p13). In plasma, it transports hormone as a homodimer. Both binding globulins determine the concentration of free hormone in the plasma, and CBG has been implicated in the selective delivery of cortisol to sites of inflammation.

If the appropriate steroid is present when either binding protein binds to its membrane receptor, rapid induction of adenylate cyclase activity and intracellular cyclic adenosine monophosphate (cAMP) accumulation follow.

STEROID RECEPTOR SUPERFAMILY

The steroid hormone receptor family includes the adrenal and sex steroid hormone receptors, vitamin D_3 receptor, thyroid hormone receptor, retinoid hormone receptor, a dioxin receptor, and a host of "orphan" receptors (putative receptor genes for which a ligand has not yet been identified) (100,230,231,305). Indeed, it is likely the largest family of transcription factors in eukaryotes.

Amino acid sequences have been determined for various steroid hormone receptors. These include the human (131,383), chicken (215), rat (206), frog (387), bovine (313), and mouse (397) estrogen receptor; the rabbit (240) and human (276) progesterone receptor; and the human vitamin D (16), glucocorticoid (162,388), and mineralocorticoid (10) receptor.

Computer studies of the amino acid sequences of these receptors have defined segments of homology (17,100,215). Computer studies of homology have accumulated circumstantial evidence for the functions of several domains, while several studies employing chimeric genes and gene deletions have demonstrated the functions of these domains (129).

The steroid hormone receptors have six domains, A–F. Region A/B is at the amino terminal and is involved in transactivation. Region C is the DNA-binding domain. This region generally has the greatest amount of homology conserved between species and types of receptor; it also contains an unusually high amount of the basic amino acids, cysteine, lysine, and arginine (215). This DNA-binding domain contains two zinc-finger regions, usually designated CI and CII. Region D is the hinge region, and homology is poorly preserved across species and receptor types. This region in the glucocorticoid receptor consists of a short stretch of basic amino acids (326), which has been implicated in nuclear localization in rat glucocorticoid receptor (302). Region E is the steroid-binding domain, which has conserved homology between species and type of receptor (100,215). Region E also plays a role in dimerization of the receptor and transcription regulation.

Laudet and colleagues (230,231) constructed phylogenic trees of the superfamily of nuclear receptors derived from two domains—the DNA-binding or steroid-binding regions—of 30 such receptor genes. Based on the C domain phylogenic tree, or DNA-binding region, three subfamilies arose. These include the thyroid hormone, retinoic acid, Rev-ErbA receptor genes (class I), most orphan receptor genes (class II), and the steroid hormone receptor and knirps genes (class III). The phylogenic tree based on the E domain, or ligand-binding domain, produced a similar tree, although two groups of receptors were placed in separate positions compared with the tree derived from the C domain. These two groups included the *Drosophila* knirps gene group, which has acquired different E domains over time, and the group composed of genes for the vitamin D receptor, ecdysone receptor, and four orphan receptor (FTZ-F1, nur 77, tailless, and HNF4).

The steroid hormones and steroid hormone receptors are the subjects of the remainder of this chapter.

STEROID HORMONES

Adrenal Steroids

Adrenal steroids exert both a glucocorticoid and a mineralocorticoid effect (356). Mineralocorticoids promote reabsorption of sodium and excretion of potassium and ammonium. Excessive sodium reabsorption and intracellular potassium exchange result in increased extracellular volume and hypertension. Glucocorticoid hormones (cortisol, cortisone, corticosterone) increase glycogenesis and gluconeogenesis, stimulate protein synthesis and lipolysis, reduce inflammation, tend to lower serum calcium concentration, and maintain the ability to excrete a water load. Cortisol is the main adrenal glucocorticoid steroid in humans (0.04–0.02 mg/mL) (67).

The middle and inner zones of the adrenal cortex (the zona fasciculata and zona reticularis) produce glucocorticoids, adrenal androgens, and estrogens (356). Aldosterone—and not glucocorticoid—is produced in the zona glomerulosa (outermost zone) of the mammalian adrenal cortex (12,115).

Estrogens

Only three estrogens are present in human female plasma: β-estradiol, estrone, and estriol. The three estrogens are all C18 steroids (vs. the C19 androgens). In natural estrogens, the A ring of the basic cyclopentano-perhydrophenanthrene structure is aromatic, there is a phenolic hydroxy group at position 3, and there is no angular methyl group at position 10 (356). The aromatic A ring appears to be responsible primarily for initiating and maintaining hormone binding. Estrogen agonists and antagonists generally exhibit similarities in the A ring and dissimilarities in the D ring (353).

There are several potential sources of exposure to estrogens (341,342): (1) endogenous hormones; (2) phytoestrogens; (3) fat and foods of livestock implanted with steroids; (4) cosmetics; (5) oral contraceptives; (6) insecticides; (7) pregnancy tests; and (8) estrogens given for medicinal purposes, including suppression of lactation, synthetic estrogens for threatened abortions, menopausal replacement, and treatment of breast or prostate cancers.

The estrogens are primarily secreted by the ovaries, where progesterone and testosterone are first made of cholesterol from the blood and coenzyme-A and subsequently converted to estrogens. The final step is conversion of testosterone to β-estradiol using aromatase (14,151). The major estrogen, β-estradiol, is normally secreted by the ovarian follicle; estrone and estriol are products of of β-estradiol metabolism (356). In pregnancy, the placenta secretes primarily estriol. Small amounts of estrone are also formed by ovarian thecal and stromal cells and by peripheral tissues from androgens originally secreted by the adrenal cortices. Nongonadal tissues such as liver, fat, muscle, and brain contain aromatases necessary for conversion of androgens to estrogens. β-Estradiol is 10–12 times more potent than estrone, and 80 times as potent as estriol (137,356). These hormones circulate in the plasma at very low concentrations (approximately 10^{-11}–10^{-7} mol/L) (66). The structural characteristic important for estrogenic activity is the presence of the two hydroxyl groups at the extreme ends of the structures (95).

The primary biological actions of estrogens include stimulation and growth of the female reproductive system, increasing circulating levels of very-low density and high-density lipoproteins, promoting closure of bony epiphyses, and stimulating hepatic synthesis of various proteins (356). Recently, estrogen has been found to promote angiogenesis (279).

There have been several case reports of genetic mutations resulting in decreased serum levels of estrogens in humans. Aromatase is involved in the conversion of testosterone to estradiol. The absence of P-450 aromatase in a female fetus and placenta resulted in increased serum androgen concentrations and decreased serum estrogen concentrations (75). The phenotype included normal female internal genitalia and partial external virilization. Two other cases were reported in which aromatase deficiency resulted in karyotypic females and psuedohermaphroditism (173,349).

Natural and synthetic estrogens have been listed as moderately toxic; 0.5–5 g/kg is the probable oral lethal dose for humans (127). Side effects noted following administration of estrogens include headache, nausea, vomiting, and sometimes vaginal bleeding (105,121, 156). Occupational exposure of males to estrogens resulted in gynecomastia and other feminizing side effects, which were reversible with removal of the estrogen (96). Absorption may occur by the oral, percutaneous, and respiratory routes.

Progesterone

Progesterone is secreted in both ovaries and adrenal glands, and by the corpus luteum in pregnancy. Secretion is controlled by gonadotropins in the ovary and adrenocorticotropic hormone (ACTH) in the adrenals. Progesterone levels vary with the menstrual cycle. This hormone has roles in ovulation and reproduction and influences the growth of the mammary gland.

The corpus luteum secretes progesterone during the second half of the menstrual cycle. One target is the endomentrium of the uterus, where it induces secretory activity necessary for implantation of the fertilized ovum. Following implantation, completion of the pregnancy requires continued progesterone presence.

Progesterone has antiovulatory action if given during the menstrual cycle from days 5 to 25. It is also immunosuppressive in pharmacologic doses and is responsible for the rise in basal body temperature in the late menstrual cycle (356).

Progesterone given intravenously (400–600 mg) induces sleep and anesthesia in humans (275) and in animals (138). In ovariectomized cats, progesterone increases the frequency of epileptic spikes from penicillin-induced epileptic foci, when given at doses comparable to pregnancy plasma levels (228). In contrast, in human females with partial epilepsy and a well-defined epileptic focus, progesterone at luteal-phase plasma levels significantly decreases the spike frequency on continuous EEG monitoring (13).

Progesterone Antagonists

Mifepristone (RU 486) used clinically at doses of 200–400 mg daily for 6–12 months has been associated with fatigue in 22 of 28 patients in one clinical trial (134). Other trials have shown fatigue, nausea, vomiting, and anorexia in 4 of 10 patients (226) and transient nausea and anorexia in 3 of 10 patients (226). Other potential symptoms include hot flashes, gynecomastia, thinning of hair, rash, cessation of menses, and diminished libido (in men) (133).

Androgens

Androgens are required for normal male phenotypic expression during embryonic development and are essential for normal male reproductive function. Androgens support gonadogenesis, affect behavior, and regulate gonadotropin secretion. They also have a protein-anabolic action in skeletal muscle (202). There is also a possible role for sex hormones, particularly testosterone, in immunologic maturation and regulation (272). A mouse strain that develops a spontaneous disorder resembling systemic lupus erythematosus was used. Pre- and postpubertal castration in male and female animals in the presence or absence of hormone treatment showed that hormonal effects on the immune system were greatest early in life. The presence of testosterone discouraged development of an autoimmune process. There is speculation that the male sex hormones may maintain suppression (suppressor T cells) of autoimmune processes compared with female sex hormones (estrogens), which may act to decrease the suppressor effects (enhance the helper cell effects). Based on this speculation, one could predict that lowering the testosterone prior to or during adolescence–such as with marijuana use–may predispose the male individual to a higher susceptibility to autoimmune disease (264).

Androgens are derived primarily from the Leydig cells and adrenals in males and ovaries and adrenals in females. Testosterone is the most important androgen produced (approximately 5 mg/day), but the testes also secrete small amounts of dehydroepiandrosterone (DHEA), androstenediol, and dihydrotestosterone (DHT). Testosterone has two possible fates: In target tissues, <10% of it acts as a pro-hormone or precursor for two other active metabolites, DHT (approximately 0.3 mg/day) and estradiol (approximately 0.02 mg/day); the remainder (90%) is metabolized to inactive metabolites in the liver (356).

Anabolic Androgenic Steroids

Anabolic androgenic steroids are synthetic derivatives designed to capitalize on the anabolic effects of testosterone in enhancing skeletal muscle rather than its masculinizing or androgenic effects. Legitimate medical uses of anabolic androgenic steroids include treatment of refractory anemias, hereditary angioedema, wound healing, male hypogonadism, some gynecologic states, and protein anabolism. They may also serve as an adjuvant in growth hormone therapy and in the treatment of osteoporosis and constitutional growth delay (80,195).

Adverse Effects of Anabolic Androgenic Steroids

Adult males may sustain a reversible testicular atrophy, urinary obstruction secondary to changes in the prostate or urethra, gynecomastia, accelerated male-pattern baldness, and decrease in sperm count. This last side effect has kept this medication active in investigations for a male contraceptive. Females may develop changes in menstrual flow, hirsutism, clitoral hypertrophy, and alopecia. Pharmacologic doses given to children result in premature fusion of epiphyseal plates and consequent short stature. Children can also undergo precocious puberty (80,195). Metabolism may also be affected by anabolic androgenic steroids, including decreased glucose tolerance (71), increased low-density lipoprotein levels, and a 30–50% reduction in high-density lipoproteins. Orally administered alkyl derivatives of anabolic androgenic steroids may produce a more deleterious effect on serum cholesterol levels than does testosterone (367). Other potential adverse effects include possible links with case reports of malignancy (82,97,158,322) and the potential for spread of blood-borne pathogens such as HIV and hepatitis via needle sharing (7,345,351).

Vitamin D

Cholecalciferol, or vitamin D_3, is formed in the skin of mammals by ultraviolet irradiation (wavelength 230–313 nm) of a precursor sterol, 7-dehydrocholesterol.

The conversion to vitamin D_3 requires approximately 36 hours at body temperature. Biological activity is subsequently conferred on cholecalciferol after two sequential hydroxylations, one at the 25 position (occurring in the liver) and the second at the 1 position (in the kidney), resulting in 1,25-dihydroxycholecalciferol ($1,25(OH)_2D_3$) (149,356).

The main function of $1,25(OH)_2D_3$ is maintenance of serum Ca^{+2} and orthophosphate (P_i). In the intestine, it facilitates calcium active transport across the intestinal epithelium brush border and stimulates the phosphate-specific carrier transport system. In bone, $1,25(OH)_2D_3$, in the presence of parathyroid hormone, acts to mobilize calcium for circulation (149,356).

Additional functions of vitamin D include stimulation of macrophage differentiation (255) and modification of T-lymphocyte activity (374).

Vitamin D Toxicity

Casual exposure to ultraviolet light in the summer months produces enough vitamin D to store for winter (140). Vitamin D toxicity may manifest as anorexia, nausea, vomiting, hypertension, and renal compromise associated with hypercalcemia in children and with the additional symptom of malaise in adults. Other symptoms may include polydipsia and polyuria, while physical signs may include subconjunctival deposits and band keratitis on slit-lamp examination (166). Altered calcium homeostasis results in hypercalcemia, hyperphosphatemia, polyuria, polydipsia, nephrolithiasis, renal failure, and vascular and ectopic calcifications (166). Exposure to greater than 10 times the recommended dose of calciferol for prolonged periods of time may result in bone demineralization and fractures in children or adults (49,356). Vitamin D intoxication may also result in soft tissue calcification and calcification of vital organs (81). Anephric patients incapable of hydroxylation to form $1,25(OH)_2D_3$ can become vitamin D intoxicated (81).

Vitamin D_3 has been marketed in the United States since 1984 under the trade names of Quintox and Rampage, and ergocalciferol (vitamin D_2) has been used as a rodenticide in both Canada and Europe since 1978. Vitamin D is listed as a moderately toxic rodenticide with an LD_{50} of 50–500 mg/kg. No serious human toxicity or deaths have yet been reported (107), despite several case reports of vitamin D intoxication from ingestion of excessively fortified milk (175) or occupational exposure (179). Treatment for moderate to severe intoxication resulting in hypercalcemia (calcium levels >11.5 mg/dL) includes intravenous hydration, cholestyramine (179), and diuresis with furosemide, prednisone, and calcitonin (see ref. 107 for details).

Vitamin D Deficiency

Without vitamin D, one would have poor calcium absorption, undermineralized bones, muscle weakness, secondary hyperparathyroidism, increased incidence of fractures, and poor growth (140). Inadequate mineralization of bone matrix results in rickets in children and osteomalacia in adults. In patients with end-stage renal disease, levels of circulating $1,25(OH)_2D_3$ are reduced or absent. This condition is reversible with renal transplantation (149).

Two clinical forms of hereditary hypocalcemic vitamin D–resistant rickets exist. Type I results in an inadequate production of $1,25(OH)_2D_3$, presumably secondary to a genetic error in 1-hydroxylase; the condition can be circumvented by supplementation of high doses of vitamin D or 25-hydroxycholecalciferol ($25(OH)D_3$). Type II is a resistance to normal levels of $1,25(OH)_2D_3$ hormone due to a genetic defect in the vitamin D receptor (148,321).

Osteomalacia is associated with patients on anticonvulsant medication, primarily phenytoin and phenobarbital. These anticonvulsants may affect calcium metabolism and cause rickets or osteomalacia (141), or this association may be merely coincidental (239). Circulating levels of $25(OH)D_3$ are reduced in many–though not all–patients on anticonvulsants (142,361). Administration of vitamin D or $25(OH)D_3$ corrects the symptoms of osteomalacia in patients on anticonvulsants (361). Anticonvulsant medications may induce suboptimal intestinal calcium absorption (78,146) or may even act in bone to inhibit calcium mobilization induced by parathyroid hormone or $25(OH)D_3$ (177).

Environmental Sources of Steroid Hormones

Endogenous Steroids

Steroid hormones or compounds with sex hormone–like activities appear in food. Estrogens are present in bovine milk and colostrum, though the colostrum does not enter food products. Low levels of estrogenic activity have also been detected in egg yolks; the levels of estrogen are too low to produce any physiologic effect (333).

Phytoestrogens

Estrogens derived from plant sources are phytoestrogens. These compounds have effects similar to animal estrogens. Phytoestrogens stimulate immature mouse uterine hypertrophy (38) and protein synthesis in the uterus of ovariectomized rats (291); they can also adversely affect the reproductive system of animals (29,337). Phytoestrogens do not, however, induce ovum implantation in ovariectomized rodents maintained on progestagen (301).

Most phytoestrogens are only weakly estrogenic. The largest group of phytoestrogens is composed of the glucoside forms of isoflavins: genistein, biochanin A, and prunetin (237). Several other phytoestrogens have also been isolated. Estrone is present in palm kernels (58); coumestrol is found in alfalfa (37); anethole is found in anise oil (414); and subterranean clover is associated with sheep sterility (337). The phytoestrogen zearalenone is a secondary metabolic product of *Fusarium graminearum* and related fungi, which can contaminate cereals; it was originally isolated during a search for an estrogenic agent responsible for sporadic hyperestrogenism in pigs consuming moldy feed (342).

Plants commonly used for food and found to have estrogenic activity in experimental animals include carrots (103); soybeans (61); wheat, rice, oats, barley, potatoes, apples, cherries, and plums (45); wheat bran, wheat germ, rice bran, and rice polish (43); and various vegetable oils including cottonseed, safflower, wheat germ, corn, linseed, peanut, olive, soybean, coconut, and refined or crude rice bran oil (43).

Asian females and vegetarians–two groups with low risk for breast cancer–have been found to have higher levels of urinary isoflavones than females consuming a Western diet, while females with breast cancer have lower levels of urinary isoflavones of all groups. From this has arisen the hypothesis that isoflavones, by an unknown mechanism, exert a protective effect against breast cancer in women (1,2). There is one animal study that supports this hypothesis (372).

Evidence of estrogen imbalance, including uterine bleeding and menstrual cycle abnormalities was detected in women consuming large quantities of tulip bulbs—which are high in estrogenic activity—during a severe food shortage near the end of World War II (222).

Derivatives of 1,25(OH)$_2$D$_3$ in Plants

Several species of plants may introduce elevated levels of glycoside derivatives of 1,25(OH)$_2$D$_3$ in grazing animals, resulting in calcinosis (385,168).

Exogenous or Xenobiotic Steroids

Estrogenic compounds have been found in chemicals used for agriculture, pesticides, and other commercial products. Implants of anabolic steroids in the form of estrogens and androgens have been used to stimulate growth and increase protein deposition during feeding periods primarily in cattle but also in sheep (62,161). Between 1954 and 1973, approximately 75% of cattle in the United States were fed diethylstilbestrol (DES), a synthetic nonsteroidal estrogen, to increase weight (333). The U.S. Food and Drug Administration prohibited DES additives to livestock feed in 1973 and implants in 1974 (91). Radioactive tracer in DES was found to remain in beef liver for up to 120 days regardless of whether it was introduced as a food additive or as an implant. Another estrogen, zeranol was developed to replace DES (341). Measurements of endogenous hormone residues in tissue exposed to exogenous hormone have been shown to be well within the physiologic range of normal steroid hormone levels for testosterone, estradiol, and progesterone. The only potential risk would be from repeated ingestion of tissue near the site of an implant; however, the site of implant is usually at a location that is discarded at slaughter—usually the ear in livestock (161).

Steroid compounds that do not naturally occur and are commonly used to increase tissue deposition in livestock include trenbolone acetate (TBA) and melengestrol acetate (MGA). TBA is a potent synthetic androgen. Following implant in livestock, approximately 80% of the drug is metabolized and excreted in the bile and feces. Analysis of tissues after exposure to TBA show the highest amount of residue in the liver, occasionally exceeded by levels in the fat (161). MGA is an orally active progestagen primarily (approximately 86%) eliminated in the feces.

The primary nonsteroidal xenobiotics include zeranol, produced by fermentation of *Gibberella zeae*, and stilbene estrogens. Use of stilbene estrogens for purposes of fattening livestock is currently prohibited worldwide. The group of stilbene estrogens includes DES and hexestrol (HEX). DES and the stilbene estrogens are potent, orally active estrogens, previously used in cattle and also sheep and swine (161). Xenobiotics, by definition, have no normal physiologic range. Xenobiotics with sex hormone activity are tumorigenic in long-term toxicity studies. No distinction is made regarding whether the compounds are carcinogenic (primary inducers) or promoters/stimulators of tissue growth (161). An association was made between adenocarcinoma of the vagina in 7 of 8 girls and treatment of their mothers with DES in the first trimester of pregnancy (154).

Three pesticides have been shown to be estrogenic: dichlorodiphenyltrichlorethane (DDT) (39,53), methoxychlor (54,277), and chlordecone (Kepone) (99,114). Lindane was shown to alter neither the estrogen receptor number nor the estrogen-dependent induction of progesterone receptor (233).

Technical grades of DDT consist of 67–85% p,p'–DDT, 8–21% o,p'–DDT, and several related compounds (25,392). Several lines of evidence support the idea that o,p'–DDT is estrogenic. DDT is uterotropic in mice, rats, mink, and birds. Both estradiol and DDT induce ornithine decarboxylase. DDT decreases the uterine cytosolic estrogen receptor and increases nuclear estrogen receptor; it does the same for cytosolic progesterone receptor (219).

Administration of o,p'–DDT (100 mg/kg) to rats and examination of uterine estrogen receptor binding reveals a decrease in uterine cytosolic estrogen receptor and concurrent increase in nuclear estrogen receptor (219).

When o,p'–DDT is administered to mature female rats, uterine cytosol progesterone receptor increases–just as it would for administration of an estrogen. The progesterone receptor that is formed shares the same sedimentation rate and affinity for [^{3}H]-progesterone as progesterone receptor from control or estradiol-treated rats (263).

Other tissues in which o,p'–DDT inhibits in vitro binding of [^{3}H]-estradiol to estrogen receptor include rat uterus cytosol (286), nuclei of rat uterus (219), rat testes cytosol (219), and human tumor cells (218). Nelson (286) found that o,p'–DDT inhibited cytosolic rat uterus estrogen receptor binding *in vitro* by 50% with 2 μmol/L (equivalent to a dose of 1 nmol/L DES). In comparison, other chlorinated biphenyl compounds also inhibited estrogen receptor binding, though to a lesser degree than o,p'–DDT; a positive correlation was seen between *in vitro* estrogen receptor binding of these compounds and an observed increase in uterus weight *in vivo*.

Methoxychlor is itself only weakly estrogenic; the estrogenic activity of this compound is likely due to a metabolite. Methoxychlor is unable to prevent tritiated estradiol binding to estrogen receptor (295). Methoxychlor incubated with rat liver microsomes becomes highly estrogenic (287). Methoxychlor is metabolized to two products, bis- and monophenol derivatives. Approximately 3% of methoxychlor is converted to the monophenol product, which has only one one-hundredth the activity of DES. Approximately 0.2% of methoxychlor is converted to the bisphenol product, and this has only one thirtieth the activity of DES (188).

Chlordecone has been shown to be estrogenic in rats (114) and in Japanese quail (99). The estrogenic properties of chlordecone were previously inferred from clinical observations of workers at a chlordecone-manufacturing plant (73).

Alkylphenol polyethoxylates (APEOs) are nonionic surfactants used in commercial products and as an additive in plastics. Nonylphenol polyethoxylates constitute approximately 80% of APEOs (>300,000 tons/year worldwide), while octylphenol polyethoxylates represent the majority of the remaining 20% of APEOs. The primary source of APEOs is detergents (396), though they are also in plastics (214,360) and are present in phenol red (32). APEOs are degraded to stable metabolites that persist in the environment; approximately 60% end up in water via sewage (308,396). Alkylphenols have been found in various freshwater sources, including groundwater (413), New Jersey tap water (69), and in fish from the Detroit River downstream from a plant producing such chemicals (348).

APEOs have been shown to demonstrate estrogenic activity in fish, bird, and mammalian cells, and although these compounds are approximately 10^3–10^4 less potent than 17β-estradiol, they mimic the effects of 17β-estradiol by binding to estrogen receptor. Biological actions of APEOs and their carboxylic acid derivatives (APECs) appear to depend on the presence of estrogen receptors. Their actions are inhibited by estrogen receptor antagonists, and they compete for binding to the estrogen receptor. Estrogenicity depends on the chain length; APEOs with greater than three ethoxylates have little, if any, estrogenic activity, and none of the compounds are toxic at doses of $<10^{-5}$M. Of the compounds studied, estrogenicity can be characterized as follows (in decreasing order): 4-tert-octylphenol > 4-nonylphenoxycarboxylic acid > 4-nonylphenol = 4-nonylphenol-diethoxylate (396). Use of these compounds in household detergents continues in Japan and the United States, and though they are no longer used in this capacity in many European countries, their use in industrial agents continues the world over (396).

STEROID HORMONE RECEPTORS

Adrenal Steroid Receptors

Mineralocorticoid Receptors

Mineralocorticoid receptors are distributed in the kidney, colon mucosa, and salivary gland ducts.

Mineralocorticoid–Mineralocorticoid Receptor Interactions

Steroids that influence renal cortex sodium absorption include the following: $9\propto$-fluorocortisol > deoxycorticosterone > cortisol = corticosterone : prednisolone (3).

Mineralocorticoid Receptor Antagonists

Although progesterone inhibits the mineralocorticoid receptor, it is not practical clinically. RU 486, originally developed as an antiglucocorticoid, has antigestational activity and does not antagonize mineralocorticoid-mediated sodium absorption. It can be used to treat hypertensive disorders mediated by glucocorticoids and can thus be used as a tool to distinguish between mineralocorticoid—or glucocorticoid-induced hypertension (3)

Synthetic spironolactones have become the agent of choice for mineralocorticoid antagonism. Their clinical use is primarily the treatment of hypertension. Addition of a methoxycarbonyl or propyl group in the 7α configuration of spironolactone results in ZK 91587 and RU 26752, respectively. These two compounds have markedly increased affinity for the mineralocorticoid receptor, relative to other mineralocorticoids (3).

Mineralocorticoid Receptor Mutations and Aldosterone Resistance

Aldosterone resistance arises from one of three known mechanisms. The first is pseudohypoaldosteronism (PHA) type I, a salt-wasting syndrome that often follows a familial pattern and is usually identified first in infants. The second known mechanism is PHA type II, resulting from an abnormality localized to the distal nephron. Aldosterone resistance may also arise secondary to other disease (210). The mineralocorticoid receptor is a single gene product from a single gene. Hippocampal mineralocorticoid receptor is identical to its renal counterpart but elutes 1–2 fractions earlier than renal mineralocorticoid receptor–a phenomenon thought to be due to a difference in associated proteins (210). The MR has an equal or perhaps even greater affinity for glucocorticoids than for aldosterone (210). There have been no mineralocorticoid receptor molecular defects described, even with PHA, and no difference has been detected in the hippocampus of persons with PHA (210).

Glucocorticoid Receptors

Glucocorticoid receptors are distributed widely in tissues of animals. Rat tissues without glucocorticoid receptor include the intermediate lobe of the pituitary; Kupffer's and endothelial cells of the liver, uterus, prostate, seminal vesicles, bladder, adipose, and jejunum; glomeruli and proximal convoluted tubules of the kidney; and acinary cells in the submaxillary glands (4). The human glucocorticoid receptor is composed of two isoforms, α (777 amino acids) and β (742 amino acids). These alternative forms are made by splicing mRNA transcribed from a single gene located on chromosome 5 (162). Although the subcellular distribution of glucocorticoid receptor remains controversial, there is morphologic and biochemical evidence that glucocorticoid receptor is associated with cytoskeletal components, likely microtubular networks, or possibly microfilaments (4).

Glucocorticoid–Glucocorticoid Receptor Interactions

Studies of human glucocorticoid receptor with point mutations in the hormone-binding domain indicate that glycine at amino acid position 567 is "crucial to ligand binding" (384).

Glucocorticoid Receptor Antagonists

RU 486 was originally developed as a potent antiglucocorticoid (278); it also inhibits the progesterone receptor (27,155). RU 486 binds to glucocorticoid receptor with higher affinity than dexamethasone (185).

Glucocorticoid and Nuclear Proto-oncogenes

Glucocorticoids tend to rapidly decrease the expression of nuclear proto-oncogenes, though the changes are tissue-specific (343).

Glucocorticoid Receptor Mutations

Three families have been described in which glucocorticoid receptor mutations resulted in glucocorticoid resistance. One case consisted of a point mutation at nucleotide 2054 causing a substitution of thymidine for adenine and resulting in a substitution of valine for aspartate at codon 641 in the glucocorticoid receptor ligand-binding domain (170). This substitution was noted to be near cysteine 638, which has been implicated in steroid binding (9).

The second case was also a point mutation, at nucleotide 2317, causing a substitution of adenine for guanine and resulting in substitution of isoleucine for valine at codon 729, also in the glucocorticoid receptor ligand-binding domain (253). In addition, deletion of four base pairs near the 3' boundary of exon 6 and intron 6 of the glucocorticoid receptor resulted in a 50% decrease in glucocorticoid receptor (189), though with normal binding of remaining glucocorticoid receptor

(225). The reduced amount of glucocorticoid receptor was thought to be secondary to reduced mRNA expression or to rapid degradation.

Chemical Modification of Glucocorticoid Receptors

The involvement of the nucleophilic residues tyrosine, serine, and histidine in the binding of dexamethasone to the human glucocorticoid receptors expressed in the baculovirus vector system has been systematically investigated (unpublished data from our laboratory). The experimental methods used were chemical modification and protection assays. Tyrosine modification did have a negative effect on binding. Tetranitromethane at a concentration of 0.5 mmol/L inhibited binding by 90%. N-Acetylimidazole (10 mmol/L) resulted in only 48% inhibition. Protection assays indicated that in both instances the modified tyrosine residues are located within the hormone-binding site. The serine protease inhibitors diisopropylfluorophosphate and phenylmethylsulfonyl fluoride, both at 5 mmol/L, reduced [^{3}H]-dexamethasone binding by 78% and 31%, respectively. Based on protection assays, the site of serine modification appears to be in or near the hormone-binding site. Histidine modification with 1 mmol/L diethylpyrocarbonate inhibited specific dexamethasone binding by 47% in a concentration-dependent manner, as was the case with tyrosine and serine.

Estrogen Receptors

Human Estrogen Receptor

The gene for the human estrogen receptor is located on the long arm of chromosome 6 (6q24-26) (248). The receptor is composed of eight exons. Exons 2 and 3 compose the DNA-binding domain, and exons 4–8 constitute the hormone-binding domain (109).

Estrogen–Estrogen Receptor Interactions

Introduction of point mutations at codon 525 in the mouse estrogen receptor so that glycine is replaced by arginine and at the methionine and/or serine at codon 521/522 essentially prevents the estrogen receptor from binding DNA and stimulating transcription (85). The decrease in affinity of estrogen receptor for estradiol does not affect the ability of tamoxifen to bind.

The human estrogen receptor cysteine at position 530 is close to the ligand-binding domain (85). A human estrogen receptor mutant was identified in which an alanine substitution for cysteine at amino acid 447, located in the hormone-binding domain, produced a thermolabile estrogen receptor with loss of DNA-binding ability (317), although mutations of the other three cysteines of the hormone-binding domain did not produce a similar result (316).

Estrogen Receptor Antagonists

Clinically, the most common use of antiestrogens is luteal deficiency giving rise to endometrial hyperplasia, myometrial hypertrophy, and myoma. However, the search for estrogen receptor antagonists has been driven by the fields of contraceptive research, and by the desire for treatment of hormone-dependent neoplasms such as breast cancer (315). Dependence on steroids by some breast cancers has been recognized for almost 100 years (28). Following the discovery of a specific cellular receptor for estrogens, variations in the levels of breast tumor estrogen receptors was reported (182,234). Detectable estrogen receptor is defined as >10 fmol receptor per milligram protein. More than 60% of breast cancer tumors with detectable estrogen receptor are responsive to endocrine therapy, while less than 5% of estrogen receptor negative tumors (<10 fmol receptor per mg protein) respond to endocrine therapy (183). Estrogen receptor antagonists are divided among steroid and nonsteroid compounds.

Progestagens are effective antiestrogens, and perhaps progesterone controls estrogen replenishment (33,34,68). Raynaud and Ojasoo (315) reviewed steroid structure and receptor-binding characteristics and surmised that effective binding of estradiol to receptor requires the hydroxy groups at C3 and C17. The former hydroxy group is thought to serve as a hydrogen bond donor and is likely involved in the first recognition step in steroid–receptor interaction.

Tamoxifen (ICI 46474), a nonsteroidal derivative of triphenylethylene, acts as an estrogen receptor antagonist (110, 145,298). However, it is capable of inducing receptor transformation and behaves as an agonist in some test systems and animal models, though the degree of agonism varies with species, tissue, or cell (110,145,298).

ICI 164384 is believed to be a pure estrogen receptor antagonist that inhibits the ability of estrogen receptor to bind to DNA, whereas tamoxifen does not. It is postulated that ICI 164384 reduces the affinity of estrogen receptor for DNA binding by interfering with estrogen receptor dimerization (102).

Estrogens and Nuclear Proto-oncogenes

The human estrogen receptor was recognized to have a high degree of homology with v-*erb* A, an oncogene encoded by avian erythroblastosis virus and capable of cooperating with truncated epidermal growth factor v-*erb* B to induce erythroleukemia in chickens (60,120,388). Once this association was made, a search began for a steroid receptor other than estrogen to have homology with c-*erb* A, the cellular proto-oncogene counterpart of v-*erb* A. The result, using low-stringency hybridization techniques, was cloning of receptors for triiodothyronine (T_3) (332,389) and $T_3R\alpha$ and β(47,117).

Estradiol increases the expression of c-*myc*, c-*jun*, and c-*fos* nuclear proto-oncogenes, which could lead to cell proliferation in a rapid, transient manner

(343). However, the effect is tissue-specific in various animal tissues or cell-culture systems.

Estrogen Receptor Mutations

Fuqua (109) suggests several possible causes for loss of functional human estrogen receptor: (1) genomic deletion of the gene; (2) mutations/rearrangements of the gene; (3) down-regulation of transcription at the promoter level; (4) methylation within the coding domain or promoter region; (5) altered message as a result of alternative splicing; and (6) aberrant human estrogen receptor function, such as a variant human estrogen receptor that is active in the absence of estrogen (dominant-positive human estrogen receptor) or a variant human estrogen receptor that is inactive and prevents the function of normal human estrogen receptor (dominant-negative human estrogen receptor).

Several types of genetic mutations have been identified that involve estrogen receptors. These first two cases illustrate gene deletion. Smith et al. (357) reported a case of estrogen resistance in a 28-year-old male who was the product of a consanguineous marriage between second cousins. He appeared to be a normal male, although he was unexpectedly tall and had delayed bone maturation and osteoporosis. Although his serum estrone, estradiol, follicle-stimulating hormone and luteinizing hormone were all elevated, he had normal male genitalia and a normal semen analysis. He was homozygous for a mutation in the human estrogen receptor gene that resulted in the absence of that receptor. The human estrogen receptor sequence from peripheral blood lymphocyte DNA demonstrated a substitution of thymine for cytosine in exon 2 of the human estrogen receptor at codon 157, which resulted in the replacement of the arginine codon (CGA) with a premature stop codon (TGA) and in a severely truncated human estrogen receptor lacking both the DNA- and hormone-binding domains. The case illustrated that total absence of the estrogen receptor is not a lethal mutation, that estrogen is not needed for male sexual development, that estrogen is critical for bone maturation in males, and that there is a role for estrogen in feedback inhibition of gonadotropin secretion in males.

A deletion in exon 5, resulting in truncated human estrogen receptor lacking the hormone-binding domain, was originally identified in estrogen receptor–negative/progesterone receptor–positive breast tumor. It was later found to be co-expressed with wild-type human estrogen receptor in a large number of estrogen receptor–positive tumors. The deletion consists of the introduction of a stop codon after amino acid 370, possibly as a result of alternative RNA splicing (109).

Chemical Modification of Estrogen Receptors

Chemical modification studies of the estrogen receptor have sought to determine the involvement of serine, tyrosine, histidine, and cysteine residues in the binding of estrogen to its receptor (203,204). In addition to binding studies conducted on the native receptor, studies were conducted on the trypsin-treated receptor (unpublished data from our laboratory). On treatment with trypsin, a 28-kd fragment was generated from the human estrogen receptor that retained hormone-binding activity and migrated with a sedimentation coefficient of 3S. Trypsin-treated receptors failed to bind to DNA. This fragment is an important tool. If hormone binding is inhibited in the presence of specific chemical agents, then one could localize the modified amino acid to the hormone-binding domain, pinpointing the location of the residue(s) important in ligand binding. On the other hand, if chemical modification does not inhibit binding to the fragment, it could be surmised that a site outside of the hormone-binding domain is responsible for inhibiting ligand binding to the intact receptor.

Inhibition of ligand binding in both the native and the trypsinized fragment was achieved with the tyrosine modifiers tetranitromethane (TNM), nitrobenzenesulfonyl (NBS), and *N*-acetylimidazole. TNM eliminated binding at 0.5 mmol/L. The serine protease inhibitors phenylmethylsulfonyl fluoride (PMSF) and diisopropylfluorophosphate (DFP) inhibited binding of [³H]-estradiol to the undigested and the digested estrogen receptor. Histidine was modified using the chemical agent diethylpyrocarbonate (DPC). In both the trypsinized and native forms, treatment with DPC reduced specific binding, confirming previous studies that found that DPC inhibited binding of hormone to the estrogen receptor (19,44).

Cysteine involvement was probed using *N*-ethylmaleimide (NEM) and *p*-chloromercuribenzoate (PCMB). Inhibition was achieved in both the native and trypsin-treated receptors. Of note, the inhibition induced by PCMB was reversed upon addition of dithiothreitol (DTT), whereas NEM formed a stable alkyl-derivative with estrogen receptor, preventing reversal with DTT.

While inhibition of hormone binding by trypsin-treated estrogen receptor suggests that there are several key residues in the hormone-binding domain, it does not exclude the possibility that an amino acid located in the DNA-binding domain or another estrogen receptor domain is indirectly involved in the binding of ligand to receptor.

Androgen Receptors

Human Androgen Receptor

The gene that encodes the androgen receptor is X-linked (Xq12) (50). The primary structure of the human androgen receptor was determined after molecular cloning and characterization of the cDNA encoding for it (63,101,242,243,368,370). The human androgen receptor protein coding region is divided over eight exons (216). The N-terminal transcriptional modulatory domain was found to be encoded entirely by exon 1 (101,216). The two DNA binding fingers were encoded by two small exons, while the information for the androgen-binding domain is contained over five exons.

Androgen–Androgen Receptor Interactions

Steroids with anabolic-androgenic potency may be divided into four groups (327): (1) steroids that bind well to receptor but poorly to sex hormone–binding globulin (SHBG); (2) steroids that bind better to SHBG than androgen receptor; (3) steroids that bind equally well to both receptor and SHBG; and (4) steroids unable to bind to either protein well.

The androgen receptor in muscle has relatively low affinity for 5α-dihydrotestosterone (DHT) compared to androgen receptor in prostate. This is thought likely to be due to rapid metabolism of DHT to inactive metabolites in muscle cytosol, which bind to SHBG but are inactive competitors of the receptor (324). The ratio of testosterone to DHT is increased in muscle compared with the prostate. Muscle does not carry out 5α-reduction of testosterone, and the 3-keto group of DHT is more easily metabolized to inactive metabolites in muscle than in the prostate (327).

Structural modification of androgenic steroids affects affinity of ligand for receptor (SHBG or androgen receptor). Removal of the 19-methyl group from testosterone increases the relative binding affinity for receptor in prostate and rabbit muscle minimally (3–4-fold) and reduces the relative binding affinity for SHBG 19-fold. Addition of a 17α-methyl group into testosterone hinders the relative binding affinity for SHBG but has little effect on relative binding affinity for androgen receptor. The relative binding affinity of 1α-methyl DHT is increased 4-fold for SHBG compared with DHT (327).

Androgen Receptor Antagonists

Precise mechanisms of antiandrogens on the androgen receptor are not known. Veldscholte et al. (381) cite several proposed mechanisms, including induction of abnormal receptor conformation (281), impaired translocation of receptor to nucleus (238,346), impaired dissociation of the nontransformed protein–receptor complex (280,346), impaired receptor dimerization and DNA binding (31,102,200), and impaired interaction between DNA-bound receptor and transcription factors (31,136,200,328). Physiologically, androgen antagonists may be divided into two groups (381): (1) the steroidal (nonpure) antiandrogens and (2) the nonsteroidal (pure) antiandrogens. Several well known drugs, including spironolactone and cimetidine have antiandrogenic action (288).

The first group of antiandrogens (the nonpure, or steroidal, antiandrogens) consists of compounds such as cyproterone acetate, megestrol acetate, medroxyprogesterone acetate, methyltrienolone (R 1881), chlormadinone acetate, and Δ^1-chlormadinone acetate. In addition to blocking androgen action, these antiandrogens have progesterone and glucocorticoid activities. Cyproterone acetate has three main properties: It is an antiandrogen, it is potent as a progestagen, and it is antigonadotrophic (288). Indications for use of cyproterone acetate include androgen-mediated skin disorders such as acne, seborrhea, hirsutism, alopecia, and other conditions, including advanced prostate carcinoma, precocious puberty, and male hypersexuality. In testotoxicosis (autonomous production of androgen from testes), therapy with an antiandrogen alone is insufficient to slow skeletal growth to a prepubertal rate. This is accomplished by including an aromatase inhibitor (232).

The latter group of nonsteroidal antiandrogens consists of compounds such as flutamide and nilutamide (RU 23908), which block androgen action and stimulate the hypothalamic–pituitary axis, leading to increased luteinizing hormone and testosterone levels (282,288,315).

Androgens and Nuclear Proto-oncogenes

Though few studies on androgen regulation of proto-oncogenes have been carried out, the existing studies all have shown an inhibition of expression of proto-oncogene (199,310,402). Levels of c-myc mRNA were reduced in the ventral prostate gland of a castrated rat by DHT (310) and by a synthetic androgen, mibolerone, in human prostate carcinoma cells (402).

Androgen Receptor Mutations

There are several categories of known androgen receptor mutations (11,270). These defects include (1) point mutations resulting in substitutions in the DNA- (132,415) or hormone-binding domains (52,88,258,259,269,270,285,320) or premature termination in exon 1 (416), 3 (256), 4 (257), 6 (329), or 7 (371); (2) gene deletions, either partial (51), or complete (247,311,312); (3) splicing defects (319); and (4) CAG trinucleotide, or glutamine, repeat polymorphisms (229).

Catagories 1–3, above, are associated with gross androgen receptor defects, and persons with these defects present with abnormal sexual development from fetal life and normal neuromuscular development. Substitution mutations in the hormone-binding domain can result in complete or incomplete testicular feminization in persons who are phenotypic females and genotypic males. These persons present with primary amenorrhea, incomplete migration of the testes, and absence of virilization (11). Milder androgen resistance presents as partial androgen insensitivity syndrome (Reifensteins'syndrome), marked by perineoscrotal or pseudovaginal hypospadias and gynecomastia with some virilization, such as axillary or pubic hair, in males (270,335).

Category 4 is represented by X-linked spinobulbar muscular atrophy (Kennedy's syndrome), a neurodegenerative disorder with selective degeneration of anterior horn cells of the spinal cord (196). Onset is in the third to fifth decade. Patients may have mental retardation, and the disease may be associated with endocrine disorders related to androgen insensitivity (196). Affected males may have gynecomastia, impaired spermatogenesis, and elevated serum gonadotropin levels in the presence of normal serum testosterone levels. This disease occurs when an expansion of an "unstable" repeat triplet (CAG) occurs in the first human androgen receptor gene exon (35,106,229). The CAG codon codes for glutamine; the normal gene codes for 11–33 glutamine residues, while the disease gene codes for 36–62 glutamines. The length of the triplet repeat expansion also accounts for the phenomenon of anticipation, in which disease can be seen earlier in succeeding generations. A similar motif has been identified in several other diseases; with the exception of fragile X syndrome and X-linked mental retardation (108,201), they are all neurodegenerative diseases. Huntington's disease (169), spinobulbar muscular atrophy (229), Machado–Joseph disease (192,205,284), spinocerebellar ataxia type 1 (143,294) and type 2 (116), and dentatorubral-pallidoluysian atrophy (205,284)–all are associated with expansions in coding regions. In contrast, myotonic dystrophy (373), fragile X syndrome (108), and X-linked mental retardation (201) are associated with expansions in noncoding regions.

The presence of the triplet repeat expansion in Kennedy's syndrome apparently interferes with androgen receptor function, affecting both gonadal and motor neuron tissue. COS-1 cells transfected with human androgen receptor cDNA from spinobulbar muscular atrophy patients and exposed to mibolerone have normal steroid-binding capacity and impaired DNA translation (250). The polyglutamine repeats in disease likely affect transcription without impairing binding of human androgen receptor to ligand. This possibility suggests a motif for other diseases with trinucleotide repeat polymorphism whose gene products are not yet known. Another proposed mechanism is formation of cross-linked products from transglutaminase action on polyglutamine substrate to cause slow, selective death of neurons (128).

In addition to the above mutations of the human androgen receptor, a single amino acid substitution point mutation has been identified in a patient with prostatic carcinoma who developed resistance to endocrine and cytotoxic therapy (84). The androgen receptor mutation was a guanine-to-adenine transition at nucleotide 2671, resulting in substitution of methionine for valine at codon 715. Adrenal androgens and progesterone resulted in a higher transactivation in the mutant receptor and may have contributed to development of resistance to endocrine treatment.

The human prostate tumor cell line LNCaP contains a single point mutation in codon 868 (threonin to alanine) of the hormone-binding domain. The resulting androgen receptor has broad specificity for other steroids, including progestagens, estradiol, and several antiandrogens. Transfection assays have established that the mutation affects both binding specificity and the induction of gene expression (381).

Chemical Modification of Androgen Receptors

The involvement of tyrosine, serine, cysteine, and histidine in androgen binding to the rat androgen receptor was investigated via covalent modification of residues in the baculovirus system (unpublished data from our laboratory). The basic binding assays were carried out with a variety of chemical agents selected for their ability to covalently modify specific residues. Chemical agents directed toward tyrosine modification, tetranitromethane (TNM) and nitrobenzenesulfonyl (NBS), drastically reduced specific androgen (R 1881) binding, though the 2 mmol/L concentration of TNM required to eliminate ligand binding was far less than the 10 mmol/L required by NBS.

Serine modification via diisopropylfluorophosphate and phenylmethylsulfonyl fluoride also demonstrated significant concentration-dependent inhibition of ligand binding. Cysteine residues provide stability to proteins via disulfide bonds and provide reactive sulfhydryl groups. The ability of N-ethylmaleimide to compromise ligand binding to the rat androgen receptor suggests that a cysteine residue is involved with androgen binding. Inhibition of steroid binding by diethylpyrocarbonate provides evidence that one or more histidine residue(s) play a role in androgen binding.

If the chemical modification agents act on residues within the hormone-binding site, it should follow that with incubation of the receptor with its ligand prior to the addition of the agent, the binding sites would be protected from inhibition. This was the case with rat androgen receptor.

Progesterone Receptors

Human Progesterone Receptor

The human progesterone receptor (hPR) maps to the long arm of chromosome 11 (11q22-23) (248).

Progesterone receptor isolated from the T47D human breast cancer cell line occurs in two distinct molecular forms (165), designated as hPR-A and hPR-B. The hPR-A is 94 kd, and the hPR-B is 116 kd. The two forms are different only at the amino terminus; there is one human progesterone receptor gene with two distinct estrogen-inducible promoters (190). There are two distinct roles for hPR-A and hPR-B (380,395): (1) hPR-B acts predominantly as an activator of progesterone-responsive genes; (2) hPR-A represses hPR-B activity and is capable of inhibiting transcriptional activity of other steroid receptors, including the glucocorticoid receptor, androgen receptor, mineralocorticoid receptor, and estrogen receptor.

Wen et al. (395) suggest two possible models to explain how hPR-A acts as a transcriptional repressor of human estrogen receptor. Both the human estrogen receptor and hPR-A may compete for a limiting factor required by human estrogen receptor for maximal transcriptional activity, or perhaps there exist distinct, noncompetitive targets for both human estrogen receptor and hPR-A for which the ratio of hPR-A to target is more important than the hPR-A to human estrogen receptor. Results of work with reconstituted systems favors the second model.

Progesterone–Progesterone Receptor Interactions

Contact of the progesterone A ring and its C4, C7, C14 surface with progesterone receptor was suggested to be close and rigid, while a more flexible association was predicted at C11, C12, and C17 (315).

GABA receptor–mediated responses are potentiated at nanomolar concentrations by 3α-hydroxy ring A—reduced pregnane steroids (171). Pregnenolone sulfate inhibits $GABA_A$-mediated responses at micromolar concentrations (251). When a series of isomeric metabolites of progesterone and deoxycorticosterone were compared for their ability to enhance GABA-evoked chloride currents in cultured hippocampal neurons, metabolites with 3-hydroxy in the α position and 5-hydroxy in the α- or β-configuration were highly effective in potentiation of GABA-evoked chloride current–and as an anticonvulsant (207). Metabolites with hydroxyl groups in the 3β position were less potent in enhancing GABA responses–and as an anticonvulsant.

Progesterone Receptor Antagonists

When the mechanism of action of several progestins and antiprogestins on the transactivating potential of progesterone receptor in extracts of T47D breast carcinoma lines was investigated, two types of antiprogestins were identified (200). Type I, a novel mechanism, was represented by ZK 98299. These compounds did not induce specific binding of progesterone receptor to progesterone-responsive elements, but competitively inhibited induction of DNA binding by progestins, as well as type II antiprogestins. The C- and D-rings of ZK 98299 are fused in the *cis*-configuration, and this compound fails to elicit structural alterations of the progesterone receptor. Type II antiprogestins induce a stable, high-affinity binding of progesterone receptor to progesterone-responsive elements and are represented by RU 486, ZK 98734, and ZK 112993. The natural *trans*-configuration of the C- and D-rings is maintained in these antiprogestins.

Progesterone and Nuclear Proto-oncogenes

Studies of the effects of progesterone on nuclear proto-oncogenes show a decrease or no effect (343).

Human Progesterone Receptor Mutations

One report of human progesterone resistance is available (194). A 23-year-old female complained of infertility. Despite a normal menstrual cycle, normal luteal phase, and normal plasma concentrations of luteinizing hormone and progesterone, the endometrium was histologically immature and suggested a defect in her ability to develop a secretory endometrium. The condition was not correctable with exogenous progesterone, and in vitro examination of her progesterone receptor concentration on day 14 of the luteal phase revealed a reduced concentration (approximately 50%). The working hypothesis was a decrease in cytosol receptors or progesterone resistance. However, a molecular mechanism was not available when this case originally presented.

Chemical Modification of Progesterone Receptor

Studies have been conducted evaluating the modulation of calf uterus progesterone receptor in relation to binding agonist (R 5020) and antagonist (RU 486) in the presence or absence of iodoacetamide, N-ethylmaleimide, β-mercaptoethanol, and dithiothreitol. Observations suggested that sulfhydryl group modifications differentially influence the properties of mammalian progesterone receptor complexed with R 5020 or RU 486.

Further studies have determined that tyrosine, serine, cysteine, and histidine residues are involved in the binding of the synthetic progestin R 5020 to human progesterone receptor expressed in a baculovirus vector system (unpublished data from our laboratory). Chemical modification of progesterone receptor with phenylmethylsulfonyl fluoride (PMSF), diisopropylfluorophosphate (DFP), tetranitromethane (TNM), nitrobenzenesulfonyl (NBS), p-chloromercuribenzoic acid (PCMB), or diethylpyrocarbonate (DPC) has been studied.

TNM and NBS, agents directed toward tyrosine residues, demonstrated high inhibition of ligand binding at low concentrations; TNM appears to be more effective. More than 90% inhibition was achieved with 0.5 mmol/L TNM; 1 mmol/L NBS inhibited binding by 64%. The serine protease inhibitors DFP and PMSF (5 mmol/L each) inhibited R 5020 binding by 48% and 50%, respectively. Modification of cysteine residues with 1 mmol/L N-ethylmaleimide (NEM) or 0.5 mmol/L PCMB resulted in 37% and 92% inhibition, respectively. The reduction in binding activity was not due to progesterone receptor degradation. Addition of 5 mmol/L dithiothreitol, a reducing agent, reversed the PCMB-induced inhibition, indicating involvement of sulfhydryl residues. One or more histidine residues appear to be involved in steroid binding; addition of DPC resulted in concentration-dependent inhibition.

Vitamin D_3 Receptor

Human Vitamin D_3 Receptor

The cholecalciferol (vitamin D_3) receptor is composed of eight exons (321) and has a molecular weight of approximately 50,000–60,000 kd. It exhibits a high affinity for 1,25-dihydroxycholecalciferol (1,25(OH)$_2$D$_3$) (148). This receptor has been shown to align with fibers thought to be microtubules or structures closely associated with microtubules (6,24).

Vitamin D_3 Receptor Mutations

In general, three types of molecular defects have been found in the vitamin D_3 receptor from fibroblasts: (1) decreased or absent 1,25(OH)$_2$D$_3$ binding; (2) decreased affinity of the vitamin D_3 receptor for DNA; and (3) defective nuclear translocation or retention.

Hereditary vitamin D–resistant rickets, first described by Albright et al. (5), illustrates reduced or absent binding of $1,25(OH)_2D_3$. It is a rare, autosomal-recessive hereditary disease. One study of four children from three families identified an ochre mutation in the vitamin D_3 receptor after DNA from the affected children was amplified and compared with that of the normal family members. A single cysteine-to-alanine base substitution in exon 7 (nucleotide 970) changed tyrosine (TAC) to a premature termination codon (TAA) at amino acid 292 and resulted in a truncated vitamin D_3 receptor with deletion of a large portion of the steroid hormone–binding domain (amino acids 292–424) (321).

Two other families have been shown to have a vitamin D_3 receptor of normal size, abundance, and affinity for $1,25(OH)_2D_3$ but with reduced affinity for DNA and an inability to activate target genes (160,254). Two distinct missense point mutations were detected in the DNA-binding domain of their vitamin D_3 receptor genes, resulting in single amino acid changes near the tip of the first zinc finger in one family and in the tip of the second zinc finger in the second family (167).

Separation of cytoplasm and nuclear fractions from fibroblasts after vitamin D exposure in two kindreds demonstrated reduced or absent nuclear localization of bound hormone, suggesting a defective transfer or defective receptor activation mechanism (236). In a second case, nuclear localization of vitamin D_3 receptor–$1,25(OH)_2D_3$ complex was absent and resulted in unresponsiveness to vitamin D. The defect was not due to a mutation in the vitamin D_3 receptor gene coding region, and transfection of cDNA from the patient to mammalian cells resulted in a normal transactivation response to vitamin D_3. This person likely had a defect in the ability to translocate the steroid-receptor complex into the nucleus. Several potential mechanisms for this included possible abnormality in an associated protein such as a heat shock protein (though one has not yet been shown to be associated with vitamin D_3 receptor), inability of vitamin D_3 receptor to dimerize, or abnormal post-translational modification of the vitamin D_3 receptor (157).

PHYSIOLOGIC AND PATHOLOGIC CONDITIONS

"Now I think I am correct in saying that the spirit of modern pathology is this–that all pathological changes are merely modified physiological ones, that there is no essential difference between the two, and that a knowledge of the forces controlling the one may sometimes give us a clue to the other."

– George Thomas Beatson, MD (28)

Toxin Interactions with Steroids or Steroid Receptors

Ethanol

Conflicting data exist regarding the effect of ethanol on glucocorticoid release in rat models in vitro (70,135,187). Acute ethanol consumption in humans results in an increase in adrenocorticoids (176,274).

Administration of ethanol to healthy volunteers at a dose of 1.5 g/kg over 3 hours raised blood alcohol levels to 25–35 mmol/L without any changes in the testosterone levels (409). However, chronic consumption of ethanol in 9 normal volunteers and 2 alcoholic volunteers for up to 24 days at a dose of 3g/kg every three hours decreased plasma testosterone by a 29–55% independent of liver disease (122). Chronic ethanol consumption results in decreased plasma testosterone levels from a decrease in production, increased metabolic clearance, and in part a decrease in nicotinamide adenine dinucleotide (NAD), which may lead to reduced conversion of pregnenolone to testosterone (124,212). Chronic use of ethanol may also directly suppress spermatogenesis via interference of vitamin A metabolism in the testes (377).

Effects of fetal alcohol syndrome on sex steroid metabolism in the brain or aromatase activity in male rats are inconclusive. Experimental evidence suggests that gonadal steroids affect the cell number, cellular growth, and synapse formation (283) or the alteration of steroid hormone receptors (144,382). The catalytic activity of hypothalamic aromatase of male rat pups of mothers fed ethanol is greater than in neonatal rats with mothers fed control diet (268). In utero exposure to ethanol ingestion does not lead to an alteration of 5α-reductase, aromatase, or their ratio in neonatal rat hypothalamic tissue (193).

Acute or chronic ethanol exposure is known to adversely affect the reproductive function of the pubertal or adult female rat (42,153,378). Acute and chronic ethanol exposure has been demonstrated to reduce the sex steroid levels in adult males (104,124,235,376). Ethanol in human females results in anovulatory cycles and persistent hyperprolactinemia (273).

Ethanol enhances metabolism of vitamin D and other compounds of similar structure, presumably via the effect ethanol has on increasing microsomal metabolism (112).

Cooperman et al. (76) described six female nondiabetic patients with seven episodes of severe ketoacidosis. All patients engaged in ethanol binges. One patient had four hospitalizations over two pregnancies, all of which were temporally related to excessive drinking. This case suggested that ovarian and placental hormones–and possibly a fetal drain on carbohydrates–might play a role in pathogenesis of alcoholic ketoacidosis. However, one would also want to consider that the diet of an alcoholic might be a risk factor for developing ketoacidosis.

Alcoholic cirrhosis in males affects gonadal function, resulting in hypogonadism (60–70%) and other signs of feminization such as gynecomastia (30–50%). Clinically, male patients present with loss of libido and sexual hair, while women present with menstrual disorders; both have vascular spiders. These findings may reflect increased estradiol and estrone levels (65). There is increased conversion of testosterone and androstenedione to estrogen (123). Neither testosterone (119) nor vitamin A (403) improves sexual function.

Tobacco

Smoking is thought to have an antiestrogenic effect, based on the association of smoking with two diseases: (1) early age at menopause (180,191,400) and (2) postmenopausal osteoporosis (23). Possible mechanisms for the association of tobacco with early menopause may be a direct toxic effect of benzo[a]pyrene, a component of cigarette smoke, on the ovaries or enhanced metabolism of steroid hormones via induction of liver microsomal enzymes by cigarette smoke components (180,191). Data suggest a modest decrease in the risk of breast cancer in women who smoke tobacco, and a greater effect in heavier smokers (>20 cigarettes per day) (292).

Nicotine and related substances in tobacco smoke inhibit several P-450 enzymes in the pathways of glucocorticoid (20,21), aldosterone (352), and sex steroid synthesis (408). There is a paucity of studies evaluating the interaction of nicotine or other tobacco products with steroid receptors.

Marijuana

A single report (309) notes inhibition of androgen receptor by tetrahydrocannibinol, the active ingredient in marijuana, though there is no follow-up. Both acute (208) and chronic (209) marijuana use decrease plasma testosterone levels, while impaired spermatogenesis is seen after more chronic use (208,209). Plasma testosterone levels decrease by 35% (from 779 ng/dL to 505 ng/dL; normal, 380–980 ng/dL) within 3 hours of smoking 1–3 marijuana cigarettes (208). The decrease in plasma testosterone level is dose-related and reversible with cessation of marijuana (209). Oligospermia (<30 million sperm/mL semen) was generally seen in 35% of individuals and was also dose-related (152,209); usually, only 10% of healthy, normal males have oligospermia. Acute alcohol use did not affect testosterone or luteinizing hormone (LH) levels (208).

The potency of various naturally occurring cannabinoids in decreasing testosterone production has been determined (57). Listed from greatest to least in testosterone-inhibiting ability, they are the following: cannabigerol > cannabidiol > cannabicyclol > cannabinol > tetrahydrocannabinol > cannabichromene.

There is one case report (77) of short stature and delayed puberty associated with extremely heavy marijuana use in a 16-year-old boy (five joints per day since age 11). Although his testicular growth was normal, his serum testosterone level was low (16–32 ng/dL), likely secondary to LH inhibition. He had normal serum growth hormone level; his bone age was 13 years. These effects were reversed after cessation of marijuana use.

Marijuana was originally thought to compete for estrogen receptor (314), although tetrahydrocannibinol (THC) was later found to bind to a fraction other than estrogens after gradient centrifugation (293,358). Subsequently, neither THC, cannabinol, nor marijuana extract was found to compete with estrogen for estrogen receptor in the primate uterus (354). Chronic marijuana use in human females has been associated with anovulatory cycles or impaired luteal phase of the menstrual cycle (264).

Animal studies with rats and mice have shown treatment-related increases in plasma corticosterone levels. However, in humans, there is no elevation in urinary cortisol excretion (83,163,164,209).

Ciguatera Toxin

The source of ciguatera toxin is primarily the blue-green algae species, *Gambierdiscus toxicus*, and possibly other species. Ciguatera fish poisoning was first noted after consumption of the turban-shell, *Livona pica*, colloquially known as ciguatera, but poisonings have also been described involving a variety of sporadically toxic fish (15). One pregnant human female near term consumed fish tainted with ciguatera toxin, experienced very active and unusual fetal movements over the next two days, and required delivery by cesarean section. The neonate suffered from facial palsy. The authors of this case report predict that the low molecular weight toxin (approximately 1000–1500 kd) might cross the placenta and suggest it may cause premature labor (300). The mother in this case also experienced pain in breast feeding.

Unleaded Gasoline

It is estimated that 110 million Americans are regularly exposed to unleaded gasoline vapors during automobile refueling (401). Selective induction of liver tumors has been reported in female–but not male–B6C3F1 mice by 2056 ppm of unleaded gasoline vapor, although the relevance of this to humans is not known (245). Subsequent studies attempted to evaluate the potential antiestrogenic potential of unleaded gasoline in female mice (246,362). Although unleaded gasoline was unable to compete for estrogen receptors, it induced estrogen metabolism in doses of 600 mg/kg/day in hepatocyte suspension when compared with control. Induction of enhanced metabolism of estrogen by unleaded gasoline is thus a plausible mechanism of antiestrogenic effects of unleaded gasoline in mice. Uterine atrophy and inhibition of endometrial cystic hyperplasia seen after exposure to unleaded gasoline is thought to have an explanation other than a direct antiestrogenic effect by unleaded gasoline (246).

Medical Illnesses Associated with Alterations in
Steroid or Steroid Receptor

Migraine

Approximately 14% of females who suffer from migraine have their symptoms exclusively at menstruation (98). The International Headache Society has defined menstrual migraine as migraine without aura that may occur almost exclusively during a particular time during the menstrual cycle. However, no generally agreed on criteria are available, and detailed epidemiologic data are lacking (150). The mechanism of hormonal influence in the etiology of menstrual migraine is unknown, although an abrupt decrease in serum estrogen concentrations before onset is strongly suspected (359).

Welch (390) recently reviewed this subject and several previously attempted treatments. Prophylaxis with percutaneous estradiol gel, applied just before and through the menses, reduced the frequency of menstrual headaches in controlled clinical trials (89,90). Women on estrogen with frequent migraine attacks may benefit by stopping or increasing the estrogen dose (391).

Although there are no controlled clinical trials using hormone antagonists or androgens in abortive or prophylactic treatment of menstrual migraine, several case reports note the use of tamoxifen (306), bromocriptine (8), or danazol, an androgen derivative that inhibits pituitary–ovarian function (334), .

Meningioma

Bickerstaff et al. (36) presented two patients and reviewed an additional nine patients with meningiomas demonstrating development and remission during and after two or more pregnancies. The locations were often similar (suprasellar, parasellar, or medial sphenoidal wing), and the symptoms usually developed in the last 4 months of pregnancy. Bickerstaff and co-workers speculated that the locations were often similar because expansion of tumor in less sensitive parts of the neuroaxis would not have so dramatic an effect as would be seen in a region near the oculomotor and optic nerves. Several etiologies were considered, including hormonal influences; however, hormonal influences were discounted in favor of water-retention of the tumor as the most likely explanation.

Schoenberg et al. (340) found an increased incidence of meningiomas in females with breast cancer. The known association of breast carcinomas with steroid receptors and the relapsing course of meningiomas with pregnancies suggested the possibility of a role for hormones or hormone receptors in meningiomas (59). Estrogen and progesterone receptors have been found in meningiomas (41,59,74,94,118,159,249,260–262,304,339,344,369,379,410), although the concentration of receptors as a criterion for the presence of receptor in tissues has not been consistently agreed on among studies (59). Review of these studies indicates the presence of estrogen receptor in a minority of meningiomas, with progesterone receptor in as many as 70% of meningiomas.

One case report (303) notes abrupt clinical progression of symptoms referable to a sphenoid wing meningioma after placement of a subcutaneous contraceptive implant containing levonorgestrel (Norplant), a progesterone agonist. Symptoms continued to progress despite removal of the implant, and no direct causal link between the two events could be proven. The case does add evidence to implicate the progesterone receptor in the growth and possible treatment of meningiomas.

One laboratory study (211) investigated the response of cultured human meningiomas cells to epidermal growth factor and modulation of the response by progesterone and RU 486. Thymidine incorporation assays suggested that progesterone in culture medium increased the sensitivity of meningioma cells to specific mitogenic stimuli (epidermal growth factor). RU 486 counteracts the stimulatory effects of progesterone on these cells in culture.

A case report of progesterone depletion with buserelin, a synthetic gonadotropin-releasing peptide, noted symptomatic relief of symptoms caused by meningioma (375). The symptoms included headache and ptosis, which fluctuated with the menstrual cycle; treatment consisted of buserelin 300 mg intranasally four times a day for one year. Headache and ophthalmic symptoms resolved with progesterone depletion; the ophthalmic symptoms recurred after cessation of treatment and again dissipated after treatment was restarted.

Grunberg (133) has reviewed several potential medical treatments, including antiprogestational agents for unresectable meningiomas. Previous use of estrogen antagonists and progesterone supplementation has not been helpful (133). Treatment of 28 patients with unresectable meningiomas with RU 486 and dexamethasone showed objective improvement with reduction of tumor size on magnetic resonance imaging or computed tomography. Visual fields were also improved in eight patients, and there was subjective improvement in extraocular muscle function or reduction in tumor-related headache in five patients (134). Another treatment trial with RU 486 (200 mg daily for up to 12 months) in ten patients resulted in meningioma regression in three patients and improvement in headache in five patients (226). Similar results were seen in a case report of two patients treated with RU 486 (200–400 mg daily for 6–8 months) and concurrent dexamethasone (1.5 mg) to compensate for antiglucocorticoid effects (139). A phase III clinical trial with RU 486 is anticipated (133).

Glucocorticoid Resistance

Glucocorticoid resistance can be primary, familial, or acquired. Persons with glucocorticoid resistance are often asymptomatic, or they complain of chronic fatigue. Signs may include hypertension or alopecia. The molecular mechanism of primary glucocorticoid resistance has been discussed (see "Glucocorticoid Receptor Mutations," above). Acquired glucocorticoid resistance was recently described in HIV-positive patients, in whom the incidence in one series was approximately 17%. The glucocorticoid receptor demonstrates reduced affinity for dexamethasone, increased receptor density, and a defective glucocorticoid-induced inhibition of [^{3}H]-thymidine incorporation (290). The same authors speculated that the reduced affinity may be due to an effect of increased interferon-α or triglycerides. Effects from interferon-α were felt to be less likely, and it is known that free fatty acids and other glyceride lipids reduce glucocorticoid receptor affinity for hormone and increase receptor density. Persons with HIV have increased serum triglyceride levels. Acquired glucocorticoid resistance has also recently been described in asthma (347), rheumatoid arthritis (338), and iatrogenically following hormonal manipulation of meningioma with RU 486 (224).

Apoptosis

Apoptosis is thought to be genetically controlled death of a cell, in which the dying cell is an active participant. Apoptosis is identified morphologically by cell shrinkage, chromatin condensation, and DNA fragmentation due to endogenous endonuclease(s), often producing a ladder pattern in the DNA, although this is not an essential feature (197).

Apoptosis is found in virtually all cell types under the right stimuli (56). Interaction of transcriptional regulators such as steroid hormones may be important in modulating inhibition or enhancement of apoptosis. Several examples exist in which steroid hormones provide such a stimulus (364).

Treatment of mothers with diethylstilbestrol (DES) seems to inhibit physiologic regression of the Müllerian duct of the fetus. Though the role of apoptosis has not been investigated, persistence of the Müllerian duct is believed to result in male genital tract malformations that resemble neoplasia (289).

Estrogen functions as an inhibitor of apoptosis in the hamster kidney estrogen-dependent tumor. Withdrawal of DES enhances apoptosis and decreases mitoses. Treatment with DES produces the opposite response (55). Testosterone also functions as a mitogen, or inhibitor, of apoptosis in the prostate (220,221).

Glucocorticoid functions as an activator of apoptosis for thymocytes and lymphocytes (67,366,398,406), is possibly mediated by Ca^{+2} activation of endogenous endonuclease responsible for chromatin cleavage (72,186,266,405,407), and depends on de novo gene transcription (72). Direct transcriptional activation of steroid-responsive genes is thought to be essential for cell death (92). Steroid hormones likely induce expression of one or more lethal genes (296), although it is possible that steroid-induced gene repression may contribute to cell death (365).

Anti-T cell receptor antibodies and glucocorticoids each induce apoptosis individually. However, when used together, they result in cell survival, unless high doses are used, and apoptosis is again observed (174,411).

REFERENCES

1. Adlercreutz H, Fotsis T, Bannwart C, et al. Determination of urinary lignans and phytoestrogen metabolites, potential antiestrogens and anticarcinogens, in urine of women on various habitual diets. *J Steroid Biochem.* 1986;25:791–797.
2. Adlercreutz H, Fotsis T, Heikkinen R, et al. Excretion of the lignans enterolactone and enterodiol and of equol in omnivorous and vegetarian postmenopausal women and in women with breast cancer. *Lancet.* 1982;2:1295–1299.
3. Agarwal MK. Perspectives in receptor-mediated mineralocorticoid hormone action. *Pharmacol Rev.* 1994;46:67–87.
4. Akner G, Wikström A-C, Gustafsson JÅ. Subcellular distribution of the glucocorticoid receptor and evidence for its association with microtubules. *J Steroid Biochem Mol Biol.* 1995;52:1–16.
5. Albright F, Butler AM, Bloomberg E. Rickets resistant to vitamin D therapy. *Am J Dis Child.* 1937;54:529–547.
6. Amizuka N, Ozawa H. Intracellular localization and translocation of 1α,25-dihydroxyvitamin D₃ receptor in osteoblasts. *Arch Histol Cytol.* 1992;55:77–88.
7. Amsel Z, Genser SG, Haverdos HW. Anabolic steroid use among male high school seniors. *JAMA.* 1989;262:207–208.

8. Andersen AN, Larsen JF, Steenstrup OR, et al. Effect of bromocriptine on the premenstrual syndrome: a double-blind clinical trial. *Baillièrre's J Obstet Gynaecol.* 1977;84:370–374.
9. Ari K, Chrousos GP. Glucocorticoid resistance. *Baillières Clin Endocrinol Metab.* 1994;8:317–331.
10. Arriza JL, Weinberger C, Cerelli G, et al. Cloning of human mineralocorticoid receptor complementary DNA: structural and functional kinship with the glucocorticoid receptor. *Science.* 1987;237:268–275.
11. Auchus RJ, Fuqua SAW. Clinical syndromes of hormone receptor mutations: hormone resistance and independence. *Semin Cell Biol.* 1994;15:127–136.
12. Ayres PJ, Gould RP, Simpson SA, Tait JF. The in vitro demonstration of differential corticosteroid production within the ox adrenal gland. *Biochem J.* 1956;63:19P.
13. Bäckström T, Zetterlund B, Blom S, Romano M. Effects of intravenous progesterone infusions on the epileptic discharge frequency in women with partial epilepsy. *Acta Neurol Scand.* 1984;69:240–248.
14. Baggett B, Engel LL, Savard K, Dorfman RI. Formation of estradiol-17β-C^{-14} from testosterone-3-C^{-14} by surviving human ovarian slices. *Fed Proc.* 1955;14:175–176.
15. Bagnis R. Ciguatera fish poisoning. In: Falconer IR, ed. *Algal Toxins in Seafood and Drinking Water.* London: Academic Press; 1993;105–115.
16. Baker AR, McDonnell DP, Hughes M, et al. Cloning and expression of full-length cDNA encoding human vitamin D receptor. *Proc Natl Acad Sci U S A.* 1988;85:3294–3298.
17. Baker ME. Computer-based search for steroid and DNA binding sites on estrogen and glucocorticoid receptors. *Biochem Biophys Res Commun.* 1986;139:281–286.
18. Baker M, Fanestil D. Diethylpyrocarbonate inhibition of estrogen binding to rat alpha feto-protein: evidence that one or more histidine residue regulates estrogen binding. *Biochem Biophys Res Commun.* 1981;98:976–982.
19. Baker ME, Sklar DH, Terry LS, Hedges MR. Diethylpyrocarbonate, a histidine selective reagent, inhibits binding to receptor protein in rat uterus cytosol. *Biochem Internat.* 1985;11:233–238.
20. Barbieri RL, Friedman AJ, Osathanondh R. Cotinine and nicotine inhibit human fetal adrenal 11β-hydroxylase. *J Clin Endocrinol Metab.* 1989;69:1221–1224.
21. Barbieri RL, York CM, Cherry ML, Ryan KJ. The effects of nicotine, cotinine and anabasine on rat adrenal 11β-hydroxylase and 21-hydroxylase. *J Steroid Biochem.* 1987;28:25–28.
22. Barker JL, Harrison NL, Lange GD, Owen DG. Potentiation of γ-aminobutyric acid-activated chloride conductance by a steroid anesthetic in cultured rat spinal neurones. *J Physiol.* 1987;386:485–501.
23. Baron JA. Smoking and estrogen-related disease. *Am J Epidemiol.* 1984;119:9–22.
24. Barsony J, McCoy W. Molybdate increases intracellular 3',5'-guanosine cyclic monophosphate and stabilizes vitamin D receptor association with tubulin-containing filaments. *J Biol Chem.* 1992;267:24,457–24,465.
25. Baselt RC, Cravey RH, eds. *Disposition of Toxic Drugs and Chemicals in Man.* 3rd ed. Chicago, Ill: Year Book Medical Publishing; 1989:241.
26. Baulieu E-E. Cell membrane, a target for steroid hormones. *Mol Cell Endocrinol.* 1978;12:247–254.
27. Baulieu E-E. Contragestion and other clinical applications of RU 486, an antiprogesterone at the receptor. *Science.* 1989;245:1351–1357.
28. Beatson GT. On the treatment of inoperable cases of carcinoma of the mamma: suggestions for a new method of treatment, with illustrative cases. *Lancet.* 1896;2:104–107.
29. Bennetts HW, Underwood EJ. The oestrogenic effects of subterranean clover (*Trifolium subterraneum*). Uterine maintenance in the ovariectomized ewe on clover grazing. *Aust J Exp Biol Med Sci.* 1951;29:249–253.
30. Berg JM. DNA binding specificity of steroid receptors. *Cell.* 1989;57:1065–1068.
31. Berry M, Metzger D, Chambon P. Role of the two activating domains of the oestrogen receptor in the cell-type and promoter-context dependent agonistic activity of the anti-oestrogen 4-hydroxy tamoxifen. *EMBO J.* 1990;9:2811–2818.
32. Berthois Y, Katzenellenbogen JA, Katzenellenbogen BS. Phenol red in tissue culture media is a weak estrogen: implications concerning the study of estrogen-responsive cells in culture. *Proc Natl Acad Sci U S A.* 1986;83:2496–2500.
33. Bhakoo HS, Katzenellenbogen BS. Progesterone antagonism of estradiol-stimulated uterine "induced protein" synthesis. *Mol Cell Endocrinol.* 1977;8:105–120.
34. Bhakoo HS, Katzenellenbogen BS. Progesterone modulation of estrogen-stimulated uterine biosynthetic events and estrogen receptor levels. *Mol Cell Endocrinol.* 1977;8:121–134.
35. Biancalana V, Serville F, Pommier J, et al. Moderate instability of the trinucleotide repeat in spinobulbar atrophy. *Hum Mol Genet.* 1992;1:255–258.
36. Bickerstaff ER, Small JM, Guest IA. The relapsing cause of certain meningiomas in relation to pregnancy and menstruation. *J Neurol Neurosurg Psychiatry.* 1958;32:89–91.

37. Bickoff EM, Booth AN. Coumestrol, a new estrogen isolated from forage crops. *Science.* 1957;126:969–970.
38. Bickoff EM, Livingston AL, Hendrickson AP, Booth AN. Relative potencies of several estrogen-like compounds found in forages. *J Agric Food Chem.* 1962;10:410–412.
39. Bitman J, Cecil HC, Harris SJ, Feil VJ. Estrogenic activity of o,p'-DDT metabolites and related compounds. *J Agric Food Chem.* 1978;26:149–152.
40. Blackmore PF, Lattanzio F. Cell surface localization of a novel non-genomic progesterone receptor on the head of human sperm. *Biochem Biophys Res Commun.* 1991;181:331–336.
41. Blankenstein MA, Blaauw G, Lamberts SWJ, Mulder E. Presence of progesterone receptors and absence of oestrogen receptors in human intracranial meningioma cytosis. *Eur J Cancer Clin Oncol.* 1983;19:365–370.
42. Bo WJ, Krueger WA, Rudeen PK, Symmes SK. Ethanol-induced alterations in the morphology and function of the rat ovary. *Anat Rec.* 1982;202:255–260.
43. Booth AN, Bickoff EM, Kohler GO. Estrogen-like activity in vegetable oils and mill by-products. *Science.* 1960;131:1807–1808.
44. Borgna JL, Scali J. Differential inhibition of estrogen and antiestrogen binding to the estrogen receptor by diethylpyrocarbonate. *J Steroid Biochem.* 1988;31:427–436.
45. Bradbury RB, White DE. The chemistry of subterranean clover, I: isolation of formononetin and genistein. *J Chem Soc.* 1951:3447–3449.
46. Brann DW, Hendry LB, Hahesh VB. Emerging diversities in the mechanism of action of steroid hormones. *J Steroid Biochem Mol Biol.* 1995;52:113–133.
47. Brent GA, Moore DD, Larsen PR. Thyroid hormone regulation of gene expression. *Annu Rev Physiol.* 1991;53:17–35.
48. Brink M, Humbel BM, De Kloet ER, Van Driel R. The unliganded glucocorticoid receptor is localized in the nucleus, not in the cytoplasm. *Endocrinology.* 1992;130:3575–3581.
49. British Paediatric Association. Hypercalcaemia in infants and vitamin D. *Br Med J.* 1956;2:149.
50. Brown CJ, Goss SJ, Lubahn DB, et al. Androgen receptor locus on the human X-chromosome: regional localization to Xq11-12 and description of a DNA polymorphism. *Am J Hum Genet.* 1989;44:264–269.
51. Brown TR, Lubahn DB, Wilson EM, et al. Deletion of the steroid-binding domain of the human androgen receptor gene in one family with complete androgen insensitivity syndrome: evidence for further genetic heterogeneity in the syndrome. *Proc Natl Acad Sci U S A.* 1988;85:8151–8155.
52. Brown TR, Lubahn DB, Wilson EM, et al. Functional characterization of naturally occurring mutant androgen receptors from patients with complete androgen insensitivity. *Mol Endocrinol.* 1990;4:1759–1772.
53. Bulger WH, Muccitelli RM. Interactions of DDT analogs with the 8S estrogen-binding protein in rat testes. Federal Proceedings [Federation of American Societies for Experimental Biology (FASEB)]. 1978;37:423. Abstract 1119.
54. Bulger WH, Muccitelli RM, Kupfer D. Studies on the in vivo and in vitro estrogenic activities of methoxychlor and its metabolites. Role of hepatic mono-oxygenase in methoxychlor activation. *Biochem Pharmacol.* 1978;27:2417–2423.
55. Bursch W, Liehr JG, Sirbasku DA, et al. Control of cell death (apoptosis) by diethylstilbestrol in an estrogen-dependent kidney tumor. *Carcinogenesis.* 1991;12:855–860.
56. Bursch W, Oberhammer F, Schulte-Hermann R. Cell death by apoptosis and its protective role against disease. *Trends Pharmacol Sci.* 1992;13:245–251.
57. Burstein S, Hunter SA, Sedor C. Further studies on inhibition of Leydig cell testosterone production by cannabinoids. *Biochem Pharmacol.* 1980;29:2153–2154.
58. Butenandt A, Jacobi H. Über die Darstellung eines Krystallisierten pflanzlichen Tokokinins (Thelykinins) und seine Identifizierung mit dem α-Follikelhormon. *Hoppe-Seyler's Z Physiol Chem.* 1933;218:104–112.
59. Cahill DW, Bashirelahi N, Soloman LW, et al. Estrogen and progesterone receptors in meningiomas. *J Neurosurg.* 1984;60:985–993.
60. Carson-Jurica MA, Schrader WT, O'Malley BW. Steroid receptor family: structure and functions. *Endocr Rev.* 1990;11:201–220.
61. Carter MW, Matrone G, Smart Jr WG. Effect of genistin on reproduction of the mouse. *J Nutr.* 1955;55:639–645.
62. Cecava MJ, Hancock DL. Effects of anabolic steroids on nitrogen metabolism and growth of steers fed corn silage and corn-based diets supplemented with urea or combinations of soybean meal and feathermeal. *J Anim Sci.* 1994;72:515–522.

63. Chang C, Kokontis J, Liao S. Structural analysis of complementary DNA and amino acid sequences of human and rat androgen receptors. *Proc Natl Acad Sci U S A.* 1988;85:7211–7215.

64. Child KJ, Currie JP, Davis B, et al. Pharmacological properties in animals of CT1341–new steroid anesthetic agent. *Br J Anaesth.* 1971;43:2–14.

65. Chopra IJ, Tulchinsky D, Greenway F. Estrogen-androgen imbalance in hepatic cirrhosis. *Ann Intern Med.* 1973;79:198–203.

66. Chrousos, GP. Radioreceptor assay of steroids and assay of receptors. In: *Hormonal Assay Techniques* (Syllabus for the 15th Training Course, April 12–16, 1989) Weintraub, B.D.,ed. Bethesda, Md: Endocrine Society; 1989:241–276.

67. Claman HN. Corticosteroids and lymphoid cells. *N Engl J Med.* 1972;287:388–397.

68. Clark JH, Hsueh AJW, Peck EJ. Regulation of estrogen receptor replenishment by progesterone. *Ann N Y Acad Sci.* 1977;286:161–179.

69. Clark LB, Rosen RT, Hartman TG, et al. Determination of alkylphenol ethoxylates and their acetic acid derivatives in drinking water by particle beam liquid chromatography/mass spectrometry. *Int J Environ Anal Chem.* 1992;47:167–180.

70. Cobb CF, Van Thiel DH, Gavaler JS, Lester R. Effects of ethanol and acetaldehyde on the rat adrenal. *Metabolism.* 1981;30:537–543.

71. Cohen JC, Hickman R. Insulin resistance and diminished glucose tolerance in powerlifters ingesting anabolic steroids. *J Clin Endocrinol Metab.* 1987; 64:960–963.

72. Cohen JJ, Duke RC. Glucocorticoid activation of a calcium-dependent endonuclease in thymocyte nuclei leads to cell death. *J Immunol.* 1984;132:38–42.

73. Cohn WJ, Boylan JJ, Blanke RV, et al. Treatment of chlordecone (Kepone) toxicity with cholestyramine. *N Engl J Med.* 1978;298:243–248.

74. Concolino G, Guiffre R, Margiotto G, et al. Steroid receptor in CNS: estradiol (ER) and progesterone (PR) receptors in human spinal cord tumors. *J Steroid Biochem.* 1984;20:491–494.

75. Conte FA, Grumbach MM, Itoh Y, Fisher CR, Simpson ER. A syndrome of female pseudo-hermaphrodism, hypergonadotropic hypogonadism, and multicystic ovaries associated with missense mutations in the gene encoding aromatase (P_{450} arom). *J Clin Endocrinol Metab.* 1994; 78:1287–1292.

76. Cooperman MT, Davidoff F, Spark R, Pallotta J. Clinical studies of alcoholic ketoacidosis. *Diabetes.* 1974;23:433–439.

77. Copeland KC, Underwood LE, Van Wyk JJ. Marihuana smoking and pubertal arrest. *J Pediatr.* 1980;96:1079–1080.

78. Corradino RA. Diphenylhydantoin: direct inhibition of the vitamin D_3-mediated calcium absorptive mechanism in organ-cultured duodenum. *Biochem Pharmacol.* 1976;25:863–864.

79. Cottrell GA, Lambert JJ, Peters JA. Modulation of $GABA_A$ receptor activity by alphaxalone. *Br J Pharmacol.* 1987;90:491–500.

80. Council on Scientific Affairs. Medical and nonmedical uses of anabolic-androgenic steroids. *JAMA.* 1990;264:2923–2927.

81. Counts SJ, Baylink DJ, Shen FH, et al. Vitamin D intoxication in an anephric child. *Ann Intern Med.* 1975;82:196–200.

82. Creagh TM, Rubin A, Evans DJ. Hepatic tumors induced by anabolic steroids in an athlete. *J Clin Pathol.* 1988;41:441–443.

83. Cruickshank EK. Physical assesment of 30 chronic cannabis users and 30 matched controls. *Ann N Y Acad Sci.* 1976;282:162–167.

84. Culig Z, Hobisch A, Cronauer MV, et al. Mutant androgen receptor detected in an advanced-stage prostatic carcinoma is activated by adrenal androgens and progesterone. *Mol Endocrinol.* 1993;7:1541–1550.

85. Danielian PS, White R, Hoare SA, et al. Identification of residues in the estrogen receptor that confer differential sensitivity to estrogen and tamoxifen. *Mol Endocrinol.* 1993;7:232–240.

86. Danielsen M, Hinck L, Ringold GM. Two amino acids within the knuckle of the first zinc finger specify DNA response element activation by the glucocorticoid receptor. *Cell.* 1989;57:1131–1138.

87. Dawson RMC, Elliott DC, Elliott WH, Jones KM, eds. *Data for Biochemical Research.* 3rd ed. Oxford, UK: Clarendon Press; 1986.

88. DeBellis A, Quigley CA, Lane MV, et al. Complete and partial androgen insensitivity syndromes due to point mutations in the androgen receptor gene. *J Cell Biochem Suppl.* 1992;16C:34. Abstract L307.

89. de Lignières B, Vincens M, Mauvais-Jarvis P, et al. Prevention of menstrual migraine by percutaneous oestradiol. *Br Med J.* 1986;293:1540.

90. Dennerstein L, Morse C, Burrows G, et al. Menstrual migraine: a double-blind trial of percutaneous estradiol. *Gynecol Endocrinol.* 1988;2:113–120.

91. DES banned again. *Nature.* 1973;243:6. Short Notes.
92. Dieken ES, Miesfeld RL. Transcriptional transactivation functions localized to the glucocorticoid receptor N terminus are necessary for steroid induction of lymphocyte apoptosis. *Mol Cell Biol.* 1992;12:589–597.
93. Distelhorst CW, Miesfeld R. Characterization of glucocorticoid receptor and glucocorticoid receptor mRNA in human leukemia cells: stabilization of the receptor by diisopropylfluorophosphate. *Blood.* 1987;69:750–756.
94. Donnell BA, Meyer GA, Donegan WL. Estrogen-receptor protein in intracranial meningiomas. *J Neurosurg* . 1979;50:499–502.
95. Duax WL, Griffin JF. Structure-activity relationships of estrogenic chemicals. In: McLachlan JA, ed. *Estrogens in the Environment. II. Influences on Development.* Amsterdam, The Netherlands: Elsevier; 1985:15–23.
96. Dunn CW. Stilbestrol-induced gynecomastia in the male. *JAMA.* 1940;115:2263–2264.
97. Edis AJ, Levit M. Anabolic steroids and colonic cancer. *Med J Aust.* 1985;142:426–427.
98. Epstein MT, Hockaday JM, Hockaday TDR. Migraine and reproductive hormones throughout the menstrual cycle. *Lancet* 1975;1:543–548.
99. Eroschenko VP. Ultrastructural changes in the cells of magnum and shell gland of Japanese quail oviduct after treatment with estradiol 17β and estrogenic insecticide Kepone. *Anatomical Record.* 1979;193:532.
100. Evans RM. The steroid and thyroid hormone receptor superfamily. *Science.* 1988;40:889–895.
101. Faber PW, Kuiper GGJM, van Rooij HCJ, van der Korput HAGM, Brinkman AO, Trapman J. The N-terminal domain of the human androgen receptor is encoded by one large exon. *Mol Cell Endocrinol.* 1989;61:257–262.
102. Fawell S, White R, Hoare S, et al. Inhibition of estrogen receptor-DNA binding by the "pure" antiestrogen ICI 164,384 appears to be mediated by impaired receptor dimerization. *Proc Natl Acad Sci U S A.* 1990;87:6883–6887.
103. Ferrando R, Guilleux MM, Guerillott-Vinet A. Oestrogen content of plants as a function of conditions of culture. *Nature.* 1961;192:1205.
104. Ficher M, Levitt DR. Testicular dysfunction and sexual impotence in the alcoholic rat. *J Steroid Biochem.* 1980;13:1089–1095.
105. Finkler RS. Toxic effects of estrogens. *JAMA.* 1949;141:738.
106. Fischbeck KH, Ionasescu V, Ritter AW, et al. Localization of the gene for X-linked spinal muscular atrophy. *Neurology.* 1986;36:1595–1598.
107. Flomenbaum NE. Rodenticides. In: LR Goldfrank, RS Weisman, NE Flomenbaum, MA Howland, eds. *Toxicologic Emergencies.* Norwalk, Conn: Appleton & Lange; 1994:1127–1139.
108. Fu Y-H, Kuhl DPA, Pizzuti A, et al. Variation of the CGG repeat at the fragile X site results in genetic instability: resolution of the Sherman paradox. *Cell.* 1991;67:1047–1058.
109. Fuqua SA. Estrogen receptor mutagenesis and hormone resistance. *Cancer.* 1994;74:1026–1029.
110. Furr BJA, Jordan VC. The pharmacology and clinical uses of tamoxifen. *Pharmacol Ther.* 1984;25:127–205.
111. Fuxe K, Wikström A-C, Okret S, et al. Mapping of glucocorticoid receptor immunoreactive neurons in the rat tel- and diencephalon using a monoclonal antibody against rat liver glucocorticoid receptor. *Endocrinology.* 1985;117:1803–1812.
112. Gascon-Barrè M. Interrelationships between vitamin D₃ and 25-hydroxy-vitamin D₃ during chronic ethanol administration in the rat. *Metabolism.* 1982;31:67–72.
113. Gee KW, Bolger MB, Brinton RE, et al. Steroid modulation of the chloride ionophore of rat brain: structure-activity requirements, regional dependence and mechanism of action. *J Pharmacol Exp Ther.* 1988;246:803–812.
114. Gellert RJ. Kepone, mirex, dieldrin, and aldrin: estrogenic activity and the induction of persistent vaginal estrus and anovulation in rats following neonatal treatment. *Environ Res.* 1978;16:131–138.
115. Giroud CJP, Stachonko J, Venning EH. Secretion of aldosterone by the zona glomerulosa of rat adrenal glands incubated in vitro. *Proc Soc Exp Biol.* 1956;92:154–158.
116. Gispert S, Twells R, Orozco G, et al. Chromosome assignment of the second locus for autosomal dominant cerebellar ataxia (SCA2) to chromosome 12q23-24.1. *Nature Genet.* 1993;4:295–299.
117. Glass CK, Holloway JM. Regulation of gene expression by the thyroid hormone receptor. *Biochim Biophys Acta.* 1990;1032:157–176.
118. Glick RP, Molteni A, Fors EM. Hormone binding in brain tumours. *Neurosurgery.* 1983;13:513–519.
119. Gluud C, Wantzin P, Eriksen J, the Copenhagen Study Group for Liver Diseases. No effect of oral testosterone on sexual dysfunction in alcoholic cirrhotic men. *Gastroenterology.* 1988;95:1582–1587.

120. Goldberg Y, Glineur C, Bosselut R, Ghysdael J. Thyroid hormone action and the *erb*A oncogene family. *Biochimie.* 1989;71:279–291.

121. Goldzieher MA, Goldzieher JW. Toxic effects of percutaneously absorbed estrogens. *JAMA.* 1949;140:1156.

122. Gordon GG, Altman K, Southren AL, et al. Effect of alcohol (ethanol) administration on sex-hormone metabolism in normal men. *N Engl J Med.* 1976;295:793–797.

123. Gordon GG, Olivo J, Rafi F, Southren AL. Conversion of androgens to estrogens in cirrhosis of the liver. *J Clin Endocrinol Metab.* 1975;40:1018–1026.

124. Gordon GG, Southren AL, Lieber CS. The effects of alcoholic liver disease and alcohol ingestion on sex hormone levels. *Alcohol Clin Exp Res.* 1978;2:259–263.

125. Gordon SG, Cross BA. A factor X-activating cysteine protease from malignant tissue. *J Clin Invest.* 1981;67:1665–1671.

126. Gorski J, Malayer JR, Gregg DW, Lundeen SG. Just where are the steroid receptors anyway? *Endocr J.* 1994;2:99–100.

127. Gosselin RE, Hodge HC, Smith RP, Gleason MN, eds. *Clinical Toxicology of Commerical Products.* Baltimore, Md: Williams & Wilkins; 1976:174.

128. Green H. Human genetic diseases due to codon reiteration: relationship to an evolutionary mechanism. *Cell.* 1993;74:955–956.

129. Green S, Chambon P. Oestradiol induction of a glucocorticoid-responsive gene by a chimaeric receptor. *Nature.* 1987;325:75–78.

130. Green S, Kumar V, Theulaz I, et al. The N-terminal DNA-binding "zinc finger" of the oestrogen and glucocorticoid receptors determines target gene specificity. *EMBO J.* 1988;7:3037–3044.

131. Green S, Walter P, Kumar V, et al. Human oestrogen receptor cDNA: sequence, expression, and homology to v-*erb*-A. *Nature.* 1986;320:134–139.

132. Griffin JE. Androgen resistance–the clinical and molecular spectrum. *N Engl J Med.* 1992;326:611–618.

133. Grunberg S. Role of antiprogestational therapy for meningiomas. *Hum Reprod.* 1994;9(suppl 1):202–207.

134. Grunberg SM, Weiss MH, Spitz IM, et al. Treatment of unresectable meningiomas with the antiprogesterone agent mifepristone. *J Neurosurg.* 1991;74:861–866.

135. Guaza C, Borrell J. Effect of ethanol on corticosterone production by dispersed adrenal cells of the rat. *Life Sci.* 1984;35:1191–1196.

136. Guiochon-Mantel A, Loosfelt H, Ragot T, et al. Receptors bound to antiprogestin form abortive complexes with hormone responsive elements. *Nature.* 1988;336:695–698.

137. Guyton AC. *Textbook of Medical Physiology.* Philadelphia, Pa: WB Saunders; 1986:876–996.

138. Gyermek L, Iriarte J, Crabbé P. Strucutre-activity relationship of some steroidal hypnotic agents. *J Med Chem.* 1968;11:117–125.

139. Haak HR, deKeizer RJW, Hagenouw-Taal JCW, et al. Successful mifepristone treatment of recurrent inoperable meningioma. *Lancet.* 1990;336:124–125.

140. Haddad JG. Vitamin D: solar rays, the milky way, or both? *N Engl J Med.* 1992;326:1213–1215.

141. Hahn TJ, Avioli LV. Anticonvulsant osteomalacia. *Arch Intern Med.* 1975;135:997–1000.

142. Hahn TJ, Hendin BA, Scharp CR, Haddad JG. Effect of chronic anticonvulsant therapy on serum 25-hydroxycalciferol levels in adults. *N Engl J Med.* 1972;287:900–904.

143. Haines JL, Schut LJ, Weitkamp LR, et al. Spinocerebellar ataxia in a large kindred: age at onset, reproduction, and genetic linkage studies. *Neurology.* 1984;34:1542–1548.

144. Handa RJ, Roselli CE, Horton L, Resko JA. The quantitative distribution of cytosolic androgen receptors in micro-dissected areas of the male rat brain: effects of estrogen treatment. *Endocrinology.* 1987;121:233–240.

145. Harper MJK, Walpole AL. A new derivative of triphenylethylene: effect on implantation and mode of action in rats. *J Reprod Fertil.* 1967;13:101–119.

146. Harrison HC, Harrison HE. Inhibition of vitamin D-stimulated active transport of calcium of rat intestine by diphenylhydantoin-phenobarbital treatment. *Proc Soc Exp Biol Med.* 1976;153:220–224.

147. Harrison NL, Simmonds MA. Modulation of the GABA receptor complex by a steroid anesthetic. *Brain Res.* 1984;323:287–292.

148. Haussler MR. Vitamin D receptors: nature and function. *Annu Rev Nutr.* 1986;6:527–562.

149. Haussler MR, McCain TA. Basic and clinical concepts related to vitamin D metabolism and action, I and II. *N Engl J Med.* 1977;297:974–978, 1041–1050.

150. Headache Classification Committee of the International Heacache Society. Classification and diagnostic criteria for headache disorders, cranial neuralgias, and facial pain. *Cephalalgia.* 1988;8(suppl 7):1–96.

151. Heard RDH, Jellinck PH, O'Donnell VJ. Biogenesis of the estrogens: the conversion of testosterone-4-C^{-14} to estrone in the pregnant mare. *Endocrinology.* 1955;57:200–204.

152. Hembree III WC, Nahas GG, Zeidenberg P, Huang HFS. Changes in human spermatozoa associated with high dose marihuana smoking. In: Nahas GG, Paton WDM, eds. *Marihuana: Biological Effects.* Oxford, UK: Pergamon Press; 1979:429–439.

153. Henderson GI, Hoyumpa Jr AM, McClain C, Schenker S. The effects of chronic and acute alcohol administration on fetal development in the rat. *Alcohol Clin Exp Res.* 1979;3:99–106.

154. Herbst AL, Ulfelder H, Poskanzer DC. Adenocarcinoma of the vagina: association of maternal stilbestrol therapy with tumor appearance in young women. *N Engl J Med.* 1971;284:878–881.

155. Herrmann W, Wyss R, Riondel A, et al. The effects of an antiprogesterone steroid in women: interruption of the menstrual cycle and of early pregnancy. *C R Acad Sci Paris.* 1982;294:933–938.

156. Hertz R. Accidental ingestion of estrogens by children. *Pediatrics.* 1958;21:203–206.

157. Hewison M, Rut AR, Kristjansson K, et al. Tissue resistance to 1,25-dihydroxyvitamin D without a mutation of the vitamin D receptor gene. *Clin Endocrinol.* 1993;39:663–670.

158. Heydenreich G. Testosterone and anabolic steroids and acne fulminans. *Arch Dermatol.* 1989;125:571–572.

159. Hinton D, Mobbs EG, Sima AA, Hanna W. Steroid receptors in meningiomas. A histochemical and biochemical study. *Acta Neuropathol (Berl).* 1983;62:134–140.

160. Hirst MA, Hochman HI, Feldman D. Vitamin D resistance and alopecia: a kindred with normal 1,25-dihydroxyvitamin D binding, but decreased receptor affinity for deoxyribonucleic acid. *J Clin Endocrinol Metab.* 1985;60:490–495.

161. Hoffman B, Evers P. Anabolic agents with sex hormone-like activities: problems of residues. In: Rico AG, ed. *Drug Residues in Animals.* New York, NY: Academic Press; 1986:111–146.

162. Hollenberg SM, Weinberger C, Ong ES, et al. Primary structure and expression of a functional human glucocorticoid receptor cDNA. *Nature.* 1985;318:635–641.

163. Hollister LE. Steroids and moods: correlations in schizophrenics and subjects treated with lysergic acid diethylamide (LSD), mescaline, tetrahydrocannibinol, and synhexyl. *J Clin Pharmacol New Drugs.* 1969;9:24–29.

164. Hollister LE, Moore F, Kanter S, Noble E. Δ^1-Tetrahydrocannibinol, synhexyl, and marijuana extract administered orally in man: catecholamine excretion, plasma cortisol levels and platelet serotonin content. *Psychopharmacologia.* 1970;17:354–360.

165. Horwitz KB, Alexander PS. In situ photolinked nuclear progesterone receptors of human breast cancer cells: subunit molecular weights after transformation and translocation. *Endocrinology.* 1983;113:2195–2201.

166. Howard JE, Meyer RJ. Intoxication with vitamin D. *J Clin Endocrinol Metab.* 1948;8:895–910.

167. Hughes MR, Malloy PJ, Kieback DG, et al. Point mutations in the human vitamin D receptor gene associated with hypocalcemic rickets. *Science.* 1988;242:1702–1705.

168. Hughes MR, McCain TA, Chang SY, et al. Presence of 1,25-dihydroxyvitamin D3-glycoside in the calcinogenic plant *Cestrum diurnum. Nature.* 1977;268:347–349.

169. Huntington's Disease Collaborative Research Group. A novel gene containing a trinucleotide repeat that is expanded and unstable on Huntington's disease chromosomes. *Cell.* 1993;72:971–983.

170. Hurley DM, Accili D, Stratakis CA, et al. Point mutation causing a single amino acid substitution in the hormone binding domain of the glucocorticoid receptor in familial glucocorticoid resistance. *J Clin Invest.* 1991;87:680–686.

171. Irwin RP, Lin S-Z, Rogawski MA, et al. Steroid potentiation and inhibition of N-methyl-D-aspartate receptor-mediated intracellular Ca^{++} responses: structure-activity studies. *J Pharmacol Exp Ther.* 1994;271:677–682.

172. Irwin RP, Maragakis NJ, Rogawski MA, et al. Pregnenolone sulfate augments NMDA receptor mediated increases in intracellular Ca^{2+} in cultured rat hippocampal neurons. *Neurosci Lett.* 1992;141:30–34.

173. Ito Y, Fisher CR, Conte FA, Grumbach MM, Simpson ER. Molecular basis of aromatase deficiency in an adult female with sexual infantilism and polycystic ovaries. *Proc Natl Acad Sci U S A.* 1993;90:11673–11677.

174. Iwata M, Hanaoka S, Sato K. Rescue of thymocytes and T cell hybridomas from glucocorticoid-induced apoptosis by stimulation via the T cell receptor/CD3 complex: a possible in vitro model for positive selection of the T cell repertoire. *Eur J Immunol.* 1991;21:643–648.

175. Jacobus CH, Holick MF, Shao Q, et al. Hypervitaminosis D associated with drinking milk. *N Engl J Med.* 1992;326:1173–1177.

176. Jenkins JS, Conolly J. Adrenocorticol response to ethanol in man. *Br J Med.* 1968;2:804–805.
177. Jenkins MV, Harris M, Wills MR. The effect of phenytoin on parathyroid extract and 25-hydroxyc-holecalciferol-induced bone resorption: adenosine 3',5' cyclic monophosphate production. *Calcif Tiss Res.* 1974;16:163–167.
178. Jensen EV, Suzuki T, Kawashima T, et al. A two-step mechanism for the interaction of estradiol with rat uterus. *Proc Natl Acad Sci U S A.* 1968;59:632–638.
179. Jibani M, Hodges NH. Prolonged hypercalcaemia after industrial exposure to vitamin D_3. *Br Med J.* 1985;290:748–749.
180. Jick H, Porter J, Morrison AS. Relation between smoking and age at menopause. *Lancet.* 1977;1:1354–1355.
181. Joab I, Radanyi C, Renoir M, et al. Common non-hormone binding component in non-transformed chick oviduct receptors of four steroid hormones. *Nature.* 1984;308:850–853.
182. Johansson H, Terenius L, Thorén L. The binding of estradiol-17β to human breast cancers and other tissues in vitro. *Cancer Res.* 1970;30:692–698.
183. Jordan VC. Biochemical pharmacology of antiestrogen action. *Pharmacol Rev.* 1984;36:245–276.
184. Jull JW. Endocrine aspects of carcinogenesis. In: Searle CE, ed. Chemical Carcinogens. Washington, DC: American Chemical Society; 1976:52–82. American Chemical Society Monograph 173.
185. Jung-Testas I, Baulieu E-E. Inhibition of glucocorticosteroid action in cultured L-929 mouse fibroblasts by RU 486, a new anti-glucocorticosteroid of high affinity for the glucocorticoid receptor. *Exp Cell Res.* 1983;147:177–182.
186. Kaiser N, Edelman IS. Calcium dependence of glucocorticoid-induced lymphocytolysis. *Proc Natl Acad Sci U S A.* 1977;74:638–642.
187. Kalant H, Hawkins RD, Czaja C. Effect of acute alcohol intoxication on steroid output of rat adrenals in vitro. *Am J Physiol.* 1963;204:849–855.
188. Kapoor IB, Metcalf RL, Nystrom RF, Sangha GK. Comparative metabolism of methoxychlor, methiochlor, and DDT in mouse, insects, and in a model ecosystem. *J Agric Food Chem.* 1970;18:1145–1152.
189. Karl M, Lamberts SWJ, Detera-Wadleigh SD, et al. Familial glucocorticoid resistance caused by a splice site deletion in the human glucocorticoid receptor gene. *J Clin Endocrinol Metab.* 1993;76:683–689.
190. Kastner P, Krust A, Turcotte B, et al. Two distinct estrogen-regulated promoters generate transcripts encoding the two functionally different human progesterone receptors forms A and B. *EMBO J.* 1990;9:1603–1614.
191. Kaufman DW, Slone D, Rosenberg L, et al. Cigarette smoking and age at menopause. *Am J Public Health.* 1980;70:420–422.
192. Kawaguchi Y, Okamoto T, Taniwaka M, et al. CAG expansions in a novel gene for Machado-Joseph disease at chromosome 14q32.1. *Nature Genet.* 1994;8:221–228.
193. Kelce WR, Ganjam VK, Rudeen PK. Effects of fetal alcohol exposure on brain 5 α-reductase/aromatase activity. *J Steroid Biochem.* 1990;35:103–106.
194. Keller DW, Wiest WG, Askin FB, et al. Psuedocorpus luteum insuffiency: a local defect of progesterone action on endometrial stroma. *J Clin Endocrinol Metab.* 1979;48:127–132.
195. Kennedy MC. Anabolic steroid abuse and toxicology. *Aust N Z J Med.* 1992;22:374–381.
196. Kennedy WR, Alter M, Sung JH. Progressive proximal spinal and bulbar muscular atrophy of late onset: a sex-linked recessive trait. *Neurology.* 1968;18:671–680.
197. Kerr JFR, Wyllie AH, Currie AR. Apoptosis: a basic biological phenomenon with wide-ranging implications in tissue kinetics. *Br J Cancer.* 1972;26:239–257.
198. King WJ, Greene GL. Monoclonal antibodies localize oestrogen receptor in the nuclei of target cells. *Nature.* 1984;307:745–747.
199. Kirkland JL, Murthy L, Stancel GM. Progesterone inhibits the estrogen-induced expression of c-*fos* messenger ribonucleic acid in the uterus. *Endocrinology.* 1992;130:3223–3230.
200. Klein-Hitpass L, Cato ACB, Henderson D, Ryffel GU. Two types of antiprogestins identified by their differential action in transcriptionally active extracts from T47D cells. *Nucleic Acids Res.* 1991;19:1227–1234.
201. Knight SJL, Flannery AV, Hirst MC, et al. Trinucleotide repeat amplification and hypermethylation of a CpG island in FRAXE mental retardation. *Cell.* 1993;74:127–134.
202. Kochakian CD. Definition of androgens and protein anabolic steroids. *Pharmacol Ther.* 1975;1:149–177.
203. Koffman B, Modarress KJ, Bashirelahi N. The effects of various serine protease inhibitors on estrogen receptor steroid binding. *J Steroid Biochem Mol Biol.* 1991;38:569–574.

204. Koffman B, Modarress KJ, Beckerman T, Bashirelahi N. Evidence for involvement of tyrosine in estradiol binding by rat uterus estrogen receptor. *J Steroid Biochem Mol Biol.* 1991;38:135–139.

205. Koide R, Ikeuchi T, Onodera O, et al. Unstable expansion of CAG repeat in hereditary dentatorubral pallidoluysian atrophy (DRPLA). *Nature Genet.* 1994;6:9–13.

206. Koike S, Sakai M, Muramatsu M. Molecular cloning and characterization of rat estrogen receptor cDNA. *Nucleic Acids Res.* 1987;15:2499–2513.

207. Kokate TG, Svensson BE, Rogawski MA. Anticonvulsant activity of neurosteroids: correlation with γ-aminobutyric acid-evoked chloride current potentiation. *J Pharmacol Exp Ther.* 1994;270: 1223–1229.

208. Kolodny RC, Lessin P, Toro G, et al. Depression of plasma testosterone with acute marihuana administration. In: Braude MC, Szara S, eds. *Pharmacology of Marihuana.* New York, NY: Raven Press; 1976:217–227.

209. Kolodny RC, Masters WH, Kolodner RM, Toro G. Depression of testosterone levels after chronic intensive marihuana use. *N Engl J Med.* 1974;290:872–874.

210. Komesaroff PA, Funder JW, Fuller PJ. Mineralocorticoid resistance. *Ballière's Clin Endocrinol Metab.* 1994;8:333–355.

211. Koper JW, Lamberts SWJ. Meningiomas, epidermal growth factor and progesterone. *Hum Reprod.* 1994;9(suppl 1):190–194.

212. Korsten MA, Lieber CS. Alcoholism: social and medical concerns. In: TN Palmer, ed. *The Molecular Pathology of Alcoholism.* New York, NY: Oxford University Press; 1991:1–59.

213. Kost SL, Smith DF, Sullivan WP, Welch WJ, Toft DO. Binding of heat shock proteins to the avian progesterone receptor. *Mol Cell Biol.* 1989;9:3829–3838.

214. Krishnan AV, Stathis P, Permuth SF, et al. Bisphenol-A: an estrogenic substance is released from polycarbonate flasks during autoclaving. *Endocrinology.* 1993;132:2279–2286.

215. Krust A, Green S, Argos P, et al. The chicken oestrogen receptor sequence: homology with v-*erb*A and the human oestrogen and glucocorticoid receptors. *EMBO J.* 1986;5:891–897.

216. Kuiper GGJM, Faber PW, van Rooij HCJ, et al. Structural organization of the human androgen receptor gene. *J Mol Endocrinol.* 1989;2:R1–R4.

217. Kumar V, Chambon P. The estrogen receptor binds tightly to its responsive element as a ligand-induced homodimer. *Cell.* 1988;55:145–156.

218. Kupfer D, Bulger W. Interaction of o,p'-DDT with the estrogen-binding protein (EBP) in human mammary and uterine tumors. *Res Commun Chem Pathol Pharmacol.* 1977;16:451–462.

219. Kupfer D, Bulger WH. Estrogenic actions of chlorinated hydrocarbons. In: Chambers JE, Yarbrough JD, eds. *Effects of Chronic Exposures to Pesticides on Animal Systems.* New York, NY: Raven Press; 1982:121–146.

220. Kyprianou N, English HF, Isaacs JT. Programmed cell death during regression of PC-82 human prostate cancer following androgen ablation. *Cancer Res.* 1990;50:3748–3753.

221. Kyprianou N, English HF, Davidson NE, Isaacs JT. Programmed cell death during regression of the MCF-7 human breast cancer following estrogen ablation. *Cancer Res.* 1991;51:162–166.

222. Labov JB. Phytoestrogens and mammalian reproduction. *Comp Biochem Physiol.* 1977;57A:3–9.

223. LaFond RE, Kennedy SW, Harrison RW, Villee CA. Immunocytochemical localization of glucocorticoid receptors in cells, cytoplasts, and nucleoplasts. *Exp Cell Res.* 1988;175:52–62.

224. Lamberts SWJ, Koper JW, de Jong FH. Familial and iatrogenic cortisol receptor resistance. *J Steroid Biochem Mol Biol.* 1992;43:385–388.

225. Lamberts SWJ, Poldermans D, Zweens M, de Jong F. Familial cortisol resistance: differential diagnostic and therapeutic aspects. *J Clin Endocrinol Metab.* 1986;63:1328–1333.

226. Lamberts SWJ, Tanghe HLJ, Avezaat CJJ, et al. Mifepristone (RU486) treatment of meningiomas. *J Neurol Neurosurg Psychiatry.* 1992;55:486–490.

227. Landers JP, Spelsberg TC. New concepts in steroid hormone action: transcription factors, proto-oncogenes, and the cascade model for steroid regulation of gene expression. *Crit Rev Eukaryot Gene Expr.* 1992;2:19–63.

228. Landgren S, Backström T, Kalistratov G. The effect of progesterone on the spontaneous interictal spike evoked by topical application of penicillin to the cat's cerebral cortex. *J Neurol Sci.* 1978;36:119–133.

229. LaSpada A, Wilson E, Lubahn D, Harding A, Fischbeck K. Androgen receptor gene mutations in X-linked spinal and bulbar muscular atrophy. *Nature.* 1991;352:77–79.

230. Laudet V, Hanni C, Coll J, et al. Evolution of the nuclear receptor gene superfamily. *J Cell Biochem Suppl.* 1992;16C:36. Abstract L317.

231. Laudet V, Hanni C, Coll J, et al. Evolution of the nuclear receptor gene superfamily. *EMBO J.* 1992;11:1003–1013.

232. Laue L, Kenigsberg D, Pescovitz OH, et al. The treatment of familial male precocious puberty with spironolactone and testolactone. *N Engl J Med.* 1989;320:496–502.

233. Laws SC, Carey SA, Hart DW, Cooper RL. Lindane does not alter the estrogen receptor or the estrogen-dependent induction of progesterone receptors in sexually immature or ovariectomized adult rats. *Toxicology.* 1994;92:127–142.

234. LeClercq G, Heuson JC, Schoenfeld R, et al. Estrogen receptors in human breast cancer. *Eur J Cancer.* 1973;9:665–673.

235. Lester R, Van Thiel DH. Gonadal function in chronic alcoholic men. *Adv Exp Med Biol.* 1977;85:399–413.

236. Liberman UA, Eil C, Marx SJ. Resistance to 1,25-dihydroxy vitamin D. Association with heterogeneous defects in cultured skin fibroblasts. *J Clin Invest.* 1983;71:192–200.

237. Liener JE. Miscellaneous toxic factors. In: Liener JE, ed. *Toxic Constituents of Plant Foodstuffs.* New York, NY: Academic Press; 1980:430–467.

238. Lindemeyer RG, Robertson NM, Litwack G. Glucocorticoid receptor monoclonal antibodies define the biological action of RU 38486 in intact B16 melanoma cells. *Cancer Res.* 1990;50:7985–7991.

239. Livingston S, Berman W, Pauli LL. Anticonvulsant drugs and vitamin D metabolism. *JAMA.* 1973;224:1634–1635.

240. Loosfelt H, Alger M, Misrahi M, et al. Cloning and sequence analysis of rabbit progesterone-receptor complementary DNA. *Proc Natl Acad Sci U S A.* 1986;83:9045–9049.

241. Lubahn DB, Brown TR, Simental JA, et al. Sequence of the intron/exon junctions of the human androgen receptor gene and identification of a point mutation in a family with complete androgen insensitivity. *Proc Natl Acad Sci U S A.* 1989;86:9534–9538.

242. Lubahn DB, Joseph DR, Sar M, et al. The human androgen receptor: complementary deoxyribonucleic acid cloning sequence analysis and gene expression in prostate. *Mol Endocrinol.* 1988;2:1265–1275.

243. Lubahn DB, Joseph DR, Sullivan PM, et al. Cloning of human androgen receptor complementary DNA and localization to the X-chromosome. *Science.* 1988;240:327–330.

244. Luisi BF, Xu WX, Otwinowski Z, et al. Crystallographic analysis of the glucocorticoid receptor with DNA. *Nature.* 1991;352:497–505.

245. MacFarland HN, Ulrich CE, Holdsworth CE, et al. A chronic inhalation study with unleaded gasoline vapor. *J Am Coll Toxicol.* 1984;3:231–248.

246. MacGregor JA, Richter WR, Magaw RI. Uterine changes in female mice following lifetime inhalation of wholly vaporized unleaded gasoline: a possible relationship to observed liver tumors? *J Am Coll Toxicol.* 1993;12:119–126.

247. Maclean HE, Warne GL, French FS, et al. Identification of a deletion in the androgen receptor gene in two siblings with androgen insensitivity syndrome. *Proc Endocr Soc Aust.* 1990;33:Abstract 1.

248. Magdelénat H, Gerbault-Seureau M, Dutrillaux B. Relationship between loss of estrogen and progesterone receptor expression and of 6q and 11q chromosome arms in breast cancer. *Int J Cancer.* 1994;57:63–66.

249. Magdelénat H, Pertuiset BF, Poisson M, et al. Progestin and oestrogen receptors in meningiomas. Biochemical characterization, clinical and pathological correlations in 42 cases. *Acta Neurochir (Wien).* 1982;64:199–213.

250. Mahtre AN, Trifiro MA, Kaufman M, et al. Reduced transcriptional regulatory competence of the androgen receptor in X-linked spinal and bulbar muscular atrophy. *Nature Genet.* 1993:184–188.

251. Majewska MD, Schwartz RD. Pregnenolone-sulfate: an endogenous antagonist of the γ-aminobutyric acid recepetor complex in brain? *Brain Res.* 1987;404:355–360.

252. Majewska MD, Harrison NL, Schwartz RD, et al. Steroid hormone metabolites are barbiturate-like modulators of the GABA receptor. *Science.* 1986;232:1004–1007.

253. Malchoff DM, Brufsky A, Reardon G, et al. A mutation in primary cortisol resistance. *J Clin Invest.* 1993;91:1918–1925.

254. Malloy PJ, Hochberg Z, Pike JW, Feldman D. Abnormal binding of vitamin D receptors to deoxyribonucleic acid in a kindred with vitamin D-dependent rickets, type II. *J Clin Endocrinol Metab.* 1989;68:263–269.

255. Mangelsdorf DJ, Koeffler HP, Donaldson CA, et al. 1,25-dihydroxyvitamin D_3-induced differentiation in a human promyelocytic leukemia cell line (HL-60): receptor-mediated maturation to macrophage-like cells. *J Cell Biol.* 1984;98:391–398.

256. Marcelli M, Tilley WD, Wilson CM, et al. Definition of the human androgen receptor gene structure permits the identification of mutations that cause androgen resistance: premature termination of the receptor protein at amino acid residue 588 causes complete androgen resistance. *Mol Endocrinol.* 1990;4:1105–1116.

257. Marcelli M, Tilley WD, Wilson CM, et al. A single nucleotide substitution introduces a premature termination codon into the androgen receptor gene of a patient with receptor-negative androgen resistance. *J Clin Invest.* 1990;85:1522–1528.

258. Marcelli M, Tilley WD, Zoppi S, et al. Androgen resistance associated with a mutation of the androgen receptor at amino acid 772 (Arg -> Cys) results from a combination of decreased messenger ribonucleic acid levels and impairment of receptor function. *J Clin Endocrinol Metab.* 1991;73:318–325.

259. Marcelli M, Zoppi S, Grino PB, et al. A mutation in the DNA-binding domain of the androgen receptor gene causes complete testicular feminization in a patient with receptor-positive androgen resistance. *J Clin Invest.* 1991;87:1123–1126.

260. Markwalder T-M, Zava DT, Goldhirsch A, Markwalder RV. Estrogen and progesterone receptors in meningiomas in relation to clinical and pathological features. *Surg Neurol.* 1983;20:42–47.

261. Martuza RL, MacLaughlin DT, Ojemann RG. Specific estradiol binding in schwannomas, meningiomas and neurofibromas. *Neurosurgery.* 1981;9:665–671.

262. Martuza RL, Miller DC, MacLaughlin DT. Estrogen and progestin binding by cytosolic and nuclear fractions of human meningiomas. *J Neurosurg.* 1985;62:750–756.

263. Mason RR, Schulte GJ. Estrogen-like effects of o,p'-DDT on the progesterone receptor of rat uterine cytosol. *Res Commun Chem Pathol Pharmacol.* 1980;29:281–290.

264. Maykut M. Health consequences of acute and chronic marihuana use. *Prog Neuropsychopharmacol Biol Psychiatry.* 1984;8(suppl):59–80.

265. McClellen MC, West NB, Tacha DE, et al. Immunocytochemical localization of estrogen receptors in the macaque reproductive tract with monoclonal antiestrophilins. *Endocrinology.* 1984;114:2002–2014.

266. McConkey DJ, Nicotera P, Hartzell P, et al. Glucocorticoids activate a suicide process in thymocytes through an elevation of cytosolic Ca^{2+} concentration. *Arch Biochem Biophys.* 1989;269:365–370.

267. McDonald RA, Gelehrter TD. Glucocorticoid regulation of amino acid transport in anucleate rat hepatoma (HTC) cells. *J Cell Biol.* 1981;88:536–542.

268. McGivern RF, Roselli CE, Handa RJ. Perinatal aromatase activity in male and female rats: effect of perinatal alcohol exposure. *Alcohol Clin Exp Res.* 1988;12:769–772.

269. McPhaul MJ, Marcelli M, Tilley WD, et al. Molecular basis of androgen resistance in a family with a qualitative abnormality of the androgen receptor and responsive to high-dose androgen therapy. *J Clin Invest.* 1991;87:1413–1421.

270. McPhaul MJ, Marcelli M, Zoppi S, et al. Mutations in the ligand-binding domain of the androgen receptor gene cluster in two regions of the gene. *J Clin Invest.* 1992;90:2097–2101.

271. Meizel S, Turner KO. Progesterone acts at the plasma membrane of human sperm. *Mol Cell Endocrinol.* 1991;77:R1–R5.

272. Melez KA, Reeves JP, Steinberg AD. Regulation of the expression of autoimmunity in NZB x NZW F_1, mice by sex hormones. *J Immunopharmacol.* 1978-1979;1:27–42.

273. Mendelson JH, Mello NK. Chronic alcohol effects on anterior pituitary and ovarian hormones in healthy women. *J Pharmacol Exp Ther.* 1988;245:407–412.

274. Merry J, Marks V. Plasma-hydrocortisone response to ethanol in chronic alcoholics. *Lancet.* 1969;1:921–923.

275. Merryman W, Boiman R, Barnes L, Rothchild I. Progesterone "anesthesia" in human subjects. *J Clin Endocrinol Metab.* 1954;14:1567–1569. Letter.

276. Misrahi M, Atger M, E'auriol L, et al. Complete amino acid sequence of the human progesterone receptor deduced from cloned cDNA. *Biochem Biophys Res Commun.* 1987;143:740–748.

277. Mitchell RH, West PR. Contamination of pesticide methoxychlor with the oestrogen chlorotrianisene. *Chem Ind.* 1978; 15:581–582.

278. Moguilewsky M, Philbert D. RU 38486: potent antiglucocorticoid activity correlated with strong binding to the cytosolic glucocorticoid receptor followed by an impaired activation. *J Steroid Biochem.* 1984;20:271–276.

279. Morales DE, McGowan KA, Grant DS, et al. Estrogen promotes angiogenic activity in human umbilical vein endothelial cells in vitro and in a murine model. *Circulation.* 1995;91:755–763.

280. Moudgil VK, Hurd C. Transformation of calf uterine progesterone receptor: analysis of the process when receptor is bound to progesterone and RU 38486. *Biochemistry.* 1987;26:4993–5001.

281. Moudgil VK, Anter MJ, Hurd C. Mammalian progesterone receptor shows differential sensitivity to sulfhydryl group modifying agents when bound to agonist and antagonist ligands. *J Biol Chem.* 1989;264:2203–2211.

282. Mowszowicz I, Bieber DE, Chung KW, Bullock LP, Bardin CW. Synandrogenic and antiandrogenic effect of progestins: comparison with nonprogestational antiandrogens. *Endocrinology.*

1974;95:1589–1599.

283. Naftolin F, MacLusky NJ, Leranth CZ, et al. The cellular effects of estrogens on neuroendocrine tissues. *J Steroid Biochem.* 1988;30:195–207.

284. Nagafuchi S, Yanagisawa H, Sato K, et al. Dentatorubral and pallidoluysian atrophy expansion of an unstable CAG trinucleotide on chromosome 12p. *Nature Genet.* 1994;6:14–18.

285. Nakao R, Haji M, Yanase T, et al. A single amino acid substitution (Met786 –> Val) in the steroid-binding domain of human androgen receptor leads to complete androgen insensitivity syndrome. *J Clin Endocrinol Metab.* 1992;74:1152–1157.

286. Nelson JA. Effects of dichlorodiphenyltrichlorethane (DDT) analogs and polychlorinated biphenyl (PCB) mixtures on 17β-[³H] estradiol binding to uterine receptor. *Biochem Pharmacol.* 1974;23:447–451.

287. Nelson JA, Struck, RF, James R. Estrogenic activities of chlorinated hydrocarbons. *J Toxicol Environ Health.* 1978;4:325–339.

288. Neumann F, Töpert M. Pharmacology of antiandrogens. *J Steroid Biochem.* 1986;25:885–895.

289. Newbold RR, Bullock BC, McLachlan JA. Müllerian remnants of male mice exposed prenatally to diethylstilbestrol. *Teratog Carcinog Mutagen.* 1987;7:377–389.

290. Norbiato G, Galli M, Righini V, Moroni M. The syndrome of acquired glucocorticoid resistance in HIV infection. *Ballières Clin Endocrinol Metab.*1994;8:777–787.

291. Noteboom WD, Gorski J. Estrogenic effect of genistein and coumestrol diacetate. *Endocrinology.* 1963;73:736–739.

292. O'Connell DL, Hulka BS, Chambless LE, et al. Cigarette smoking, alcohol consumption, and breast cancer risk. *J Natl Cancer Inst.* 1987;78:229–234.

293. Okey AB, Bondy GP. Δ⁹-Tetrahydrocannabinol and 17β-estradiol bind to different macromolecules in estrogen target tissues. *Science.* 1978;200:312–314.

294. Orr HT, Chung M-Y, Banfi S, et al. Expansion of an unstable trinucleotide CAG repeat in spinocerebellar ataxia type 1. *Nature Genet.* 1993;4:221–226.

295. Ousterhout JM, Struck RF, Nelson JA. Estrogenic properties of methoxychlor metabolites. *Fed Proc Fed Am Soc Exp Biol.* 1979;38:537. Abstract 1625.

296. Owens GP, Hahn WE, Cohen JJ. Identification of mRNAs associated with programmed cell death in immature thymocytes. *Mol Cell Biol.* 1991;11:4177–4188.

297. Papavassiliou AG. Molecular medicine: transcription factors. *N Engl J Med.* 1995; 332:45–47.

298. Patterson J, Furr B, Wakeling A, Battersby L. The biology and physiology of "Nolvadex" (tamoxifen) in the treatment of breast cancer. *Breast Cancer Res Treat.* 1982;2:363–374.

299. Paul SM, Purdy RH. Neuroactive steroids. *FASEB J.* 1992;6:2311–2322.

300. Pearn JH, Harvey P, DeAmbrosis W, et al. Ciguatera and pregnancy. *Med J Aust.* 1982;1:57–58. Letter.

301. Perel E, Lindner HR. Dissociation of uterotrophic action from implantation-inducing activity in two non-steroidal oestrogens (coumestrol and genistein). *J Reprod Fertil.* 1970;21:171–175.

302. Picard D, Yamamoto KR. Two signals mediate hormone-dependent nuclear localization of glucocorticoid receptor. *EMBO J.* 1987;6:3333–3340.

303. Piper JG, Follett KA, Fantin A. Sphenoid wing meningioma progression after placement of a subcutaneous progesterone agonist contraceptive implant. *Neurosurgery.* 1994;34:723–725.

304. Poisson M, Pertuiset BF, Hauw J-J, et al. Steroid hormone receptors in human meningiomas, gliomas and brain metastases. *J Neurooncol.* 1983;1:179–189.

305. Poland A, Glover E, Kende A. Stereospecific, high affinity binding of 2,3,7,8-tetrachlorodibenzo-*p*-dioxin by hepatic cytosol. *J Biol Chem.* 1976;251:4936–4946.

306. Powles TJ. Prevention of migrainous headaches by tamoxifen. *Lancet* 1986;2:1344.

307. Previero A, Barry L-G, Coletti-Previero M-A. Specific O-acylation of hydroxylamino acids in presence of free amino groups. *Biochim Biophys Acta.* 1972;263:7–13.

308. Purdom CE, Hardiman PA, Bye VJ, et al. Estrogenic effects of effluents from sewage treatment works. *Chem Ecol.* 1994;8:275–285.

309. Purohit V, Ahluwahlia BS, Vigersky RA. Marijuana inhibits dihydrotestosterone binding to the androgen receptor. *Endocrinology.* 1980;107:848–850.

310. Quarmby VE, Beckman WC, Wilson EM, French FS. Androgen regulation of c-*myc* messenger ribonucleic acid levels in rat ventral prostate. *Mol Endocrinol.* 1987;1:865–874.

311. Quigley CA, Evans BAJ, Simental JA, et al. Complete androgen insensitivity due to deletion of exon C of the androgen receptor gene highlights the functional importance of the second zinc finger of the androgen receptor in vivo. *Mol Endocrinol.* 1992;6:1103–1112.

312. Quigley CA, Friedman KJ, Johnson A, et al. Complete deletion of the androgen receptor gene: definition of the null phenotype of the androgen insensitivity syndrome and determination of the carri-

er status. *J Clin Endocrinol Metab.* 1992;74:927–933.

313. Ratajcazk T, Brockway MJ, Hahnel R, et al. Chemical characterization by protein sequence analysis of the bovine estrogen receptor. *Biochem Biophys Res Commun.* 1988;156:116–124.

314. Rawitch AB, Schultz GS, Ebner KE, Vardaris RM. Competition of Δ^9-tetrahydrocannabinol with estrogen in rat uterine estrogen receptor binding. *Science.* 1977;197:1189–1191.

315. Raynaud J-P, Ojasoo T. The design and use of sex-steroid antagonists. *J Steroid Biochem.* 1986;25:811–833.

316. Reese JC, Katzenellenbogen BS. Mutagenesis of cysteines in the hormone binding domain of the human estrogen receptor. *J Biol Chem.* 1991;266:10,880–10,887.

317. Reese JC, Katzenellenbogen BS. Characterization of a temperature-sensitive mutation in the hormone binding domain of the human estrogen receptor. Studies in cell extracts and intact cells and their implications for hormone-dependent transcriptional activation. *J Biol Chem.* 1992;267:9868–9873.

318. Revelli A, Modetti M, Piffaretti-Yanez A, et al. Steroid receptors in human spermatozoa. *Hum Reprod.* 1994;9:760–766.

319. Ris-Stalpers C, Kuiper GGJM, Faber PW, et al. Aberrant splicing of androgen receptor mRNA results in the synthesis of a nonfunctional receptor protein in a patient with androgen insensitivity. *Proc Natl Acad Sci U S A.* 1990;87:7866–7870.

320. Ris-Stalpers C, Trifiro MA, Kuiper GGJM, et al. Substitution of aspartic acid-686 by histidine or asparagine in the human androgen receptor leads to a functionally inactive protein with altered hormone-binding characteristics. *Mol Endocrinol.* 1991;5:1562–1569.

321. Ritchie HH, Hughes MR, Thompson ET, et al. An ochre mutation in the vitamin D receptor gene causes hereditary 1,25-dihydroxyvitamin D_3-resistant rickets in three families. *Proc Natl Acad Sci U S A.* 1989;86:9783–9787.

322. Roberts JT, Essenhigh DM. Adenocarcinoma of prostate in 40-year-old body-builder. *Lancet.* 1986;2:742.

323. Rosner W. Plasma steroid-binding proteins. In: Strauss III JF, ed. *Steroid Hormones. Endocrino Metab Clin North Am.* 1991;20:697–720.

324. Rossini GP, Malaguti C. The subcellular distribution of glucocorticoid-receptor complexes as studied by chemical crosslinking of intact HTC cells. *J Steroid Biochem Mol Biol.* 1994;48:517–521.

325. Rossini GP, Malaguti C. Nanomolar concentrations of untransformed glucocorticoid receptor in nuclei of intact cells. *J Steroid Biochem Moled Biol.* 1994;51:291–298.

326. Rusconi S, Yamamoto KR. Functional dissection of the hormone and DNA binding activities of the glucocorticoid receptor. *EMBO J.* 1987;6:1309–1315.

327. Saartok T, Dahlberg E, Gustafsson J-Å. Relative binding affinity of anabolic-androgenic steroids: comparison of the binding to the androgen receptors in skeletal muscle and in prostate, as well as to sex hormone-binding globulin. *Endocrinology.* 1984; 114:2100–2106.

328. Sabbah M, Gouilleux F, Sola B, Redeuilh G, Baulieu E-E. Structural differences between the hormone and antihormone estrogen receptor complexes bound to the hormone response element. *Proc Natl Acad Sci U S A.* 1991;88:390–394.

329. Sai TJ, Seino S, Chang CS, et al. An exonic point mutation of the androgen receptor gene in a patient with complete androgen insensitivity. *Am J Hum Genet.* 1990;46:1095–1100.

330. Sanchez ER, Faber LE, Henzel WJ, Pratt WB. The 56 kDa protein in the nontransformed fllucocorticoid receptor is a unique protein that exists in cytosol in a complex with both the 70 kDa and 90 kDa heat shock proteins. *Biochemistry.* 1990;29:5145–5152.

331. Sanchez-Bueno A, Sancho MJ, Cobbold PH. Progesterone and oestradiol increase cytosolic Ca^{2+} in single rat hepatocytes. *Biochem J.* 1991;280:273–276.

332. Sap J, Munoz A, Damm K, et al. The c-*erb*-A protein is a high-affinity receptor for thyroid hormone. *Nature.* 1986;324:635–640.

333. Sapeika N. Meat and dairy products. In: Liener IE, ed. *Food Science and Technology.* New York, NY: Academic Press; 1974:1–32.

334. Sarno Jr AP, Miller Jr EJ, Lundblad EG. Premenstrual syndrome: beneficial effects of periodic, low-dose danazol. *Obstet Gynecol.* 1987;70:33–36.

335. Saunders PTK, Padayachi T, Tincello DG, Shalet SM, Wu FCW. Point mutations detected in the androgen receptor gene of three men with partial androgen insensitivity syndrome. *Clin Endocrinol.* 1992;37:214–220.

336. Schena M, Freedman LP, Yamamoto KR. Mutations in the glucocorticoid receptor zinc finger region that distinguish interdigitated DNA binding and transcriptional enhancement activities. *Genes Dev.* 1989;3:1590–1601.

337. Schinckel PG. Infertility in ewes grazing subterranean clover pastures. Observations on breeding behavior following transfer to "sound" country. *Aust Vet J.* 1948;24:289–294.
338. Schlaghecke R, Kornely E, Wollenhaupt J, Specker C. Glucocorticoid receptors in rheumatoid arthritis. *Arthritis Rheum.* 1992;35:740–744.
339. Schnegg J-F, Gomez F, Le Marchang-Beraud T, de Tribolet N. Presence of sex steroid hormone receptors in meningioma tissue. *Surg Neurol.* 1981;15:415–418.
340. Schoenberg BS, Christine BW, Whisnant JP. Nervous system neoplasms and primary malignancies of other sites. The unique association between meningiomas and breast cancer. *Neurology.* 1975;25:705–712.
341. Schoental R. Carcinogens in plants and microorganisms. In: Searle CE, ed. *Chemical Carcinogens.* Washington, DC: American Chemical Society; 1976:626–689. Monograph 173.
342. Schoental R. Fusarial mycotoxins and cancer. In: Searle CE, ed. *Chemical Carcinogens.* 2nd ed. Washington, DC: American Chemical Society; 1984:1137–1170. American Chemical Society Monograph 182.
343. Schuchard M, Landers JP, Sandhu NP, Spelsberg TC. Steroid hormone regulation of proto-oncogenes. *Endocr Rev.* 1993;14:659–669.
344. Schwartz MR, Randolph RL, Cech DA, et al. Steroid hormone binding macromolecules in meningiomas. Failure to meet criteria of specific receptors. *Cancer.* 1984;53:922–927.
345. Scott MJ, Scott MJ. HIV infection associated with injections of anabolic steroids. *JAMA.* 1989;262:207–208.
346. Segnitz B, Gehring U. Mechanism of action of a steroidal antiglucocorticoid in lymphoid cells. *J Biol Chem.* 1990;265:2789–2796.
347. Sher ER, Leung DYM, Surs W, et al. Steroid-resistant asthma. Cellular mechanism contributing to inadequate response to glucocorticoid therapy. *J Clin Invest.* 1994;93:33–39.
348. Shiraishi H, Carter DS, Hites RA. Identification and determination of tert-alkylphenols in carp from the Trenton channel of the Detroit River, Michigan, USA. *Biomed Environ Mass Spectr.* 1989;18:478–483.
349. Shozu M, Akasofu K, Harada T, Kubota Y. A new cause of female pseudohermaphroditism: placental aromatase deficiency. *J Clin Endocrinol Metab.* 1991;72:560–566.
350. Simons S, Thompson E. Dexamethasone 21-mesylate: an affinity label of glucocorticoid receptors from rat hepatoma tissue cells. *Proc Natl Acad Sci U S A.* 1981;78:3541–3545.
351. Sklarek HM, Mantovani RP, Erens E, et al. AIDS in a body-builder using anabolic steroids. *N Engl J Med.* 1984;311:1701.
352. Skowronski RJ, Feldman D. Inhibition of aldosterone synthesis in rat adrenal cells by nicotine and related constituents of tobacco smoke. *Endocrinology.* 1994;134:2171–2177.
353. Sluyser M, ed. *Interaction of Steroid Hormone Receptors with DNA.* Chichester, UK: Ellis Horwood; 1985.
354. Smith CG, Smith MT, Besch NF, et al. Effect of Δ^9-tetrahydrocannabinol (THC) on female reproductive function. In: Nahas GG, Paton WDM, eds. *Marihuana: Biological Effects.* Oxford, UK: Pergamon Press; 1979:449–467.
355. Smith DF, Faber LE, Toft DO. Purification of unactivated progesterone receptor and identificiation of novel receptor-associated proteins. *J Biol Chem.* 1990;265:3996–4003.
356. Smith EL, Hill RL, Lehman IR, et al, eds. *Principles of Biochemistry.* New York, NY: McGraw-Hill; 1983.
357. Smith EP, Boyd J, Frank GR, et al. Estrogen resistance caused by a mutation in the estrogen-receptor gene in a man. *N Engl J Med.* 1994;331:1056–1061.
358. Smith RG, Besch NF, Besch PK, Smith CG. Inhibition of gonadotropin by Δ^9-tetrahydrocannabinol: mediation by steroid receptors? *Science.* 1979;204:325–327.
359. Somerville BW. Estrogen-withdrawal migraine, I: duration of exposure required and attempted prophylaxis by premenstrual estrogen administration. *Neurology.* 1975;25:239–244.
360. Soto AM, Justicia H, Wray JW, Sonnenschein C. p-Nonyl-phenol: an estrogenic xenobiotic released from "modified" polystyrene. *Environ Health Perspect.* 1991;92:167–173.
361. Stamp TCB, Round JM, Rowe DJF, et al. Plasma levels and therapeutic effect of 25-hydroxycholecalciferol in epileptic patients taking anticonvulsant drugs. *Br Med J.* 1972;4:9–12.
362. Standeven AM, Blazer III DG, Goldsworthy TL. Investigation of antiestrogenic properties of unleaded gasoline in female mice. *Toxicol Appl Pharmacol.* 1994;127:233–240.
363. Sullivan WP, Vroman BT, Bauer VJ, et al. Isolation of steroid receptor binding protein from chicken oviduct and production of monoclonal antibodies. *Biochemistry.* 1985;24:4214–4222.
364. Thompson CB. Apoptosis in the pathogenesis and treatment of disease. *Science.* 1995;267:1456–1462.
365. Thompson EB, Nazareth LV, Thulasi R, et al. Glucocorticoids in malignant lymphoid cells: gene reg-

ulation and the minimum receptor fragment for lysis. *J Steroid Biochem Mol Biol.* 1992;41:273–282.

366. Thompson EB, Norman MR, Lippman ME. Steroid hormone actions in tissue culture cells and cell hybrids–their relation to human malignancies. *Recent Prog Horm Res.* 1977;33:571–615.

367. Thompson PD, Cullinane EM, Sady SP, et al. Contrasting effects of testosterone and stanozolol on serum lipoprotein levels. *JAMA.* 1989;261:1165–1168.

368. Tilley WD, Marcelli M, Wilson JD, McPhaul MJ. Characterization and expression of a c-DNA encoding the human androgen receptor. *Proc Natl Acad Sci U S A.* 1989;86:327–331.

369. Tilzer LL, Plapp FV, Evans JP, et al. Steroid receptor proteins in human meningiomas. *Cancer.* 1982;49:633–636.

370. Trapman J, Klaassen P, Kuiper GGJM, et al. Cloning, structure and expression of a cDNA encoding the human androgen receptor. *Biochem Biophys Res Commun.* 1988;153:241–248.

371. Trifiro M, Prior RL, Sabbaghian N, et al. Amber mutation creates a diagnostic Mae I site in the androgen receptor gene of a family with complete androgen insensitivity. *Am J Med Genet.* 1991;40:493–499.

372. Troll W, Wiesner R, Shellabarger CJ, et al. Soybean diet lowers breast cancer incidence in irradiated rats. *Carcinogenesis.* 1980;1:469–472.

373. Tsilfidis C, MacKenzie AE, Gabrielle M, et al. Correlation between CTG trinucleotide repeat length and frequency of severe congenital myotonic dystrophy. *Nature Genet.* 1992;1:192–195.

374. Tsoukas CD, Provvedini DM, Manolagas SC. 1,25-Dihydroxyvitamin D_3: a novel immunoregulatory hormone. *Science.* 1984;224:1438–1440.

375. Van Seters AP, van Dulken H, de Keizer RJW, Vielvoye GJ. Symptomatic relief of meningioma by buserelin maintenance therapy. *Lancet.* 1989;1:564–565. Letter.

376. Van Thiel DH, Lester R. Alcoholism: its effect on hypothalamic pituitary function. *Gastroenterology.* 1976;71:318–327.

377. Van Thiel DH, Gavaler JS, Lester R. Ethanol inhibition of vitamin A metabolism in the testes: possible mechanism for sterility in alcoholics. *Science.* 1974;186:941–942.

378. Van Thiel DH, Gavaler JS, Lester R, Sherins RJ. Alcohol-induced ovarian failure in the rat. *J Clin Invest.* 1978;61:624–632.

379. Vaquero J, Marcos ML, Martinez R, Bravo G. Estrogen- and progesterone-receptor proteins in intracranial receptors. *Surg Neurol.* 1983;19:11–13.

380. Vegeto E, Shahabaz M, Wen DX, et al. Human progesterone receptor A form is a cell- and promoter-specific repressor of human progesterone receptor B function. *Mol Endocrinol.* 1993;7:1244–1255.

381. Veldscholte J, Berrevoets CA, Ris-Stalplers, et al. The androgen receptor in LNCaP cells contains a mutation in the ligand binding domain which affects steroid binding characteristics and response to antiandrogens. *J Steroid Biochem Mol Biol.* 1992;41:665–669.

382. Vito CC, Fox TO. Androgen and estrogen receptors in embryonic and neonatal rat brain. *Dev Brain Res.* 1982;2:97–110.

383. Walter PS, Green G, Greene A, et al. Cloning of the human estrogen receptor cDNA. *Proc Natl Acad Sci U S A.* 1985;82:7889–7893.

384. Warriar N, Yu C, Govindan MV. Hormone binding domain of human glucocorticoid receptor. Enhancement of transactivation function by substitution mutants M565R and A573Q. *J Biol Chem.* 1994;269:29,010–29,015.

385. Wasserman RH, Henion JD, Haussler MR, et al. Calcinogenic factor in *Solanum malacoxylon:* evidence that it is 1,25-dihydroxy-vitamin D_3-glycoside. *Science.* 1976;194:853–855.

386. Webster JC, Jewell CM, Sar M, Cidlowski JA. The glucocorticoid receptor: maybe not all steroid receptors are nuclear. *Endocr J.* 1994;2:967–969.

387. Weiler IJ, Lew D, Shapiro DJ. The *Xenopus laevis* estrogen receptor: sequence homology with human and avian receptors and identification of multiple estrogen messenger ribonucleic acids. *Mol Endocrinol.* 1987;1:355–362.

388. Weinberger C, Hollenberg SM, Rosenfeld MG, Evans RM. Domain structure of human glucocorticoid receptor and its relationship to the v-*erb*-A oncogene product. *Nature.* 1985;318:670–672.

389. Weinberger C, Thompson CC, Ong ES, et al. The c-*erb*-A gene encodes a thyroid hormone receptor. *Nature.* 1986;324:641–646.

390. Welch KMA. Drug therapy of migraine. *N Engl J Med.* 1993;329:1476–1483.

391. Welch KMA, Darnley D, Simkins RT. The role of estrogen in migraine: a review and a hypothesis. *Cephalalgia.* 1984;4:227–236.

392. Welch RM, Levin W, Conney AH. Estrogenic action of DDT and its analogs. *Toxicol Appl Pharmacol.* 1969;14:358–367.

393. Welshons WV, Krummel BM, Gorski J. Nuclear localization of unoccupied receptors for glucocorticoids, estrogens, and progesterone in GH$_1$ cells. *Endocrinology.* 1985;117:2140–2147.

394. Welshons WV, Lieberman ME, Gorski J. Nuclear localization of unoccupied estrogen receptor. *Nature.* 1984;307:747–749.

395. Wen DX, Xu Y-F, Mais DE, et al. The A and B isoforms of the human progesterone receptor operate through distinct signaling pathways within target cells. *Mol Cell Biol.* 1994;14:8356–8364.

396. White R, Jobling S, Hoare SA, et al. Environmentally persistent alkylphenolic compounds are estrogenic. *Endocrinology.* 1994;135:175–182.

397. White R, Lees JA, Needham M, et al. Structural organization and expression of the mouse estrogen receptor. *Mol Endocrinol.* 1987;1:735–744.

398. Wielckens K, Delfs T. Glucocorticoid-induced cell death and poly [adenosine diphosphate (ADP)-ribosyl]ation: increased toxicity of dexamethasone on mouse S49.1 lymphoma cells with the poly (ADP-ribosyl)ation inhibitor benzamide. *Endocrinology.* 1986;119:2383–2392.

399. Wikström A-C, Bakke O, Okret S, et al. Intracellular localization of the glucocorticoid receptor: evidence for cytoplasmic and nuclear localization. *Endocrinology.* 1987;120:1232–1242.

400. Willett W, Stampfer MJ, Bain C, et al. Cigarette smoking, relative weight, and menopause. *Am J Epidemiol.* 1983;117:651–658.

401. Wixtrom RN, Brown SL. Individual and population exposure to gasoline. *J Expo Anal Environ Epidemiol.* 1992;2:23–78.

402. Wolf DA, Kohlhuber F, Schulz P, Fittler F, Eick D. Transcriptional down-regulation of c-*myc* in human prostate carcinoma cells by synthetic androgen mibolerone. *Br J Cancer.* 1992;65:376–382.

403. Worner TM, Gordon GG, Leo MA, Lieber CS. Vitamin A treatment of sexual dysfunction in male alcoholics. *Am J Clin Nutr.* 1988;48:1431–1435.

404. Wu FS, Gibbs TT, Farb DH. Pregnenolone sulfate: a positive allosteric modulator at the *N*-methyl-D-aspartate receptor. *Mol Pharmacol.* 1991;40:333–336.

405. Wyllie AH. Glucocorticoid-induced thymocyte apoptosis is associated with endogenous endonuclease activation. *Nature.* 1980;284:555–556.

406. Wyllie AH, Kerr JFR, Currie AR. Cell death: the significance of apoptosis. *Int Rev Cytol.* 1980;68:251–300.

407. Wyllie AH, Morris RG, Smith AL, Dunlop D. Chromatin cleavage in apoptosis: association with condensed chromatin morphology and dependence on macromolecular synthesis. *J Pathol.* 1984;142:67–77.

408. Yeh J, Barbieri RL, Friedman AJ. Nicotine and cotinine inhibit rat testis androgen biosynthesis in vitro. *J Steroid Biochem.* 1989;33:627–630.

409. Ylikahri R, Huttunen M, Härkönen M, et al. Acute effects of alcohol on anterior pituitary secretion of the tropic hormones. *J Clin Endocrinol Metab.* 1978;46:715–720.

410. Yu Z-Z, Wrange O, Haglund B, et al. Estrogen and progestin receptors in intracranial meningiomas. *J Steroid Biochem.* 1982;16:451–456.

411. Zacharchuk CM, Mercép M, Chakraborti P, et al. Programmed T lymphocyte death: cell-activation and steroid-induced pathways are mutually antagonistic. *J Immunol.* 1990;145:4037–4045.

412. Zhang SJ, Jackson MB. Neuroactive steroids modulate GABA$_A$ receptors in peptidergic nerve terminals. *J Neuroendocrinol.* 1994;6:533–538.

413. Zoller U. Groundwater contamination by detergents and polycyclic aromatic hydrocarbons–a global problem of organic contaminants: is the solution locally specific? *Water Sci Technol.* 1993;27:187–194.

414. Zondek B, Bergmann E. Phenol methyl ethers as oestrogenic agents. *Biochem J.* 1938;32:641–645.

415. Zoppi S, Marcelli M, Deslypere J-P, et al. Amino acid substitutions in the DNA-binding domain of the human androgen receptor are a frequent cause of receptor-positive androgen resistance. *Mol Endocrinol.* 1992;6:409–415.

416. Zoppi S, Wilson CM, Harbison MD, et al. Complete testicular feminization caused by an amino terminal truncation of the androgen receptor with downstream initiation. *J Clin Invest.* 1993. 91:1105–1112.

Endocrine Toxicology, 2nd ed.,
Edited by J. A. Thomas and H. D. Colby
Copyright © 1997 Taylor & Francis

7

Xenoestrogens and Estrogen Receptor Action

Kenneth S. Korach, Vicki L. Davis, Sylvia W. Curtis,
and Wayne P. Bocchinfuso

*Receptor Biology Section, Laboratory of Reproductive and Developmental Toxicology,
National Institute of Environmental Health Sciences, National Institutes of Health,
Research Triangle Park, North Carolina 27709-2233*

INTRODUCTION

Estrogens are a class of steroid hormones that influence development, sexual differentiation, fertility, and control of female reproductive tract organ responsiveness (50,74). Endogenous estrogens are formed by aromatization of androgens by steroidogenic enzymes primarily in the gonads, as well as in extragonadal sites including the placenta, brain, and adipose tissue. In addition, a group of exogenous chemicals called xenoestrogens can display estrogen-like functions that influence the growth and development of female reproductive tissues. The source of xenoestrogens can be dietary in nature including phytoestrogens (eg, coumestrol, genistein), or exist as environmental pollutants (eg, o,p'-DDT, PCBs) produced as pesticides or waste from manufacturing processes. A noticeable feature of these estrogenic agents is their structural diversity (Fig. 1). Although a phenolic ring is required for estrogen-like activity, the array of chemical structures and substitutions found in many environmental compounds make prediction of estrogenic potency difficult. Estrogen elicits its biologic actions in certain tissues by interacting with the estrogen receptor, which resides within the nucleus of target cells. Thus, xenoestrogens can interact with the estrogen receptor, inducing a response that mimics endogenous estrogen stimulation. Alternatively, the receptor can bind the xenoestrogens, producing an inactive receptor–ligand complex that inhibits endogenous estrogen function. Either type of interference by xenoestrogens may result in aberrant reproductive function as a result of altered organ physiology or toxicity.

There is a strong association between estrogen exposure and breast cancer. Whether estrogens act as initiators and/or promoters of breast cancers has not been determined. Since many breast tumors, as well as nonmalignant reproductive tract diseases such as endometriosis, are hormonally responsive, environmental estrogen exposure may be an important component of their etiology (113).

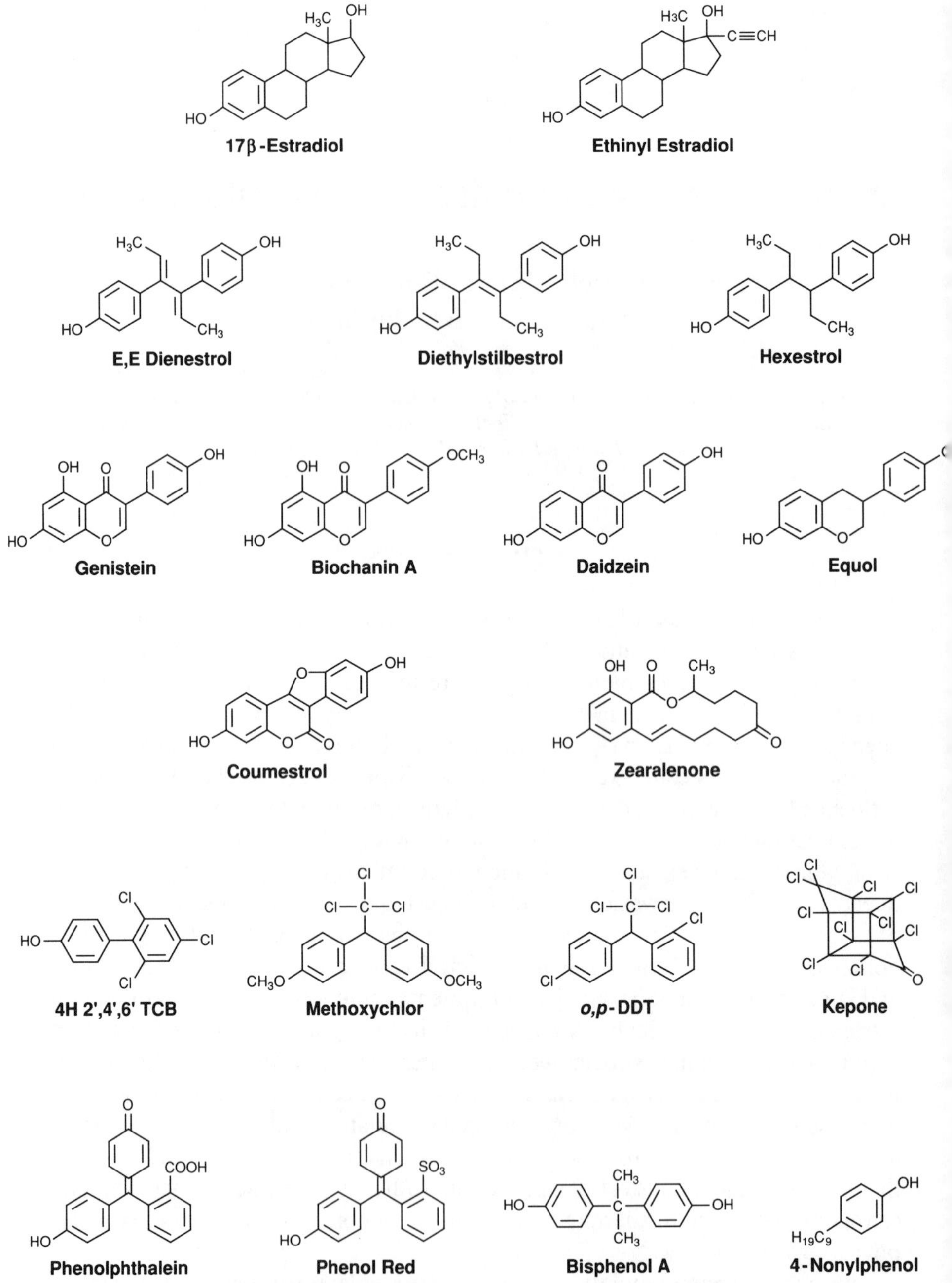

FIG. 1. Chemical structures of a variety of estrogenic compounds.

Furthermore, prenatal estrogen exposure is known to produce hypospadias and cryptorchidism in human males. Recent reports have hypothesized a link between an increase in testicular tumors and low sperm counts in humans with possible prenatal and neonatal estrogen exposure (123). Since the role(s) of estrogen in male reproductive physiology is not well understood, the effect of neonatal estrogen exposure on males is difficult to evaluate.

In addition to side effects of environmental estrogen exposure in humans, there are reported estrogenic effects on fertility and sexual development in wildlife populations (33). Most notably, wildlife exposed to the pesticide DDT exhibited hypospadias and male infertility resulting from low sperm counts, and these observations were confirmed by experimental studies of rats and mice treated with o,p'-DDT (144). Other types of alkyl substituted phenols (eg, 4-octylphenol, 4-nonylphenol), exist as nonionic surfactants present in detergents and were shown to persist in contaminated waters affecting fish populations (108). Estrogenic xenobiotics not only are found in the environment but are by-products (eg, nonylphenol, bisphenol A) of laboratory plasticware. In some cases, compounds used in the synthesis of plastics were found to alter the growth of MCF-7 breast cancer cells due to their estrogenic activity (77,129). The biological activities of these agents are weak; however, large amounts of alkylphenol polyethoxylates are introduced into the environment each year, which could result in significant estrogen exposure.

The impact of environmental estrogens on the development of human disease is not well defined. Although wildlife populations have been affected, analyses on the incidence of cancer in the exposed animal populations are lacking. Furthermore, epidemiologic studies will be required to evaluate the effects of these exposures in human populations.

The bioavailability, lipophobicity, metabolism, and pharmacokinetics of environmental compounds must be considered when evaluating their estrogenic potency. These biological properties have not been determined for many structurally different compounds, which will likely differ from steroidal estrogens. A single estrogenic agent may have minimal biological activity, but mixtures of compounds that exist in the environment may result in a synergistic effect. In fact, it has been reported that some sources of drinking water contain as many as 20 chemically related alkylphenolic compounds (30). Therefore, in addition to the chemical and pharmacologic properties of individual xenoestrogens, the biological activity of a mixture of compounds and the effect of persistent exposure require further study.

This chapter provides a general review of the biochemical and molecular mechanism of estrogen action within target cells. In addition, suspected xenoestrogens are discussed with respect to their activities and structures.

CHEMISTRY, STRUCTURE, METABOLISM

Estrogens are steroid hormones that contain the cyclopentanoperhydrophenanthrene chemical ring structure. They differ from other classes of steroid hormones in that the estrane steroid nucleus contains a phenolic A ring rather than the nonaromatic cyclohexane ring that is part of the androgen or progestin steroid nucleus. The presence of the phenolic ring imparts unique chemical properties to estrogens. In fact, both the phenolic ring and the C17 hydroxyl group are required for biological activity, which is mediated by binding to the estrogen receptor (discussed in a later section).

The biological activity of estrogens is determined by assessing the ability of the hormone to stimulate or increase the weight of the rodent uterus. Other assays evaluated the ability of estrogens to induce vaginal cornification or estrus in rats or mice, which provided the basis for the name *estrogen*. Of the endogenous estrogens, 17β-estradiol has the greatest biological activity, which is reduced approximately 10-fold when metabolized to estrone. Liver metabolism of estrogen involves sulfation or glucuronidation of the phenolic A ring hydroxyl group, thereby imparting increased solubility for excretion in the urine. In addition, these metabolites of estrogen do not bind the estrogen receptor and, therefore, cannot generate an estrogen response. Catechol estrogens are formed in certain tissues, notably the brain, liver, and placenta, and it is hypothesized that specific cell populations generate these metabolites, which exhibit autocrine/paracrine function (143). Most biologically active estrogens have similar effects on the major target tissues in different species. However, synthetic estrogen compounds are being identified that elicit tissue-specific effects, such as bone-specific agonists with minimal side effects in the uterus. Therefore, such compounds could be used to treat a tissue or organ directly without generating a toxic effect on other estrogen-responsive tissues in the body.

Pharmacologic techniques have been used to alter the biological activity of a number of compounds. The potency of estradiol has been enhanced by introducing chemical derivatives such as pentyl or benzoyl groups via an ester linkage to the C17 hydroxy, which alters the pharmacokinetics of the estrogen. Therefore, by reducing the metabolic clearance rate of estrogenic compounds, their biological effects may persist in the body.

The phenolic ring structure is unique to estrogens; therefore, a number of synthetic compounds with phenolic rings have been found to mimic estrogens. These include stilbene estrogens such as diethylstilbestrol (DES), hexestrol, and E,E-dienestrol (99). Similarities to steroidal estrogens arise from a composite diphenolic ring structure as shown in Fig. 1, and the biological potencies vary between different isomeric forms of the same compounds. For instance, E,E-dienestrol is an active estrogen while the Z,Z-dienestrol isomer is relatively inactive (73), even though Z,Z-dienestrol has been shown to be highly toxic in some tests. The stilbene ring structure of DES is also found in several triphenylethylene compounds, which possess antiestrogenic activity (66). Metabolism of DES, a highly potent synthetic estrogen, involves conjugation as well as oxidation (99), which has been purported to create reactive intermediates that may be responsible for the toxic and carcinogenic properties of this compound (98).

Most of the synthetic compounds described above as well as natural compounds, including the phytoestrogens (genistein, coumestrol, biochanin A) or mycotoxins (zearalenone and a synthetic derivitive, zearalanol), contain various phenolic ring substitutions. Most phytoestrogens are isoflavanoids or coumestans, and their biological activities vary depending on their chemical stability and interaction with the estrogen receptor (90). Two of the resorcylic acids, zearalanol and zearalenone, have potent estrogenic activity, and they differ by containing either a ketone or an aliphatic hydroxyl attached to the phenolic ring. It is likely that the oxygen moiety on the carbon backbone influences the biological activity and receptor-binding affinity. In the case of zearalanol, estrogen receptor binding is higher than in other environmental compounds (43).

Chlorination of compounds has been used to minimize their metabolism, but this chemical change can also influence estrogenicity of the compound. For instance o,p'-dichlorodiphenyltrichloroethane (DDT) has been shown in several reports to be estrogenic (144). However, the estrogenicity appears related to the positions of the chlorine atoms since o,p'-DDT is more estrogenic than the p,p' DDT (115). Hormonal activity of the chlorinated compounds is related to stereospecific differences in binding affinities for the estrogen receptor (76). Metabolic hydroxylation of DDT and o,p'-dichlorodiphenylethylene (DDE) produces compounds containing a phenolic hydroxyl that is similar to other compounds described in Fig. 1. Pesticides such as methoxychlor were shown to be estrogenic in vivo but had low estrogen receptor–binding activity in vitro (15). Subsequent studies by Kupfer and Bulger (16) indicated that the methoxychlor was being demethylated in vivo, thereby producing a compound with a phenolic ring that permitted interaction with the estrogen receptor. Kepone, a highly chlorinated chlordecone with reported weak estrogenic activity (17) is structurally unrelated to any of the known estrogens.

Recently, another group of compounds called polychlorinated biphenyls (PCBs) were demonstrated to have estrogenic activity (49). As with the biphenyl methane compounds (eg, DDT), there appear to be certain structural requirements, which correlate with estrogen receptor binding and estrogenic activity. One of the more active compounds, 4H2',4',6'TCB (Fig. 2), illustrates the need for a phenolic hydroxyl and chlorination of certain carbons on the opposing aromatic ring. Molecular modeling studies have shown that the chlorine atoms can arrange the two aromatic rings in a twisted conformation that approximates the shape of estradiol (92).

Mueller and colleagues had described the binding of simple phenols to the estrogen receptor in 1980 (102). Nonylphenol is an alkylphenol reported to be estrogenic (129). The nature of the alkyl side chain confers some specificity, since side chains with fewer than eight carbon atoms retain less estrogenic activity. In addition, side chains in the ortho position result in different estrogen receptor binding and activity from side chains in the para position. However, molecular modeling of these compounds, which might confirm these observations with respect to interaction with the estrogen receptor, has not been performed. Although

STRUCTURE	NAME	C_{50}
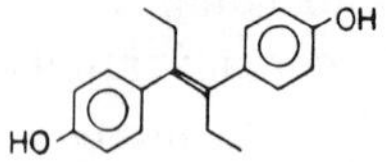	DES	0.4
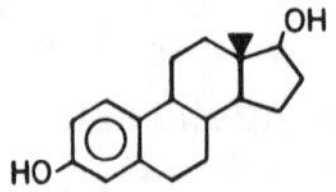	ESTRADIOL	1.0
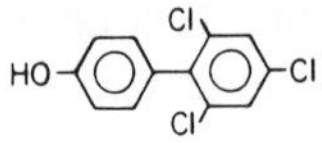	4-hydroxy, 2',4',6'-trichloro biphenyl (4H2',4',6'TCB)	42
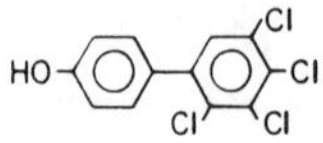	4-hydroxy, 2',3',4',5'-tetrachloro biphenyl (4H2',3',4',5'TCB)	95
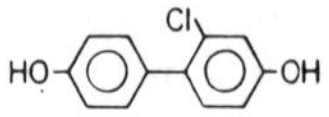	4,4' dihydroxy 2'-chloro biphenyl (4,4'DH 2'CB)	90
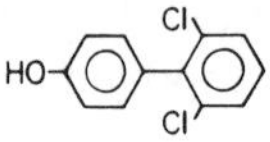	4-hydroxyl 2',6'-dichloro biphenyl (4H2',6'DCB)	388
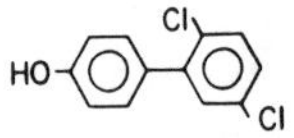	4-hydroxy 2',5' dichloro biphenyl (4H2',5'DCB)	506
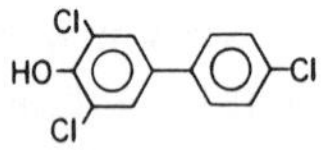	4-hydroxy 3,5,4'-trichloro biphenyl (4H3,5,4'TCB)	1000
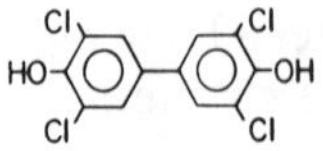	4,4'-dihydroxy 3,5,3',5'-tetrachloro biphenyl (4,4'DH3,5,3',5'TCB)	1354
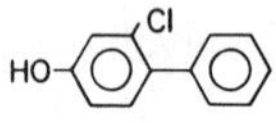	4-hydroxy 2-chloro biphenyl (4H2CB)	2500
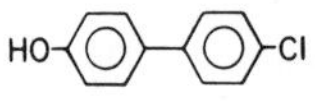	4-hydroxy 4'-chloro biphenyl (4H4'CB)	3900
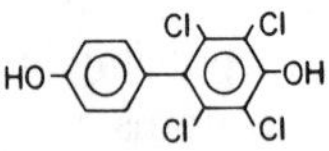	4,4'-dihydroxy 2',3',5',6'-tetrachloro biphenyl (4,4'DH2',3',5',6'TCB)	5000
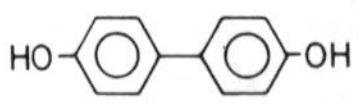	4,4'-dihydroxy biphenyl (4,4'DHB)	>5000
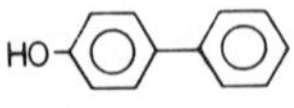	4-hydroxy biphenyl (4HB)	>5000

FIG. 2. Receptor binding and estrogenic activity of hydroxylated polychlorinated biphenyls. (From ref. 19, with permission.)

the nonylphenol compound has a phenolic ring required for binding to the estrogen receptor, it may be possible that the carbon side chain could fulfill the remaining spatial requirements of the ligand-binding site in the receptor. Furthermore, an additional oxygen distinct from the phenolic ring is also required for biological potency, and it may be possible that the alkylphenol compounds are subsequently metabolized by addition of an aliphatic hydroxyl to the side chain. Until the crystal structure of the estrogen receptor ligand–binding domain is deduced, it will be mere speculation as to how the estrogen receptor binds to such a diverse group of compounds with resulting biological activity.

MECHANISMS OF ESTROGEN ACTION

The actions of estrogens are mediated via the estrogen receptor, which is a member of the nuclear hormone receptor superfamily. This group includes the receptors for steroid hormones, thyroid hormones, vitamin D, and retinoic acid, as well as orphan receptors that are thought to have unidentified ligands (25,136). The estrogen receptor is composed of six functional domains, designated A–F (Fig. 3). The DNA binding domain (C) contains two zinc fingers, the first of which contains an α-helical region that determines the specificity of DNA binding (25,136). The estrogen receptor binds with high affinity to a specific, 13-base-pair DNA palindrome called the estrogen-response enhancer (ERE). The consensus sequence for the ERE is an inverted repeat 5'GGTCAnnnTGACC, with the three central nucleotides acting as a spacer between the palindromic half-sites of the ERE. ERE half-sites that contain one or two nucleotide changes, creating an imperfect palindrome, are still recognized by the estrogen receptor. Fig. 4 shows several known EREs that regulate various genes and, with the exception of the

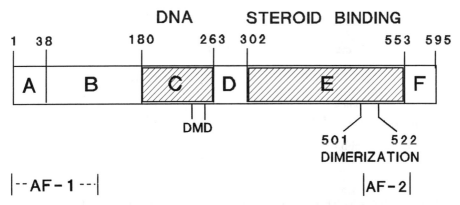

FIG. 3. The domains of the estrogen receptor. Transcriptional activation occurs through either the AF-1 in the A/B domain or the hormone-dependent AF-2 region in the E domain. Dimerization is mediated through regions of the C and E domains. The C domain contains the zinc finger DNA-binding motif, and the E domain contains the steroid-binding site.

vitellogenin A2 ERE, contain one or two variations from the consensus sequence (10,36,67,70,85,111,126,142). EREs have been identified within gene promoters but also occur in introns, as in the case of the rat calbindin gene (36). The estrogen receptor binds to the ERE as a homodimer, with each estrogen receptor monomer interacting with one ERE half-site. The two regions of the estrogen receptor that are involved in dimerization are located within the DNA- (C) and ligand-binding (E) domains (see Fig. 2). However, in vitro studies indicate that dimerization can occur prior to ligand or DNA binding (69) and that binding to the ERE can occur without ligand (35).

The estrogen receptor acts as an inducible transcription factor that can modulate expression of target genes after binding the estrogenic ligand. The estrogen receptor resides in the nucleus of target cells, and the hydrophobic estrogens enter the nucleus where they bind with high affinity to the ligand-binding domain of the estrogen receptor (Fig. 5). The estrogen–estrogen receptor complex is able to modulate gene transcription; however, the mechanism of gene regulation is still unclear. The estrogen receptor is thought to interact indirectly with RNA polymerase II through other proteins in the transcription complex. In a model developed using an in vitro transcription system, the estrogen receptor acts by either stabilizing or inducing the formation of the preinitiation complex. The preinitiation complex consists of RNA polymerase II and several transcription factors (TF) including, TF-IID, TF-IIA, TF-IIB, and TF-IIF, which assemble in a sequential manner (136).

VIT A2	G G T C A c a g T G A C C
NRE	G A̲ T C A c a g T G A̲ T̲ C
PS2	G G T C A c g g T G G̲ C C
human OXYTOCIN	G G T G̲ A c c t T G A C C
human c-FOS	C̲ G G̲ C A g c g T G A C C
CALBINDIN	G G T C A g g g T G A T̲ C
mouse LACTOFERRIN	G G T C A a g g T A̲ A C C
rabbit UTEROGLOBIN	G G T C A g c g T G C̲ C C

FIG. 4. Estrogen response elements (EREs) from estrogen-regulated genes. The canonical palindrome was discovered in the vitellogenin A2 gene. Bases that vary from the consensus sequence are underlined, and the three-base spacer is shown in lower case letters. The NRE is a synthetic element that has been shown to be nonresponsive to estrogen receptor and glucocorticoid receptor (From ref. 29, with permission.)

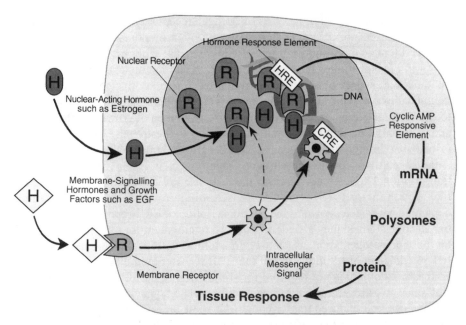

FIG. 5. Receptor-mediated activation mechanisms in target cells. (From ref. 49, with permission.)

Transcriptional activation is modulated by two activation functions (AFs), AF1 and AF2, which are localized in the A/B and E domains of the estrogen receptor, respectively (see Fig. 3) (54). Deletion analysis and construction of chimeric estrogen receptor proteins have demonstrated that the AF2 is estrogen-dependent (82,135). AF1 may be involved in basal promoter activity of ERE-containing genes, since deletion of AF2 region produces a protein that is constitutively active and functions independent of hormone (82,135). The ability of the estrogen receptor to activate selective genes may result from interactions between either the AF1 or AF2 regions and other transcription factors that are promoter- or cell type–specific (97,135,137). The structural variations between estrogenic ligands can influence slight conformational changes in the estrogen receptor that result in differential activation of the AF domains (97). This mechanism may account for the incomplete agonist activity observed with many of the xenoestrogens and for variations in their ability to activate estrogen-responsive genes.

Estrogen target tissues contain the estrogen receptor, and their sensitivity to estrogen varies with respect to the levels of receptor. Furthermore, the estrogen receptor level in an individual tissue varies during development (29,53). For instance, in adult rodents, estrogen receptor message and protein levels are very high in the uterus and oviduct. In contrast, estrogen receptor mRNA is low in ovarian tissue and detectable only with very sensitive procedures, such as RT-PCR. The estrogen receptor is present in mammary gland, pituitary, testis, prostate, and liver, but at much lower levels than in the uterus. Other adult tissues that contain detectable estrogen receptor levels include spleen, bone, and brain (29). Other species also exhibit similar patterns of estrogen receptor expression. In addition, the estrogen receptor protein can be detected by immunohistochemistry in the male and female reproductive tracts of day-10 mouse embryos (53).

Several recent studies have indicated that growth factors can mimic estrogen action via cross-talk between the estrogen receptor and other intracellular signaling pathways. For example, administration of epidermal growth factor (EGF) to ovariectomized mice stimulates the uterine responses of growth, proliferation, and differentiation that are normally associated with estrogen (104). This effect is mediated through the estrogen receptor because treatment with ICI 164384, an antiestrogen that depletes the estrogen receptor protein levels (51) and prevents transcriptional activation, decreases the response to EGF. Furthermore, insulin-like growth factor I (IGF-I), EGF, transforming growth factor-α (TGF), and dopamine have been shown to induce transcription of ERE-reporter genes in cell transfection studies; they also demonstrate a requirement for the estrogen receptor, but not estrogen agonists (26,61). In addition, estrogen antagonists, such as ICI 164384, can block induction of the ERE-reporter by the cytokines. However, the AF2 domain is not required for stimulation of the ERE-reporter expression since an estrogen receptor mutant with a deleted ligand-binding domain can still mediate EGF-induced transcription (61). These observations raise the prospect that molecules other than estrogen agonists can activate the estrogen receptor. Therefore, molecules that are not estrogen receptor ligands, but elicit estrogenic responses by interacting with the N-terminal half of the estrogen receptor to activate growth factor pathways, may be considered xenoestrogens. Recently, a transgenic mouse model that lacks functional estrogen receptor was developed (72,86); it may be a useful tool in dissecting the relative importance of estrogen receptor in cytokine pathways and xenoestrogen action.

Possible Mechanisms of Xenoestrogen Action

Xenoestrogens differ widely in their affinities for the estrogen receptor as well as their ability to transactivate the estrogen receptor. Estrogen-responsive promoters may also vary in their sensitivity to a xenoestrogen–estrogen receptor complex. In addition, the environmental estrogens may also influence estrogen action through other mechanisms not related to estrogen receptor activation. Circulating sex steroid hormones are predominantly bound to albumin or sex hormone–binding globulin (SHBG), which reduces their effective free concentration in plasma and decreases their clearance rate from the bloodstream (41,125). In contrast, synthetic and dietary estrogens have lower affinities for these plasma proteins, and therefore their availability to target tissues may be enhanced due to an increased relative free concentration in plasma. Increased plasma concentrations of xenoestrogens may also affect the activity or production of steroidogenic enzymes and thus alter the rate of synthesis and metabolism of endogenous estrogens.

The effects of pharmaceutical estrogens, most notably DES, on the fetus have been well established (94). During normal development, there are two fetal duct systems present, the Müllerian and Wolffian ducts, which are the female and male genital precursors, respectively. As normal fetal growth and differentiation continues the wolffian duct in the female or the müllerian duct in the male regresses. However, DES exposure causes the retention of both duct systems in either sex, as well as other structural and functional defects of the reproductive tract. Normally, alpha-fetoprotein (AFP) binds estrogen and protects the fetus and neonate from an estrogen-rich environment. Alternatively, the developing fetus may be exposed to elevated levels of DES since this reproductive toxin is not sequestered by AFP. Other xenoestrogens with reduced affinity for this serum protein may influence critical developmental stages and cause similar pathologies. Indeed, neonatal exposure of mice to the phytoestrogens zearalenone and coumestrol results in developmental abnormalities similar to those seen with DES treatment (19–21,150).

Assays for Estrogenic Hormone Activity

Several assays are available to measure the activity of suspected xenoestrogens. Affinity of a ligand for the estrogen receptor can be measured using a competitive-binding assay (60). Our laboratory uses mouse uterine cytosol or receptor-enriched preparations as a source for estrogen receptor, but bacculovirus-expressed or in vitro–translated estrogen receptor is also suitable. The samples containing estrogen receptor are incubated with [^{3}H]-estradiol; then the tracer is competed with increasing amounts of unlabeled ligand in order to determine the concentration required to displace 50% of the [^{3}H]-estradiol from the estrogen receptor. The affinity of a ligand for the estrogen receptor is not necessarily predictive of its biological activity; consequently, other functional assays are recommended.

In vitro techniques are useful for determining whether environmental estrogens can induce specific estrogenic responses. For example, MCF-7 cells, a human mammary carcinoma cell line that contains estrogen receptor, has been used to screen potential compounds for the known estrogen responses of cell proliferation and induction of pS2 and progesterone receptor levels (65,131). Tissue culture expression systems can also be useful for analyzing estrogenicity, antiestrogenicity, and estrogen receptor–dependence of possible estrogens. Dose-response curves can be generated by treatment of estrogen receptor–positive cells transfected with an estrogen-responsive reporter gene, such as chloramphenicol acetyltransferase (CAT), to determine the level of agonist activity of the compound in question. Antiestrogenicity can be similarly assessed by the ability of the test compound to block estradiol stimulation of reporter expression. In addition, expression systems are important tools for proving that xenoestrogens require the estrogen receptor to transactivate estrogen-responsive genes. This can be achieved by co-transfecting estrogen receptor–negative cells with a reporter construct and an estrogen receptor–expression plasmid or control plasmid lacking the estrogen receptor gene, followed by estrogen treatment. If no induction is detected in the absence of estrogen receptor or in the presence of a "pure" antiestrogen, such as

ICI 164384, the estrogen response is mediated through estrogen receptor mechanisms. To prevent background estrogen activity, it is essential that cell culture experiments be performed in the absence of serum or with charcoal-stripped serum to remove endogenous steroids. Phenol red should also be excluded from the media, as it has been shown to contain an estrogenic component (11). Furthermore, another source of estrogen contamination is found in some plastics used in tissue culture that shed the xenoestrogen, nonylphenol (129).

Estrogen receptor–expression plasmids and estrogen-responsive β-galactosidase reporter constructs can also be co-transfected into yeast to screen ligands for estrogenic activity. For example, some biphenolic compounds are capable of inducing β-galactosidase expression in yeast, at half-maximal concentrations that are 25- to 10,000-fold greater than DES (Fig. 6). Interestingly, these compounds induce transcriptional activity at levels comparable with or better than their receptor-binding affinities. In yeast expression systems, all antiestrogens display some agonist activity and no antagonist activity, with the exception of nafoxidine, which exhibits partial antagonism (71). Therefore, compounds exhibiting agonist activity in the yeast system need to be screened in a mammalian system as well.

Potential xenoestrogens should also to be tested in vivo to account for their metabolism, bioavailability, and differential activities that are cell-type- and promoter-dependent. The rodent uterotropic bioassay is a suitable method for screening possible estrogens. A 3-day treatment regime is used to determine the dose required to double the wet weight of an ovariectomized or immature rodent uterus. Other estrogenic responses, such as progesterone receptor induction, can also be measured in the rodent uterus. However, chemical treatments in vivo can appear to produce estrogenic effects, which are actually occurring through indirect mechanisms. For example, carbon tetrachloride was initially shown to be estrogenic in immature rats; however, further study revealed that carbon tetrachoride was hepatotoxic. The liver toxicity altered the metabolism of endogenous estrogens, resulting in elevated estrogen levels and in the subsequent hormonal response (83). Transgenic mice that lack a functional estrogen receptor (72) could help in elucidating whether xenoestrogenic effects in vivo are mediated by the estrogen receptor.

In summary, xenoestrogens that enter into the signaling mechanisms normally reserved for endogenous estrogens may have profound effects on development and reproduction via interaction with and activation of the estrogen receptor.

XENOESTROGENS

The two major types of xenoestrogens are the natural dietary estrogens and the synthetic chemical pollutants. Both sources of xenoestrogens are prevalent in the environment, reach human and animal populations mainly via food and water intake, and must be considered when assessing total estrogen exposure. In addition, both types can bind the estrogen receptor and produce estrogenic and/or antiestrogenic effects in humans, wildlife, livestock, laboratory animals, and cultured

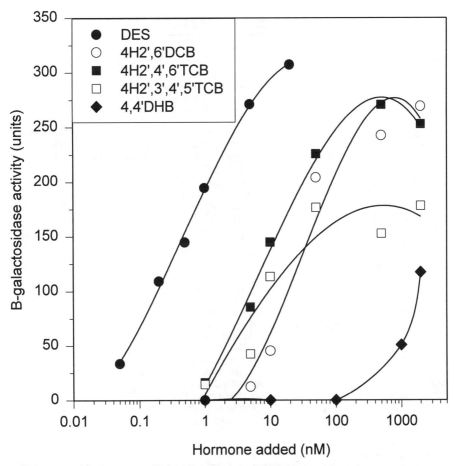

FIG. 6. Transcriptional activation of an estrogen-responsive β-galactosidase reporter gene by DES and various biphenolic compounds. Yeast cells transfected with a mouse estrogen receptor–expression plasmid and a β-galactosidase reporter gene construct were treated with increasing amounts of different compounds for 2 hours prior to measurement of β-galactosidase activity in cellular extracts. Abbreviations are defined as in Fig. 2.

cells, which are summarized below. The chemical structures of some xenoestrogens are shown in Fig. 1 and their classifications are given in Table 1.

Dietary Estrogens

Dietary estrogens are naturally occurring estrogenic compounds found in plants or in fungal contamination of stored grains. These include the lignans, mycoestrogens, and the major family of flavonoids or phytoestrogens.

TABLE 1. *Xenoestrogens.*

Natural	Synthetic
Flavonoids (phytoestrogens)	Organochlorines
Flavanones	Polychorinated biphenyls (PCB)
4',7-Dihydroxyflavanone	2',5'-Dichloro-4-hydroxybiphenyl
Naringenin	2',4',6'-Trichloro-4-hydroxybipheyl
Flavones	2',3',4',5'-Tetrachloro-4-hydroxybiphenyl
Apigenin	Polychlorinated dibenzo-*p*-dioxins (PCDD or dioxins)
4',5-Dihydroxyflavone	2,3,7,8-Tetrachlorodibenzo-p-dioxin (TCDD)
4',6-Dihydroxyflavone	Polychlorinated dibenzofurans (PCDF or furans)
Flavonols	2,3,7,8-Tetrachlorodibenzofuran
Kaempferol	2,3,4,7,8-Pentchlorodibenzofuran
Hydroxychalcones	Dichlorodiphenylethanes
Phloretin	o,p'-DDT
Isoliquiritigenin	o,p'-DDE
4,4'-Dihydroxychalcone	o,p'-DDD
Isoflavonoids	Methoxychlor
Isoflavones	Hexachlorocyclohexanes
Genistein	Lindane
Daidzein	Cyclodienes
Formononetin	Chlordecone (Kepone)
Biochanin A	Dieldrin
β-Sitosterol	Alkylphenols
O-Desmethylangolensin	4-Nonylphenol
Isoflavans	4-Octylphenol
Equol	4-Butylphenol
Coumestans	4-Nonylphenol-diethoxylate (NP2EO)
Coumestrol	4-Nonylphenoxycarboxylic acid (NP1EC)
Lignans	Synthetic Estrogens
Enterlactone	Ethinyl estradiol
Enterodiol	Diethylstilbestrol (DES)
Mycoestrogens	Hexestrol
Zearalenone	
Zearalenol	
Zearalanol (zeranol)	

Lignans

Generally, lignans are composed of a dibenzylbutane skeleton. Precursors of estrogenic lignans are found in whole grains, legumes, vegetables, and fruits, with the highest levels found in oilseeds, especially flaxseed (134). The two major lignans are enterolactone and enterodiol, which are metabolized from plant precursors by bacterial enzymes in the intestinal tract. Both enterolactone and enterodiol have been isolated in human urine. These two lignans bind with weak affinity to the estrogen receptor, stimulate some estrogenic responses (4), including (SHBG) synthesis (6), and inhibit estrogen biosynthesis in vitro (5). Compared with the other dietary estrogens, there is little information on the possible in vivo effects of the lignans.

Mycoestrogens

The resorcylic acid lactone, zearalenone, is produced by *Fusarium* species. This mycotoxin is generally found in improperly stored grains, and therefore the levels of zearalenone found in food sources varies according to the level of fungal contamination. Zearalenol is a metabolite of zearalenone, and zearalanol (zeranol) is a synthetic derivative that is used as an anabolic agent in beef cattle. Their relative order of affinities for the estrogen receptor is as follows: α-zearalanol > α-zearalenol > β-zearalanol > zearalenone > β-zearalenol (79). These mycoestrogens can induce multiple biological responses in vivo (79). Zearalenone exhibits higher uterotropic activity than would be expected from in vitro binding studies, possibly due to its conversion to the more active metabolite, zearalenol. In addition, zearalenone, zearalenol, and zearalanol have been shown to be potent estrogen agonists in vitro (88,91,130). Of all the dietary estrogens and the synthetic pollutants (except for the pharmaceutical estrogens), the mycotoxins are the most estrogenic.

Flavonoids

Many of the flavonoid classes, including hydroxychalcones, flavanones, flavonols, flavones, and isoflavonoids, are estrogenic. Flavonoids, natural products formed by all plant families, can be isolated from most plant tissues including stems, seeds, roots, flowers, and leaves (100). These compounds are believed to act as insect deterrents and natural fungicides (phytoalexins) and are synthesized in response to stress, such as fungal infections, pesiticide treatment, and injury (146).

The isoflavonoid class, which comprises isoflavones, isoflavans, and coumestans, represents the most prevalent of the phytoestrogens. The isoflavonoids are found in limited plant families, with the highest levels found in soybeans and other legumes (46). The isoflavones formononetin and biochanin A are metabolized by the normal intestinal flora to daidzein and genistein, respectively, which are more potent estrogens compared with the plant precursors. Daidzein is further metabolized to equol, an isoflavan. Equol is responsible for the majority of the estrogenic activity in ruminants (1). The main source of isoflavonoids in the human diet is soybeans and soy products. The major phytoestrogens detected in human urine include equol, daidzein, and genistein. Although the affinity of these dietary estrogens for the estrogen receptor is low, normal dietary intake can produce circulating levels of the phytoestrogens that are several orders of magnitude higher than the more potent endogenous estrogens (146). In addition, some compounds like coumestrol are thought to have a cumulative effect, by which diets low in coumestrol do not induce uterine growth in rats over short time periods but can be uterotropic over extended time periods (147). Coumestrol is the major coumestan and exhibits the highest potency of the isoflavonoids in mouse uterotropic assays and in vitro analysis; it is followed in relative estrogenic potency by genistein, daidzein, biochanin A, and formononetin (88,91,100). Besides the isoflavonoids, estrogenic activity has been demonstrated for some compounds in the other flavonoid classes. For example, isoliquiritigenin (a hydroxychalcone), 4',7-dihydroxflavanone and naringenin (flavanones), kaempferol (a flavonol), and 4',5- and 4',6'-dihydroxyflavone and apigenin (flavones) were estrogen agonists in an in vitro assay (100). In addition, these various classes of flavonoids are estrogenic in vivo using uterotropic bioassays (91,146).

Member compounds from all of the flavonoid classes are able to bind to the estrogen receptor, with the isoflavonoids having the highest affinity (100,101,146). These compounds can also induce transcription of an estrogen-responsive reporter gene in cells co-transfected with the estrogen receptor, but they require higher concentrations compared with 17β-estradiol (88,100,101). Pure antiestrogens can block their estrogenic response and the flavonoids cannot induce the reporter gene without the presence of the estrogen receptor (88,101). Therefore, phytoestrogens, like the mycoestrogens, can stimulate estrogen-responsive pathways directly through classical estrogen receptor–mediated mechanisms.

Environmental Effects from Dietary Estrogens

Animals

Livestock that has grazed in red clover or alfalfa pastures, which are rich in isoflavonoids, develop reproductive dysfunction and can become permanently infertile after prolonged exposure (see ref. 1 for review). Isoflavonoids have been isolated from alfalfa and clover extracts, which proved to be highly estrogenic in a uterotropic assay (121). However, grazing in these pastures may also be beneficial for beef cattle, since phytoestrogens may act as an anabolic agent to improve meat quality (28,103). The reproductive potential of captive and wild animals may be affected by the phytoestrogen content in their diets. For example, attempts to breed the cheetah in captivity to prevent extinction have been hindered because of a high incidence of infertility and liver disease. The commercial diet for cheetahs that is used in North American zoos may be responsible for these disorders, since the feed is high in isoflavones and extracts proved to be estrogenic in the uterotropic bioassay (122).

Certain species may be more susceptible to phytoestrogen exposure. More pronounced reproductive disorders are observed in sheep compared with cattle that have grazed in pastures rich in isoflavonoids (105). Differential sensitivity to zearalenone is also found in the various species of farm animals, with swine being especially susceptible compared with cattle and poultry being resistant (79). These data illustrate the difficulty in generalizing the predicted effects of dietary estrogens between species.

Humans

High fiber/low fat diets that are rich in soy are associated with lower incidences of breast and prostate cancer (see ref. 4 for review). High fiber foods, including cereal brans, whole grains, fruits, legumes, vegetables, and oilseeds, contain phytoestrogens and lignans (46,134). Therefore, it has been posulated that the diphenolic dietary estrogens may act as chemotherapeutic agents (see refs. 3,4,7,8,116 for reviews). Although these compounds have been shown to be weak estrogen agonists, this protective effect from hormone-dependent cancers would also support antiestrogenic activity. However, since only agonist activity has been demonstrated in vitro (88), other in vivo mechanisms are being examined. One postulated mechanism for this cancer-preventive effect is the stimulation of sex hormone–binding globulin (SHBG) synthesis in the liver. Enterolactone, genistein, and daidzein can stimulate SHBG synthesis in cultured hepatocytes (4). Therefore, increasing SHBG levels would reduce the bioavailability of circulating endogenous estrogens and testosterone and possibly influence the etiology of hormonal carcinogenesis. Furthermore, high SHBG levels correlate positively in humans with vegetarian diets and elevated levels of phytoestrogens in urine. Cancer-preventive effects of dietary estrogens may be associated with other mechanisms important in carcinogenesis, including malignant cell proliferation, tumor promotion, and angiogenesis (see refs. 4,46 for reviews). The estrogenic activities of these compounds may be distinct from the cancer prevention properties. For example, genistein, a predominant isoflavone, is able to inhibit tumor cell growth in the absence of estrogen receptor, and therefore the chemotherapeutic effects of genistein may be related to its nonestrogenic activities as a tyrosine kinase inhibitor (8) or antioxidant (141). However, genistein administered to neonatal rats prevents chemically induced mammary tumors and alters the ontogeny of mammary development (80). The modified development of the gland may be a direct result of the estrogenic activity of genistein and therefore may contribute to the decreased susceptibility to the carcinogen.

Since estrogens may act as antiandrogens in the male, they can elicit feminizing effects, such as gynecomastia (140), possibly by activating neuroendocrine pathways. Alcoholic men often display evidence of feminization. Interestingly, phytoestrogen congeners isolated from bourbon and beer, β-sitosterol, biochanin A, genistein, and daidzein can bind the estrogen receptor and induce estrogenic biological responses (48,117). Estrogenic activity was also detected in wine (48). However, when intake is not excessive, these xenoestrogens are associated with a decreased incidence of prostate cancer, indicating a beneficial role for the dietary estrogens in males.

The effects of the dietary estrogens on the developing reproductive tract have been investigated with regard to DES, a known reproductive toxin (see ref. 62 for review). Neonatal administration of coumestrol can elicit many, but not all, of the female reproductive abnormalities associated with DES treatment (18,95,96). It can also alter neuroendocrine development in male rats (148). The effects of prenatal exposure to genistein were inconsistent with those of DES or estradiol (84). Equol also elicited responses not characteristic of estrogenic or antiestrogenic actions in the uterus (95,96). These data indicate that phytoestrogens can influence development but that they are incomplete agonists. The developmental effects of dietary estrogens on humans, livestock, and wildlife are unknown.

Data indicating possible effects of dietary estrogens on human fertility, implantation, and pregnancy are lacking; however, these xenoestrogens have not been excluded as potential agents relating to the decline in sperm counts in the last five decades (23,123). Conceivably, these dietary estrogens may also influence other estrogen-dependent disorders, including osteoporosis and cardiovascular disease. It has been suggested that the phytoestrogens found in soy diets may be responsible for reduction of cholesterol levels in patients with hyperlipidemias, for protection against the development of coronary artery atherosclerosis and coronary heart disease, and for prevention of postmenopausal bone loss (see ref. 31 for review).

Chemical Contaminants

Synthetic compounds showing estrogenic and/or antiestrogenic activity include organochlorine compounds, alkylphenols, and synthetic estrogens developed for pharmaceutical use. Animals and humans are exposed to these pollutants through food, water, air, and skin contact. These chemicals have extremely long half-lives and bioaccumulate in adipose tissue, thereby increasing the level of exposure over time.

Organochlorines

The organochlorines include polychlorinated compounds such as dichlorodiphenylethanes, hexachlorocyclohexanes, cyclodienes, polychlorinated biphenyls (PCBs), polychlorinated dibenzo-*p*-dioxins (PCDDs or dioxins), and polychlorinated dibenzofurans (PCDFs or furans). PCDD and PCDF are compounds that are industrial by-products of commercial products ranging from insecticides to fire retardants. Estrogenic activity has been associated with many members of these classes of synthetic pollutants.

Over 200 PCB congeners have been synthesized for use as heat transfer fluids, adhesives, plasticizers, paint additives, dedusting agents, laminating agents, dielectric fluids for capacitors and transformers, fire retardants, and waxes (118). The thermal-stable properties that make PCBs useful also explains their persistence in the environment. Several PCB congeners are able to bind to the estrogen receptor with varying affinities less than that of 17β-estradiol (76). Furthermore, many of the congeners were able to induce proliferation of the estrogen-responsive MCF-7 cell line. Of the PCBs showing agonist activity, none were coplanar in structure (131); however, antiestrogenicity was observed with several coplanar

PCBs in an in vitro assay (63). The most potent PCB agonists were 2',5'-dichloro-4-hydroxybiphenyl, 2',4',6'-trichloro-4-hydroxybiphenyl, and 2',3',4',5'-tetrachloro-4-hydroxybiphenyl (131). Uterotropic assays also indicate that some PCB compounds are estrogen agonists; however, one congener displayed only estrogen antagonism in this assay (63,76).

The chlorinated cyclodiene insecticides include chlordane, aldrin, mirex, dieldrin, and chlordecone. Chlordecone (Kepone) binds to the estrogen receptor at approximately 0.1% the affinity of 17β-estradiol, and it can elicit estrogen-dependent responses in vivo, such as increases in uterine weight, uterine DNA synthesis, and progesterone receptor synthesis (15,109). In an in vitro xenobiotic screening assay, chlordecone also displayed significant estrogen agonist activity (130). The other cyclodienes show little estrogenicity in vivo (15). However, dieldrin has been shown in vitro to have estrogenic properties (131). Mirex did not demonstrate estrogenicity in this same assay, although one of its degradation products is chlordecone (24). Therefore, environmental exposure to mirex may induce estrogenic responses via the potent chlordecone product.

Hexachlorocyclohexanes (or benzene hexachlorides), also produced as insectides, have shown estrogenic activity in rats. However, one isomer in the insecticide lindane has displayed both estrogenic and antiestrogenic activities in vivo (133) but did not show estrogenic activity in an in vitro assay (131).

Dichlorodiphenylethanes, another class of insectides, includes DDT, DDD, DDE, and methoxychlor. The o,p' isomers of DDT, DDD, and DDE and the methoxy analog of DDT, methoxychlor, have been shown to be the most estrogenic of the DDT-related chemicals in uterotropic and other in vivo assays, in vitro, and in estrogen receptor–binding assays (15,130,131). Endosulfan and methoxychlor are two insecticides that are still in use in the United States and other countries, mainly because their persistence in the environment and potential for bioaccumulation is lower than the others mentioned above (47). Endosulfan, like methoxychlor, has shown estrogenic effects both in vivo and in vitro (131).

PCDD and PCDF Compounds

There are 75 PCDDs (dioxins) and 135 PCDF (furans) congeners that originate as by-products from the manufacture of industrial and agricultural chemicals such as herbicides, PCBs, and naphthalenes. In the environment, they are also found in paper- and pulp-bleaching effluent, emmisions from hospital incinerators and steel foundries, municipal waste, and vehicle exhausts (120,133). The most potent dioxin, 2,3,7,8-tetrachlorodibenzo-p-dioxin (TCDD), does not bind to the estrogen receptor, and agonist activity has not been reported; however, TCDD displays antiestrogenic activity both in vivo and in vitro. Antiestrogenic properties are mediated through the aryl hydrocarbon (Ah) receptor, for which TCDD is an agonist, although the mechanism of antagonism is unknown (119). Several furans compounds also demonstrate antiestrogenicity in vitro. Their relative antiestrogenic potencies are TCDD > 2,3,7,8-tetrachlorodibenzofuran >

2,3,4,7,8-pentachlorodibenzofuran > 1,2,3,7,9-pentachlorodibenzofuran > 1,3,6,8-tetrachlorodibenzofuran (78). In general, the affinity of these compounds for the Ah receptor parallels their activity as an estrogen antagonist. Other Ah-receptor agonists have also been shown to act as antiestrogens in culture, including polynuclear aromatic hydrocarbons and PCBs (27,78).

Alkylphenols

The alkylphenols, another group of weak estrogens found in the environment, arise from the degradation of nonionic surfactants (alkylphenol polyethoxylates, APEOs) during sewage treatment. Massive quantities of APEOs are used as detergents in the textile and paper industries. The alkylphenols exhibit estrogenic activity in vitro and bind to the estrogen receptor (64,130,131,145). The two alkylphenols with the highest levels of estrogenicity are 4-octylphenol and then 4-nonylphenol. In order to evoke an estrogen response in vitro, the alkylphenol must be composed of an alkyl chain of at least three carbons and the backbone chain must contain C–C bonds (versus C–O bonds) (130). Some APEOs with short ethoxy side chains also display estrogenic properties in vitro (64,145). Trout placed in the effluent from sewage treatment plants exhibited elevated levels of vitellogenin, an estrogen-responsive gene product. The suspected estrogenic agents in the polluted water are the aklylphenol and APEO compounds as well as ethinyl estradiol, the synthetic estrogen in oral contraceptives (108).

Butylated hydroxyanisole (BHA) is another antioxidant, not related to the alkylphenols, that displays estrogenic activity in a xenobiotic screening assay (131). This compound is used as a preservative in many prepared foods and consequently is another possible dietary source of xenoestrogens.

Pharmaceutical Estrogens

Estrogens that have been synthesized for therapeutic purposes have also become environmental contaminants. There is concern that ethinyl estradiol, an estrogen used in oral contraceptives, may enter waste waters and rivers from urinary excretion and from waste during its manufacture; however, only limited amounts have been detected in rivers and sewage (2,112). Beef cattle were treated with DES, until its ban in the 1970s, to increase production of lean meat and improve the efficiency of converting feed to beef (68). Currently, zearalanol (zeranol), the synthetic derivative of zearalenone, is used as an anabolic agent in cattle (36). Another concern is that plants fertilized with manure from DES-treated cattle have also been found to contain DES residues (42). Therefore, human exposure to these anabolic estrogens may occur not only from ingestion of beef also but possibly plants. In addition, steroidal estrogens excreted from humans and animals were detected in sewage treatment facilities and lake water in Israel (124). Therefore, these potent estrogens must also be considered as environmental pollutants.

Environmental Effects from Synthetic Xenoestrogens

Humans

Organochlorine residues are lipophilic and are stored in adipose tissue. The major DDT metabolite, DDE, was detected in breast adipose tissue of women undergoing biopsy for breast cancer. Women with estrogen receptor–positive breast cancer had significantly higher levels of DDE in their tissues than women with estrogen receptor–negative breast cancer or benign breast disease (39). Furthermore, the mean level of DDE detected in plasma was elevated in breast cancer patients compared with control subjects (152). Another human study linked the incidence of malignant disease with increased concentrations of DDE and PCBs in breast adipose tissue (44,151). These studies indicate that bioaccumulation of these estrogenic organochlorines in humans may be important in the etiology of mammary carcinogenesis. In vivo experimental evidence also supports that xenoestrogen exposure can induce or promote breast cancer (see ref. 37 for review).

Endometriosis is a prevalent disorder in women, characterized by the abnormal and hormone-dependent growth of the uterine endometrial cells. The etiology of endometriosis is unknown, but immunologic factors may contribute to the disease process (40,59). Steroidal and environmental estrogens are known to influence a variety of immunologic responses (see ref. 87 for review); therefore, xenoestrogens may influence both the immunologic and hormonal aspects of this reproductive disorder. In rhesus monkeys, a direct correlation exists between exposure to dioxin and the incidence of endometriosis. Moreover, disease severity was shown to be dependent on dioxin dosage (113,114). Another simian study showed similar associations with exposure to PCBs (22). Although dioxin or PCB exposure has not been correlated with the incidence of endometriosis in humans, this indicates that other hormone-dependent disorders in humans may also be influenced by organochlorines.

Transgenic mice that lack a functional estrogen receptor have abnormal testicular development and marked reduction in sperm production, indicating that, at least in mice, estrogen is crucial for male reproduction (72). In addition, estrogens in the male act as antiandrogens, and consequently administration of additional estrogenic agents during sexual development is associated with feminization of the male reproductive tract in numerous species (93). Therefore, it is plausible that male, as well as female reproduction may be adversely affected by the presence of these environmental estrogens. During the past 50 years, the incidence of male reproductive tract developmental disorders has doubled, the incidence of testicular cancer has increased, and sperm counts have declined; these abnormalities may be related to xenoestrogen exposure during development and/or adulthood (23,123). The production of synthetic estrogenic compounds and their contamination of the environment has also been prominent during this half century. Animal studies with these estrogenic contaminants also revealed decreases in male fertility and altered reproductive tract development (see ref. 140 for review).

The fact that these compounds are stored in mammary adipose tissue is especially important during lactation. The levels of the lipophilic chemicals can be 10–40-fold higher to the nursing infant than the daily intake for an adult (149). Therefore, preventing exposure to xenoestrogens during critical periods of development, when the sensitivity to these chemicals may be increased, may be paramount to maintaining reproductive integrity. Prenatal exposure is also a concern because these compounds have little or no affinity for alpha-fetoprotein, which would result in increased exposure to the developing fetus. Diverse developmental defects in humans and animals have been associated with perinatal exposure to xenoestrogens (see refs. 12,13,52,106,128 for reviews). In addition, in Puerto Rico during the 1970s and 1980s, there was a high incidence of precocious puberty and premature thelarche in children 6 months to 8 years old. Multiple dietary sources for estrogenic contamination were investigated, but no causative agent was precisely identified (58). Whether exposure occurred pre- or postnatally, this indicates that estrogenic pollutants may alter the onset of sexual development in humans.

Wildlife

The effects of estrogenic contaminants in the environment and their impact on the reproductive potential of wildlife is relevant for protecting endangered species and maintaining balanced ecosystems. In addition, human exposure to these pollutants is increased by consumption of many species that store these xenoestrogens in their adipose tissue. There are multiple examples of reproductive dysfunctions that occur in fish, birds, marine animals, and reptiles in the wild after exposure to environmental pollutants (32,38,45,81,110,120). Evidence of detrimental effects in wildlife, as in humans, is predominately indirect; however, some in vivo data are now available to indicate a direct correlation with exposure.

Juvenile male alligators living in Lake Apopka in Florida, which is contaminated with DDT and other chemicals from agricultural and sewage waste, displayed abnormalities in testes development, as well as substantially depressed testosterone levels. Female alligators had excessive levels of estradiol and abnormal ovarian morphology (57). These reproductive defects have resulted in a sharp decline in the adult alligator population at Lake Apopka compared with unpolluted lakes. Estrogens can have a profound effect on sex determination in many species of reptiles. The sex of alligators and turtles, which is determined by egg incubation temperature, can be reversed by treating the eggs with estrogens. Therefore, estrogenic contaminants could alter sex ratios or produce intersex animals, especially feminized males, which could devastate the reproductive potential of the species in contaminated locales. Alligator eggs were treated with DDE at levels comparable with those detected in eggs from Lake Apopka and were incubated at temperatures that would normally produce 100% males. DDE treatment resulted in reproductive defects, including sex reversal, modified sex hormone levels, and intersexual gonads, similar to those observed in alligators living at the contaminated lake (55,56).

In a study investigating the effect of PCB exposure on sex determination in turtle eggs, treatment with two PCB compounds could also induce the estrogen-dependent sex reversal at the incubation temperature required for male hatchlings. Both 2',4',6'-trichloro-4-biphenylol and 2',3',4,'5'-tetrachloro-4-biphenylol were able to induce male-to-female sex reversal or partial sex reversal (9,34). This species of turtle, living in Lake Apopka, exhibited phenotypes similar to those observed with the alligators (56). These studies indicate that the reproductive abnormalities seen in wildlife can be directly linked to exposure to xenoestrogenic toxins and that sex determination in reptile eggs can possibly be used as a bioassay for the detection of environmental estrogen contamination. In addition, these data indicate that the period of fetal or neonatal development is the most sensitive to xenoestrogen exposure, which can result in profound alterations in development and reproductive potential.

Common Properties

In general, both the dietary and synthetic xenoestrogens are weakly estrogenic, with activities and binding affinities ranging from approximately 10- to 1000-fold lower compared with endogenous 17β-estradiol, with the exception of the potent pharmaceutical estrogens. The estrogenicity of the individual compound can also vary depending on the type of assay, the response tested, and the host or estrogen receptor species used. Although these xenoestrogens can elicit estrogenic responses in nature and in the laboratory, individually they are incapable of inducing the full spectrum of responses credited to endogenous estrogens. The differential responses mediated by the environmental estrogens may be related to the diverse structural properties that cause slight variations in the conformation of the estrogen receptor; thereby some promoters containing estrogen-response enhancers are not activated by the estrogen receptor–xenoestrogen complex or are only partially induced. Differential activation has been observed in our laboratory with various DES metabolites and analogs (75). Different patterns of activation were also reported with estradiol analogs (107,138,139). Therefore, the toxicity of the xenoestrogens may, in part, arise from the differential pattern of activation of estrogen-responsive genes by the environmental estrogens relative to the endogenous estrogens (132).

Another possible reason for the differential responses between xenoestrogens may be related to an activity or toxicity, not mediated by the estrogen receptor, that may counteract estrogenic responses. Many of these compounds are known to activate other signaling pathways. For example, genistein has multiple activities, including those as a tyrosine kinase inhibitor and an antioxidant (8,141); and PCBs, PCDDs, and PCDFs bind to the aryl hydrocarbon receptor, which can modulate its own response elements in target genes (118). Therefore, these nonestrogenic activities may account for the differential responses seen in the laboratory and in nature.

The potency of environmental estrogens in vitro does not always represent their efficacy in vivo. This may occur for multiple reasons:

1. The xenobiotic may be metabolized by enzymes in the liver or the intestinal flora to a more potent, weaker, or inactive estrogen.

2. These compounds can affect the metabolism of endogenous estrogens, which can modify the hormonal milieu of the host. The activity of steroidogenic enzymes important for estrogen metabolism can be influenced by both phytoestrogens (5,89) and organochlorines (14).

3. The bioavailability of endogenous and environmental estrogens can be modified with plasma steroid-binding proteins. Phytoestrogens can increase SHBG levels, which would reduce the levels of free endogenous estrogens (3). In addition, the xenoestrogens do not bind to binding proteins, such as SHBG and alpha-fetoprotein, which can result in their increased availability to the estrogen receptor. For example, the inability of alpha-fetoprotein to bind these estrogens can leave the fetus vulnerable to an estrogen-rich environment during crucial times of development.

4. In the environment, xenoestrogen potency must also be related to their long-term stability and to the bioaccumulation of these lipophilic substances in adipose tissue.

5. Furthermore, each individual may be exposed to many xenoestrogens during his or her lifetime. The mixed levels of these compounds, combined with their reduced clearance rates, can increase the estrogen body burden. Even though the exposure to any one chemical may be low, the cumulative levels of environmental estrogen exposure may act synergistically to induce estrogenic responses and/or cause reproductive toxicity.

Effects on reproduction have been associated with many chemicals that are not considered xenoestrogens. Some compounds may act as antiandrogens, which are becoming recognized as another class of environmental hormones. Antiandrogens can produce biological responses that mimic estrogens, although they exert their effects through the androgen receptor. Other toxins can influence reproduction via other mechanisms not directly related to estrogen or the estrogen receptor per se. For example, tetrahydrocannabinol (THC) found in marihuana is not considered an estrogen agonist, but it produces estrogen-like effects, possibly through neuroendocrine pathways (127).

The natural and synthetic xenoestrogens are prevalent in our environment. Generally, fewer adverse affects have been associated with the dietary estrogens compared with the synthetic compounds. Indeed, the dietary estrogens may provide beneficial properties, such as protection against certain types of cancer. In contrast, exposure to the synthetic estrogen pollutants is associated with negative repercussions for humans and wildlife. Whether the beneficial properties of the dietary estrogens can counter possible detrimental effects from these contaminants is not known. It is clear that additional experimental and epidemiologic evaluations of exposed populations will have to be conducted before a more direct and causative relationship can be drawn.

REFERENCES

1. Adams NR. Organizational and activational effects of phyotestrogens on the reproductive tract of the ewe. *Proc Soc Exp Biol Med.* 1995;208:87–91.
2. Aherne GW, English J, Marks V. The role of the immunoassay in the analysis of microcontaminants in water samples. *Ecotoxicol Environ Safety.* 1985;9:79–83.
3. Aldercreutz H. Western diet and Western diseases: some hormonal and biochemical mechanisms and associations. *Scand J Clin Lab Invest.* 1990;50(suppl 201):3–23.
4. Aldercreutz H. Phytoestrogens: epidemiology and a possible role in cancer protection. *Environ Health Perspect.* In press.
5. Aldercreutz H, Bannwart C, Wahala K, et al. Inhibition of human aromatase by mammalian lignans and isoflavonoid phytoestrogens. *J Steroid Biochem Mol Biol.* 1993;44:147–153.
6. Aldercreutz H, Mousavi Y, Clark J, et al. Dietary phytoestrogens and cancer: in vitro and in vivo studies. *J Steroid Biochem Mol Biol.* 1992;41:331–337.
7. Aldercreutz H, Mousavi Y, Hockerstedt K. Diet and breast cancer. *Acta Oncol.* 1992;31:175–181.
8. Barnes S, Peterson TG. Biochemical targets of the isoflavone genistein in tumor cell lines. *Proc Soc Exp Biol Med.* 1995;208:103–108.
9. Bergeron JM, Crews D, McLachlan JA. PCBs as environmental estrogens: turtle sex determination as a biomarker of environmental contamination. *Environ Health Perspect.* 1994;102:780–781.
10. Berry M, Nunez AM, Chambon P. Estrogen-responsive element of the human pS2 gene is an imperfectly palindromic sequence. *Proc Natl Acad Sci U S A.* 1989;86:1218–1222.
11. Berthois Y, Katzenellenbogen JA, Katzenellenbogen BS. Phenol red in tissue culture media is a weak estrogen: implications concerning the study of estrogen-responsive cells in culture. *Proc Natl Acad Sci U S A.* 1986;83:2496–2500.
12. Birnbaum LS. Endocrine effects of prenatal exposure to PCBs, dioxins, and other xenobiotics: implications for policy and future research. *Environ Health Perspect.* 1994;102:676–679.
13. Birnbaum LS. Developmental effects of dioxins. *Environ Health Perspect.* In press.
14. Bradlow HL, Davis DL, Lin G, Sepkovic D, Tiwari R. Effects of pesticides on the ratio of $16\alpha/2$-hydroxyestrone: A biological marker of breast cancer risk. *Environ Health Perspect.* In press.
15. Bulger WH, Kupfer D. Estrogenic activity of pesticides and other xenobiotics on the uterus and male reproductive tract. In: Thomas JA, Korach KS, McLachlan JA, eds. *Endocrine Toxicology.* New York, NY :Raven Press; 1985:1–33.
16. Bulger WH, Muccitelli RM, Kupfer D. Studies on the in vivo and in vitro estrogenic activities of methoxychlor and its metabolites. Role of hepatic mono-oxygenase in methoxychlor activation. *Biochem Pharmacol.* 1978;27:2417–2423.
17. Bulger WH, Muccitelli RM, Kupfer D. Studies on the estrogenic activity of chlordecone (Kepone) in the rat: effects on uterine estrogen receptor. *Mol Pharmacol.* 1979;15:515–524.
18. Burroughs CD. Long-term reproductive tract alterations in female mice treated neonatally with coumestrol. *Proc Soc Exp Biol Med.* 1995;208:78–81.
19. Burroughs CD, Bern HA, Stokstad EL. Prolonged vaginal cornification and other changes in mice treated neonatally with coumestrol, a plant estrogen. *J Toxicol Environ Health.* 1985; 15:51–61.
20. Burroughs CD, Mills KT, Bern HA. Long-term genital tract changes in female mice treated neonatally with coumestrol. *Reprod Toxicol.* 1990;4:127–135.
21. Burroughs CD, Mills KT, Bern HA. Reproductive abnormalities in female mice exposed neonatally to various doses of coumestrol. *J Toxicol Environ Health.* 1990;30:105–122.
22. Campbell JS, Wong J, Tryphonas L, et al. Is simian endometriosis an effect of immunotoxicity? Presented at the Ontario Association of Pathologists, 48th Annual Meeting; 1985; London, Ontario, Canada.
23. Carlsen E, Giwercman A, Keiding N, Skakkebaek NE. Declining semen quality and increasing incidence of testicular cancer. Is there a common cause? *Environ Health Perspect.* In press.
24. Carlson DA, Konyha KD, Wheeler WB, Marshall GP, Zaylskie RG. Mirex in the environment: its degradation to Kepone and related compounds. *Science.* 1976;194:939–941.

25. Carson-Jurica MA, Schrader WT, O'Malley BW. Steroid receptor family: structure and functions. *Endocr Rev.* 1990;11:201–220.

26. Chalbos D, Philips A, Rochefort H. Cross-talk between the estrogen receptor and growth factor regulatory pathways in estrogen target tissues. *Semin Cancer Biol.* 1994;5:361–368.

27. Chaloupka K, Krishnan V, Safe S. Polynuclear aromatic hydorcarbon carcinogens as antiestrogens in MCF-7 human breast cancer cells: role of the Ah receptor. *Carcinogenesis.* 1992;13:2233–2239.

28. Cheng E, Story CD, Yoder L, Hale WH, Burroughs W. Estrogenic activity of isoflavone derivatives extracted and prepared from soybean oil meal. *Science.* 1953;118:164–165.

29. Ciocca DR, Vargas-Roig LM. Estrogen receptors in human nontarget tissues:biological and clinical implications. *Endocr Rev.* 1995;16:35–56.

30. Clark LB, Rosen RT, Hartman TG, et al. Determination of alkylphenol ethoxylates and their acetic acid derivatives in drinking water by particle beam liquid chromatography mass spectrometry. *Int J Environ Anal Chem.* 1992;47:167–180.

31. Clarkson TB, Anthony MS, Hughes Jr CL. Estrogenic soybean isoflavones and chronic disease: risks and benefits. *Trends Endocrinol Metab.* 1995;6:11–16.

32. Colborn T, vom Saal FS, Soto AM. Developmental effects of endocrine-disrupting chemicals in wildlife and humans. *Environ Health Perspect.* 1993;101:378–384.

33. Colburn T, Clement C, eds. *Chemically Induced Alterations in Sexual and Functional Development: The Wildlife/Human Connection.* Princeton, NJ: Princeton Scientific Publishing; 1992.

34. Crews D, Bergeron JM, McLachlan JA. The role of estrogen in turtle sex determination and the effect of PCBs. *Environ Health Perspect.* In press.

35. Curtis SW, Korach KS. Uterine estrogen receptor-DNA complexes: effects of different ERE sequences, ligands, and receptor forms. *Mol Endocrinol.* 1991;5:959–966.

36. Darwish H, Krisinger J, Furlow JD, Smith C, Murdoch FE, DeLuca HF. An estrogen responsive element mediates the transcriptional regulation of calbindin D-9K gene in rat uterus. *J Biol Chem.* 1991;266:551–558.

37. Davis DL, Bradlow HL, Wolff M, Woodruff T, Hoel DG, Anton-Culver H. Medical hypothesis: xenoestrogens as preventable causes of breast cancer. *Environ Health Perspect.* 1993;101:372–377.

38. Davis WP, Bortone SA. Effects of kraft mill effluent on the sexuality of fishes: an environmental early warning? In: Colburn T, Clement C, eds. *Chemically Induced Alterations in Sexual and Functional Development: The Wildlife/Human Connection.* Princeton, NJ: Princeton Scientific Publishing; 1992:113–127.

39. Dewailly E, Dodin S, Verreault R, et al. High organochlorine body burden in women with estrogen receptor-positive breast cancer. *J Natl Cancer Inst.* 1994;86:232–234.

40. Dmowski WP, Braun D, Gebel H. The immune system in endometriosis. In: Thomas EJ, Rock JA, eds. *Modern Approaches to Endometriosis.* Boston, Ma: Kluwer Academic; 1991:97–111.

41. Dunn JF, Nusula BC, Rodbard D. Transport of steroid hormones: binding of 21 endogenous steroids to both testosterone-binding globulin and corticosteroid-binding globulin in human plasma. *J Clin Endocrinol Metab.* 1981;53:58–68.

42. Ferrando R, Valette J-P. Absorption du diethystilboestrol (DES) par les plantes. Dangers d'utilisation dur fumier d'animaux traitesDES. *Eur J Toxicol.* 1976;9:335–338.

43. Fitzpatrick DW, Picken CA, Murphy LC, Buhr MM. Measurement of the relative binding affinity of zearalenone, alpha-zearalenol and beta-zearalenol for uterine and oviduct estrogen receptors in swine, rats and chickens: an indicator of estrogenic potencies. *Comp Biochem Physiol C.* 1989;94:691–694.

44. Flack Jr F, Ricci Jr A, Wolff MS, Godbold J, Deckers P. Pesticides and polychlorinated biphenyl residues in human breast lipids and their relation to breast cancer. *Arch Environ Health.* 1992;47;143–146.

45. Fox GA. Epidemiological and pathobiological evidence of contaminant-induced alterations in sexual development in free-living wildlife. In: Colburn T, Clement C, eds. *Chemically Induced Alterations in Sexual and Functional Development: The Wildlife/Human Connection.* Princeton, NJ: Princeton Scientific Publishing; 1992:147–158.

46. Franke AA, Custer LJ, Cerna CM, Narala K. Rapid HPLC analysis of dietary phytoestrogens from legumes and from human urine. *Proc Soc Exp Biol Med.* 1995;208:18–26.

47. Fry DM. Reproductive effects in birds exposed to pesticides and industrial chemicals. *Environ Health Perspect.* In press.

48. Gavaler JS, Rosenblum ER, Deal SR, Bowie BT. The phytoestrogen congeners of alcoholic beverages: current status. *Proc Soc Exp Biol Medicine.* 1995;208:98–102.

49. Gellert RJ. Utertropic activity of polychlorinated biphenyls (PCB) and induction of precocious reproductive aging in neonatally treated female rats. *Environ Res.* 1978;16:123–130.

50. George FW, Wilson JD. Sex determination and sex differentiation. In: Knobil E, Neil JD, Ewing LL, Greenwald GS, Markert CL, Pfaff DW, eds. *The Physiology of Reproduction.* New York, NY: Raven Press; 1988:3–26.

51. Gibson MK, Nemmers LA, Beckman Jr W, Davis VL, Curtis SW, Korach KS. The mechanism of ICI 164,384 antiestrogenicity involves rapid loss of estrogen receptor in uterine tissue. *Endocrinology.* 1991;129:2000–2010.

52. Gray Jr LE. Chemical-induced alterations of sexual differentiation: a review of effects in humans and rodents. In: Colburn T, Clement C, eds. *Chemically Induced Alterations in Sexual and Functional Development: The Wildlife/Human Connection.* Princeton, NJ: Princeton Scientific Publishing; 1992:203–230.

53. Greco TL, Duello TM, Gorski J. Estrogen receptors, estradiol, and diethylstilbestrol in early development: the mouse as a model for the study of estrogen receptors and estrogen sensitivity in embryonic development of male and female reproductive tracts. *Endocr Rev.* 1993;14:59–71.

54. Gronemeyer H. Control of transcription activation by steroid hormone receptors. *FASEB J.* 1992;6:2524–2529.

55. Gross TS, Guillette LJ. Pesticide induction of developmental abnormalities of the reproductive system of alligators (*Alligator mississippiensis*) and turtles (*Trachemys scripta*). Presented at the Estrogens in the Environment III: Global Health Implications meeting; 1994; Washington, DC.

56. Guillette Jr LJ, Crain DA, Rooney AA, Pickford DB. Organization versus activation: the role of endocrine-disrupting contaminants (EDCs) during embryonic development in wildlife. *Environ Health Perspect.* In press.

57. Guillette Jr LJ, Gross TS, Masson GR, Matter JM, Percival HF, Woodward AR. Developmental abnormalities of the gonad and abnormal sex hormone concentrations in juvenile alligators from contaminated and control lakes in Florida. *Environ Health Perspect.* 1994;102:680–688.

58. Haddock L, Lebron G, Martinez R, et al. Premature sexual development in Puerto Rico: Background and current status. In: McLachlan JA, ed. *Estrogens in the Environment II: Influences on Development.* New York, NY: Elsevier; 1985:358–375.

59. Hill JA. Immunological factors in endometriosis and endometriosis-associated reproductive failure. *Infertil Reprod Med Clin North Am.* 1992;3:583–596.

60. Hughes MR, Schrader WT, O'Malley BW, eds. *Laboratory Manual for Hormone Action and Molecular Endocrinology.* Houston, Texas: Houston Biological Associates, Inc; 1990.

61. Ignar-Trowbridge DM, Nelson KG, Bidwell MC, et al. Coupling of dual signaling pathways: epidermal growth factor action involves the estrogen receptor. *Proc Natl Acad Sci U S A.* 1992;89:4658.

62. Iguchi T. Cellular effects of early exposure to sex hormones and antihormones. *Int Rev Cytol.* 1992;139:1–57.

63. Jansen HT, Cooke PS, Porcelli J, Liu T-C, Hansen LG. Estrogenic and antiestrogenic actions of PCBs in the female rat: in vitro and in vivo studies. *Reprod Toxicol.* 1993;7:237–248.

64. Jobling S, Sumpter JP. Detergent components in sewage effluent are weakly oestrogenic to fish: an in vitro study using rainbow trout (*Oncorhynchus mykiss*) hepatocytes. *Aquatic Toxicol.* 1993;27:361–372.

65. Jordan VC, ed. *Estrogen/Antiestrogen Action and Breast Cancer Therapy* Madison, Wis: University of Wisconsin Press; 1986.

66. Jordan VC, Lieberman ME, Cormier E, Koch R, Bagley JR, Ruentiz PC. Structural requirements for the pharmacological activity of nonsteroidal antiestrogens in vitro. *Mol Pharmacol.* 1984;26:272–278.

67. Jost JP, Seldran M, Geiser M. Preferential binding of estrogen-receptor complex to a region containing the estrogen-dependent hypomethylation site preceding the chicken vitellogenin II gene. *Proc Natl Acad Sci U S A.* 1984;81:429–433.

68. Jukes TH. Diethylstilbestrol in beef production: what is the risk to consumers? *Prev Med.* 1976;5:438–453.

69. King R. Effects of steroid hormones and related compounds on gene transcription. *Clin Endocrinol.* 1992;36:1–14.

70. Klock G, Strahle U, Schutz G. Oestrogen and glucocorticoid responsive elements are closely related but distinct. *Nature.* 1987;329:734–736.

71. Kohno H, Gandini O, Curtis SW, Korach KS. Anti-estrogen activity in the yeast transcription system: estrogen receptor mediated agonist response. *Steroids.* 1994;59:572–578.

72. Korach KS. Insights from the study of animals lacking functional estrogen receptor. *Science.* 1994;266:1524–1527.

73. Korach KS, Metzler M, McLachlan JA. Estrogenic activity in vivo and in vitro of some diethystilbestrol metabolites and analogs. *Proc Natl Acad Sci U S A.* 1978;75:468–471.

74. Korach KS, Migliaccio S, Davis VL. Estrogens. In: Munson PL, ed. *Principles of Pharmacology: Basic Concepts and Clinical Applications.* New York, NY :Chapman and Hall; 1995:809–826.

75. Korach KS, Fox-Davies C, Quarmby VE, Swaisgood MH. Diethylstilbestrol metabolites and analogs. Biochemical probes for differential stimulation of uterine estrogen responses. *J Biol Chem.* 1985;260:15420–15426.

76. Korach KS, Sarver P, Chae K, McLachlan JA, McKinney JD. Estrogen receptor binding activity of polychlorinated hydroxybiphenyls: conformationally restricted structural probes. *Mol Pharmacol.* 1988;33:120–126.

77. Krishnan AV, Starbis P, Permuth SF, Tokes L, Feldman D. Bisphenol-A: an estrogenic substance is released from polycarbonate flasks during autoclaving. *Endocrinology.* 1993;132:2279–2286.

78. Krishnan V, Safe S. Polychlorinated biphenyls (PCBs), dibenzo-*p*-dioxins (PCDDs), dibenzofurans (PCDFs) as antiestrogens in MCF-7 human breast cancer cells: quantitative structure-activity relationships. *Toxicol Appl Pharmcol.* 1993;120:55–61.

79. Kuiper-Goodman T, Scott PM, Watanabe H. Risk assessment of the mycotoxin zearalenone. *Regul Toxicol Pharmacol.* 1987;7:253–306.

80. Lamartiniere CA, Moore J, Holland M, Barnes S. Neonatal genistein chemoprevents mammary cancer. *Proc Soc Exp Biol Med.* 1995;208:120–123.

81. Leatherland JF. Endocrine and reproductive function in Great Lakes salmon. In: Colburn T, Clement C, eds. *Chemically Induced Alterations in Sexual and Functional Development: The Wildlife/Human Connection.* Princeton, NJ: Princeton Scientific Publishing; 1992:129–145.

82. Lees JA, Fawell SE, Parker MG. Identification of two transactivation domains in the mouse oestrogen receptor. *Nucleic Acids Res.* 1989;17:5477–5488.

83. Levin W, Welch RM, Conney AH. Effect of carbon tetrachloride and other inhibitors of drug metabolism on the metabolism and action of estradiol-17 and estrone in the rat. *J Pharmacol Exp Ther.* 1970;173:247–255.

84. Levy JR, Faber KA, Ayyash L, Hughes Jr CL. The effect of prenatal exposure to phytoestrogen genistein on sexual differentiation in rats. *Proc Soc Exp Biol Med.* 1995;208:60–66.

85. Liu Y, Teng CT. Estrogen response module of the mouse lactoferrin gene contains overlapping chicken ovalbumin upstream promoter transcription factor and estrogen receptor-binding elements. *Mol Endocrinol.* 1992;6:355–364.

86. Lubahn DB, Moyer JS, Golding TS, Couse JS, Korach KS, Smithies O. Alteration of reproductive function but not prenatal sexual development after insertional disruption of the mouse estrogen receptor gene. *Proc Natl Acad Sci U S A.* 1993;90:11162–11166.

87. Luster MI, Pfeifer RW, Tucker AN. Influence of sex hormones on immunoregulation with specific reference to natural and environmental estrogens. In: Thomas JA, Korach KS, McLachlan JA, eds. *Endocrine Toxicology.* New York, NY: Raven Press: 1985:67–83.

88. Makela S, Davis VL, Tally WC, et al. Dietary estrogens act through estrogen receptor-mediated processes and show no antiestrogenicity in cultured breast cancer cells. *Environ Health Perspect.* 1994;102:572–578.

89. Makela S, Poutanen M, Lehtimaki J, Kostian M-L, Santti R, Vihko R. Estrogen specific 17fl-hydroxysteroid oxidoreductase type 1 (E.C. 1.1.1.62) as a possible target for the action of phytoestrogens. *Proc Soc Exp Biol Med.* 1995;208:51–59.

90. Martin PM, Horwitz KB, Ruyan DS, McGuire WL. Phytoestrogen interaction with estrogen receptors in human breast cancer cells. *Endocrinology.* 1978;103:1860–1867.

91. Mayr U, Butsch A, Schneider S. Validation of two in vitro test systems for estrogenic activities with zearalenone, phytoestrogens and cereal extracts. *Toxicology.* 1992;74:135–149.

92. McKinney JD, Gottschalk KE, Pederson L. A theoretical investigation of the conformation of polychlorinated biphenyls (PCB's). *J Mol Struct.* 1983;104:445–450.

93. McLachlan JA. Functional toxicology: a new approach to detect biologically active xenobiotics. *Environ Health Perspect.* 1993;101:386–387.

94. McLachlan JA, Newbold RR. Estrogens and development. *Environ Health Perspect.* 1987;75:25–27.

95. Medlock KL, Branham WS, Sheehan DM. Effects of coumestrol and equol on the developing reproductive tract of the rat. *Proc Soc Exp Biol Med.* 1995;208:67–71.

96. Medlock KL, Branham WS, Sheehan DM. The effects of phytoestrogens on neonatal rat uterine growth and development. *Proc Soc Exp Biol Med.* 1995;208:307–313.

97. Metzger D, Losson R, Bornert JM, Lemoine Y, Chambon P. Promoter specificity of the two transcriptional activation functions of the human oestrogen receptor in yeast. *Nucleic Acids Res.* 1992;20:2813–2817.

98. Metzler M. Metabolic activation of carcinogenic diethylstilbestrol in rodents and humans. *J Toxicol Environ Health*. 1976;(suppl 1):21.

99. Metzler M. The metabolism of diethylstilbestrol. *Crit Rev Biochem*. 1981;10:171–212.

100. Miksicek R. Estrogenic flavonoids: structural requirements for biological activity. *Proc So Exp Biol Med*. 1995;208:44–50.

101. Miksicek RJ. Commonly occurring plant flavonoids have estrogenic activity. *Mol Pharmacol*. 1993;44:37–43.

102. Mueller GC, Kim UH. Displacement of estradiol from estrogen receptors by simple alkyl phenols. *Endocrinology*. 1978;102:1429–1435.

103. Murphy PA. Phytoestrogen content of processed soybean products. *Food Tech (Champaign)*. 1982;34:60–64.

104. Nelson KG, Takahashi T, Bossert NL, Walmer DK, McLachlan JA. Epidermal growth factor replaces estrogen in the stimulation of female genital-tract growth and differentiation. *Proc Natl Acad Sci U S A*. 1991;88:21–25.

105. Nwannenna AI, Madej A, Lundh TJ-O, Fredriksson G. Effects of oestrogenic silage on some clinical and endocrinological parameters in ovariectomized heifers. *Acta Vet Scand*. 1994;35: 173–183.

106. Peterson RE, Moore RW, Mably TA, Bjerke DL, Goy RW. Male reproductive system ontogeny: effects of perinatal exposure to 2,3,7,8-tertachlorodibenzo-*p*-dioxin. In: Colburn T, Clement C, eds. *Chemically Induced Alterations in Sexual and Functional Development: The Wildlife/Human Connection*. Princeton, NJ: Princeton Scientific Publishing; 1992:175–193.

107. Pilat MJ, Hafner MS, Kral LG, Brooks SC. Differential induction of pS2 and cathepsin D mRNAs by structurally altered estrogens. *Biochemistry*. 1993;32:7009–7015.

108. Purdom CE, Hardiman PA, Bye VJ, Eno NC, Tyler CR, Sumpter JP. Estrogenic effects of effluents from sewage treatment works. *Chem Ecol*. 1994;8:275–285.

109. Reel JR, Lamb IV JC. Reproductive toxicology of chlordecone (Kepone). In: Thomas JA, Korach KS, McLachlan JA, eds. *Endocrine Toxicology*. New York, NY: Raven Press; 1985:357–392.

110. Reijnders PJH, Brasseur SMJM. Xenobiotic induced hormonal and associated disorders in marine organisms and related effects in humans: an overview. In: Colburn T, Clement C, eds. *Chemically Induced Alterations in Sexual and Functional Development: The Wildlife/Human Connection*. Princeton, NJ: Princeton Scientific Publishing; 1992:159–174.

111. Richard S, Zingg HH. The human oxytocin gene promoter is regulated by estrogens. *J Biol Chem*. 1990;265:6098–6103.

112. Richardson ML, Bowron JM. The fate of pharmaceutical chemicals in the aquatic environment. *J Pharm Pharmacol*. 1985;37:1–12.

113. Rier SE, Martin DC, Bowman RE, Becker JL. Immunoresponsiveness in endometriosis: implications of estrogenic toxins. *Environ Health Perspect*. In press.

114. Rier SE, Martin DC, Bowman RE, Dmowski WP, Becker JL. Endometriosis in rhesus monkeys (*Macaca mulatta*) following chronic exposure to 2,3,7,8-tetrachlordibenzo-*p*-dioxin. *Fundam Appl Toxicol*. 1993;21:433–441.

115. Robison AK, Schmidt WA, Stancel GM. Estrogenic activity of DDT: estrogen receptor profiles and the responses of individual uterine cell types following o,p¥-DDT administration. *J Toxicol Environ Health*. 1985;16:493–508.

116. Rose DP. Diet, hormones, and cancer. *Annu Rev Public Health*. 1993;14:1–17.

117. Rosenblum ER, Stauber RE, Van Thiel DH, Campbell IM, Gavaler JS. Assessment of the estrogenic activity of phytoestrogens isolated from bourbon and beer. *Alcholol Clin Exp Res*. 1993;17:1207–1209.

118. Safe S. Polychlorinate biphenyls (PCBs), dibenzo-*p*-dioxins (PCDDs), dibenzofurans (PCDFs), and related compounds: environmental and mechanistic considerations which support the development of toxic equivalency factors (TEFs). *Crit Rev Toxicol*. 1990;21:51–88.

119. Safe S, Astroff B, Harris M, et al. 2,3,7,8-Tetrachlorodibenzo-*p*-dioxin (TCDD) and related compounds as antioestrogens: characterization and mechanism of action. *Pharmacol Toxicol*. 1991;69:400–409.

120. Safe SH. Comparative toxicology and mechanism of action of polychlorinated dibenzpo-*p*-dioxins and dibenzofurnas. *Annu Rev Pharmacol Toxicol*. 1986;26:371–399.

121. Saloniemi H, Wahala K, Nykanen-Kurki P, Kallel K, Saastamoinen I. Phytoestrogen content and estrogenic effect of legume fodder. *Proc Soc Exp Biol Med*. 1995;208:13–17.

122. Setchell KDR, Gosselin SJ, Welsh MB, et al. Dietary estrogensóa probable cause of infertility and liver disease in captive cheetahs. *Gastroenterology*. 1987;93:225–233.

123. Sharpe RM, Skakkebaek NE. Are oestrogens involved in falling sperm counts and disorders of the male reproductive tract? *Lancet.* 1993;341:1392–1395.
124. Shore LS, Gurevitz M, Shemesh M. Estrogen as an environmental pollutant. *Bull Environ Contam Toxicol.* 1993;51:361–366.
125. Siiteri PK, Murai JT, Hammond GL, Nisker JA, Raymoure WJ, Kuhn RW. The serum transport of steroid hormones. *Recent Prog Horm Res.* 1982;38:457–510.
126. Slater EP, Redeuihl G, Theis K, Suske G, Beato M. The uteroglobin promoter contains a noncanonical estrogen responsive element. *Mol Endocrinol.* 1990;4:604–610.
127. Smith RG, Besch NF, Besch PK, Smith CG. Inhibition of gonadotropin by delta+9 tetrahydrocannabinol: mediation by steroid receptors. *Science.* 1979;204:325–327.
128. Solomon GL. Extra ingredients: hormones in food. *Environ Health Perspect.* 1994;102:632–635.
129. Soto AM, Justica H, Wray JW, Sonnenschein C. *p*-Nonphenol: an estrogenic xenobiotic released from "modified" polystyrene. *Environ Health Perspect.* 1991;92:167–173.
130. Soto AM, Lin T-M, Justicia H, Silvia RM, Sonnenschein C. An "in culture" bioassay to assess the estrogenicity of xenobiotics (E-SCREEN). In: Colburn T, Clement C, eds. *Chemically Induced Alterations in Sexual and Functional D evelopment: The Wildlife/Human Connection.* Princeton, NJ: Princeton Scientific Publishing; 1992:295–309.
131. Soto AM, Sonnenschein C, Chung KL, Fernandez MF, Olea N, Serrano FO. The E-SCREEN assay as a tool to identify estrogens: an update on estrogenic environmental pollutants. *Environ Health Perspect.* In press.
132. Stancel GM, Boettger-Tong HL, Chiappetta C, et al. The toxicity of endogenous and environmental estrogens: what is the role of elemental interactions? *Environ Health Perspect.* In press.
133. Thomas KB, Colburn T. Organochlorine endocrine disruptors in human tissue. In: Colburn T, Clement C, eds. *Chemically Induced Alterations in Sexual and Functional Development: The Wildlife/Human Connection.* Princeton, NJ: Princeton Scientific Publishing; 1992:365–394.
134. Thompson LU, Robb R, Serraino M, Cheung F. Mammalian lignan production from various foods. *Nutr Cancer.* 1991;16:43–52.
135. Tora L, White J, Brou C, et al. The human estrogen receptor has two independent nonacidic transcriptional activation functions. *Cell.* 1989;59:477–487.
136. Tsai MJ, O'Malley BW. Molecular mechanisms of action of steroid/thyroid receptor superfamily members. *Annu Rev Biochem.* 1994;63:451–486.
137. Tzukerman MT, Esty A, Santiso-Mere D, et al. Human estrogen receptor transactivational capacity is determined by both cellular and promoter context and mediated by two functionally distinct intramolecular regions. *Mol Endocrinol.* 1994;8:21–30.
138. VanderKuur JA, Wiese T, Brooks SC. Influence of estrogen structure on nuclear binding and progesterone receptor induction by the receptor complex. *Biochemistry.* 1993;32:7002–7009.
139. VanderKuur JA, Hafner MS, Christman JK, Brooks SC. Effects of estradiol-17 analogues on activation of estrogen response element regulated chloramphenicol acetyltransferase expression. *Biochemistry.* 1993;32:7016–21.
140. Waller DP, Killinger JM, Zaneveld LJD. Physiology and toxicology of the male reproductive tract. In: Thomas JA, Korach KS, McLachlan JA, eds. *Endocrine Toxicology.* New York, NY: Raven Press; 1985:269–333.
141. Wei H, Bowen R, Cai Q, Barnes S, Wang Y. Antioxidant and antipromotional effects of the soybean isoflavone genistein. *Proc Soc Exp Biol Med.* 1995;208:124–130.
142. Weisz A, Rosales R. Identification of an estrogen response element upstream of the human c-fos gene that binds the estrogen receptor and the AP-1 transcription factor. *Nucleic Acids Res.* 1990;18:5097–5106.
143. Weisz J. Metabolism of estrogens by target cells: diversification and amplification of hormone action and the catecholestrogen hypothesis. In: Hochberg RB, Naftolin F, eds. *New Biology of Steroid Hormones.* New York, NY: Raven Press; 1991;74:101–112.
144. Welch RM, Levin W, Conney AH. Estrogenic action of DDT and its analogs. *Toxol Appl Pharmacol.* 1969;14:358–367.
145. White R, Jobling S, Hoare SA, Sumpter JP, Parker MG. Environmentally persistent alkylphenolic compounds are estrogenic. *Endocrinology.* 1994;135:175–182.
146. Whitten PL, Naftolin F. Dietary estrogens: a biologically active background for estrogen action. In: Hochberg RB, Naftolin F, eds. *New Biology of Steroid Hormones.* New York, NY: Raven Press; 1991;74:155–167.
147. Whitten PL, Russell E, Naftolin F. Effects of a normal human-concentration phytoestrogen diet on rat uterine growth. *Steroids.* 1992;57:98–106.

148. Whitten PL, Lewis C, Russell E, Naftolin F. Phytoestrogen influences on the behavior and gonadotropin function. *Proc Soc Exp Biol Med*. 1995;208:82–86.
149. WHO. *Levels of PCBs, PCDDs, and PCDFs in Breast Milk*. Copenhagen, Denmark: World Health Organization Regional Office for Europe; 1989.
150. Williams BA, Mills KT, Burroughs CD, Bern HA. Reproductive alterations in female C57BL/Crgl mice exposed neonatally to zearalenone, an estrogenic mycotoxin. *Cancer Lett*. 1989;46:225–230.
151. Wolff MS, Toniolo PG. Environmental organochlorine exposure as a potential etiologic factor in breast cancer. *Environ Health Perspect*. In press.
152. Wolff MS, Toniolo PG, Lee EW, Rivera M, Dubin N. Blood levels of organochlorine residues and risk of breast cancer. *J Natl Cancer Inst*. 1993;85:648–652.

Endocrine Toxicology, 2nd ed.,
Edited by J. A. Thomas and H. D. Colby
Copyright © 1997 Taylor & Francis

8

Cellular and Molecular Effects of Androgenic-Anabolic Steroids

Arun K. Roy, Robert L. Vellanoweth,
Myeong H. Jung, and Bandana Chatterjee

Department of Cellular and Structural Biology, The University of Texas Health Science Center at San Antonio, San Antonio, Texas 78284-7762

HISTORICAL BACKGROUND

In 1849 Professor Berthold at the University of Göttingen made the landmark observation that the characteristic male plumage of cockerels can be maintained in the caponized birds by simply implanting a testis in the abdominal cavity. This observation started the search for the blood-borne chemical mediator later called "the internal secretions" by Claude Bernard and ushered in the beginning of endocrinology. Forty years later, the French physician Brown-Sèquard again startled the scientific community by announcing at the age of 72 that he had succeeded in a dramatic self-rejuvenation by injecting himself with an extract of dog testicles. During the next 50 years, the claim of Brown-Sèquard and supporting statements found in ancient medical texts, such as the Ayurveda of Susruta (c. 1000 BC) recommending animal testicles as a remedy for impotence, may have led to the rush for both homologous and heterologous testicular transplants in men desirous of improving their sexual ability or regaining their youthful vigor (17). At the beginning of the twentieth century one of the major proponents of the testicular transplant, Dr. Serge Voronoff, traveled all around the world to perform heterologous transplantation of monkey testes into older men. Unfortunately, much of the initial excitement of the dramatic therapeutic claims of the testicular extracts and testicular transplants did not survive careful scientific scrutiny. However, interest in the subject was strong enough to generate working hypotheses and experimental designs that eventually resulted in the isolation and characterization of testosterone, the male sex hormone. Later studies revealed that testosterone exerts profound physiologic effects not only on the reproductive organs but also on the skeletal muscle and can even influence animal behavior. The initial report of Kochakian that the androgenic component of human male urine causes positive nitrogen balance and increases the body weight of castrated dogs was immediately confirmed in humans (22,23). These observations led to the view that the anabolic or myotropic action of androgens is distinctly different from its well known reproductive actions.

ANDROGENIC VS. ANABOLIC ACTIONS
OF THE MALE SEX HORMONE

Androsterone and testosterone were initially isolated and characterized from male urine by Butenandt in 1931 and from testes by David and Laquer in 1935, respectively. Since then a large number of steroid analogs with different biological potencies for reproductive stimulation (androgenic) and myotropic function (anabolic) have been synthesized. Before the discovery of the steroid hormone receptors and understanding of the molecular mechanism of steroid hormone action, the prevailing hypothesis favored separate androgenic and anabolic domains of the steroid molecule. Strong commercial incentives resulted in the synthesis and testing of about 2000 androgen analogs with the hope of identifying a pure anabolic hormone. Although we now know that no such steroid can be created, these studies have produced a number of steroidal compounds with a high ratio of anabolic (myotropic) to androgenic (reproductive) actions. As discussed later, differences in the anabolic and androgenic potencies of synthetic steroids appear to be due to the tissue-specific expression of steroid-metabolizing enzymes, most importantly the enzyme 5α-reductase.

Hormonal steroids, including androgens, are not only inactivated in the liver through oxido-reduction and conjugation reactions but also undergo both enzymatic inactivation/activation and conversion within the target cell (15,35). The major pathways for the enzymatic modification of androgenic steroids are presented in Fig. 1.

Both sulfurylation and glucuronidation convert the androgen to its receptor-inactive form and make the steroid more hydrophilic, thereby enhancing its clearance through the kidney. Formation of androstenediol and androstanediol by the enzyme hydroxysteroid dehydrogenase facilitates their sulfo- and glucu-conjugation. However, 5α-reduction of testosterone in target cells provides a physiologic mechanism for the amplification of the androgenic signal (2,7). 5α-Dihydrotestosterone (DHT) possesses about a one order of magnitude higher binding affinity for the androgen receptor, which not only enhances the signal transduction at the level of gene transcription but also protects the receptor from proteolytic degradation (51). The enzyme 5α-reductase is rather widely expressed among both reproductive and nonreproductive targets of androgenic steroids (40). Reproductive tissues, especially the prostate and seminal vesicle, contain the highest levels of 5α-reductase, and the skeletal muscle appears to be one of the few tissues that contain the lowest level of this enzyme (50). Such a large difference in the cellular levels of 5α-reductase between the reproductive tissues and the muscle seems to be the reason for the high myotropic and low reproductive actions of certain androgen analogs such as 19-nortestosterone. Both testosterone

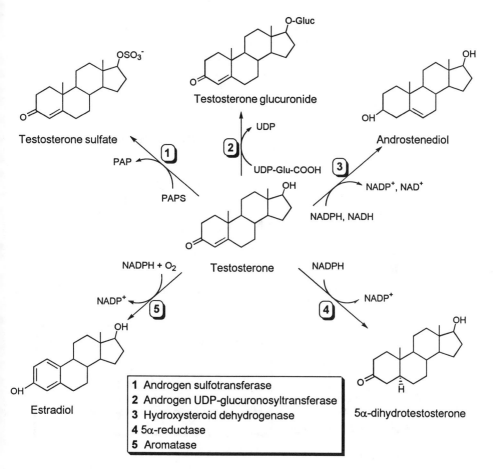

FIG 1. Major pathways for the enzymatic modification of testosterone.

and 19-nortestosterone can serve as substrates for 5α-reductase that produce DHT and 5α-dihydronortestosterone (DHN). Nortestosterone itself is one half to one third as effective as testosterone in its ability to bind to the androgen receptor in reproductive and nonreproductive tissues. However, when it is converted to its 5α derivative (DHN), its ability to interact with androgen receptor is markedly diminished (approximately 3-fold). Thus, tissues such as the prostate and seminal vesicles with high levels of 5α-reductase show a low response to nortestosterone due to its rapid conversion to DHN, while skeletal muscle, with its nearly complete absence of 5α-reductase activity, continues to utilize the steroid for the activation of the androgen receptor (45).

Much of the steroid administered orally has to pass through the liver and thus is subject to enzymatic inactivation before reaching the peripheral targets. Synthetic chemists have produced a number of androgen derivatives that can escape

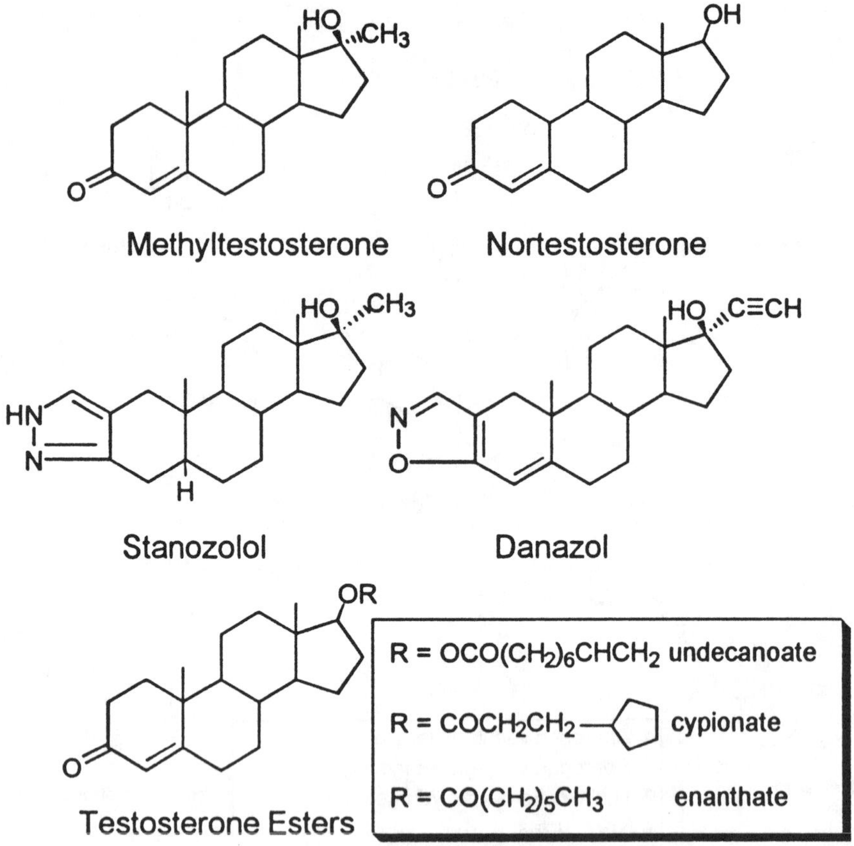

FIG 2. Structures of commonly used anabolic androgens.

the hepatic inactivation. The addition of alkyl groups on the 17α position retards the hepatic catabolism of androgenic steroids, allowing them to reach the systemic circulation. Alkylation at position 1 also serves the same purpose. Another approach to making orally effective androgens is to attach a highly hydrophobic side chain on the 17β position. For example, testosterone undecanoate is so nonpolar that after its intestinal absorption most of the steroid is partitioned to the intestinal lymph, bypassing the hepatic portal circulation. One disadvantage of the orally effective androgens for long-term treatment is the high turnover rate requiring more than one intake per day. This problem can be circumvented by parenteral administration of various carboxylic esters of testosterone. These esters are highly nonpolar and fat-soluble and are slowly released from the site of injection (21). Testosterone cypionate and testosterone enanthate need to be administered only once every 2-3 weeks to maintain high circulating levels of the hormone during the time between the injections. The chemical structures of some of the orally effective and long-acting anabolic androgens are presented in Fig. 2.

ANDROGEN RECEPTOR AND ANDROGEN RESPONSE ELEMENTS

In order to appreciate the androgenic-anabolic actions of the androgenic steroids, a concise review of the androgen receptor and the androgen response element is essential (37). The androgen receptor is a member of the superfamily of transcription factors that includes the steroid, thyroid, retinoic acid receptors (11,19). In the absence of ligand, the androgen receptor exists in the cytoplasm in a hypophosphorylated state complexed with heat shock proteins (46). When bound to the androgens, it undergoes a conformational change that facilitates receptor phosphorylation and its dissociation from heat shock proteins. The ligand-bound activated receptor translocates to the nucleus and binds as a homodimer to the target gene at the androgen response element (ARE). The AREs are generally localized to the promoter region of the target gene, although examples of intragenic AREs are also known. It is presumed that the DNA-bound receptor interacts with the component proteins of the basal transcription machinery, either directly or via specific bridging factors, and modulates the rate of target gene transcription (30). Additional regulatory processes involving DNA bending at the receptor-binding site, nucleosome displacement, recruitment of coregulators, and displacement of an activator/repressor from the binding site can also influence the androgenic response (1,31–33). For this article, it is important to note that certain structural features of the androgenic steroid may play critical roles in mediating the tissue-specific response that is central to the anabolic and androgenic functions. For example, both testosterone and DHT are capable of activating the receptor protein. However, the testosterone–androgen receptor complex exhibits 3-fold faster dissociation kinetics than the DHT–androgen receptor complex, and the unliganded but activated androgen receptor is rapidly degraded (51). Thus, certain steroid derivatives may only provide a transient effect, while others with slower dissociation kinetics can prolong the hormone action.

Similar to other members of the steroid receptor superfamily, the androgen receptor protein is segmented into several functional domains. The amino acid sequences of the centrally located DNA-binding domain and the C-terminal hormone-binding domain of the androgen receptor are highly homologous to similar domains in other steroid receptors (9). The amino-terminal sequence of the androgen receptor, on the other hand, is not conserved. The DNA-binding domain of 66 amino acids contains nine conserved cysteine residues, eight of which form two zinc-coordinated stem-loop structures, known as type II zinc fingers, that can intercalate into the DNA duplex. The DNA-binding domain of the androgen receptor displays the strongest sequence homology (79–82%) to the progesterone receptor and the glucocorticoid/mineralocorticoid receptor. As a consequence, the androgen receptor, progesterone receptor, and glucocorticoid/mineralocorticoid receptor all recognize the 15-base pair (15-bp) steroid response element (and its minor variations), which has the following nucleotide sequence:5'-GG (A/T)ACAnnnTGTTCT-3', where *n* represents nonspecific bases. The first zinc finger in the receptor structure directs target gene specificity, and the second zinc finger stabilizes receptor–DNA interactions (4,48). The hormone binding domain of the androgen receptor comprises 258 amino acids at the carboxy terminus. An approximately 500-amino-acid-long amino terminal domain seems to have an essential role in the transactivating function of the androgen receptor (20,39,42). Interaction between the amino terminus and steroid-binding regions of the androgen receptor also plays an important role in the transcriptional regulatory function of the androgen receptor (42). The receptor is encoded by a single-copy gene localized over approximately 90 kilobase (kb) pairs of the human chromosome at Xq11-q12 (6,12).

As mentioned earlier, a 15-bp consensus androgen response element/progesterone response element/glucocorticoid response element (ARE/GRE/PRE) binds to androgen receptor, progesterone receptor, and glucocorticoid/mineralocorticoid receptor with almost equal affinity in vitro, and all of these receptors can mediate reporter gene expression in transfected cells directed by this consensus element. This observation raises the issue of the mechanism of hormonal specificity for androgen, progesterone and glucocorticoid action. One way to maintain the physiologic specificity for each class of steroid hormones is through tissue-specific, differential expression of the receptor gene. However, multiple types of hormone receptors are simultaneously expressed in the same cell. Under these circumstances, protein–protein interactions involving the DNA-bound receptor and auxiliary factors, which bind to DNA sequences overlapping or neighboring the androgen response element, can impose specificity in steroid–receptor interactions with the core transcription machinery. For most naturally occurring androgen regulated genes, such as the rat probasin and human prostate-specific antigen, the androgen response elements do not exactly conform to the consensus ARE/GRE/PRE sequence (27,30,32,34). These minor sequence variations within the consensus element may also contribute to the receptor specificity for the target genes.

TISSUE-SPECIFIC EFFECTS OF ANDROGENIC-ANABOLIC STEROIDS

It has already been emphasized that androgenic and anabolic designations of male sex hormones are merely operational terms that are determined by the tissue-specific metabolism of these hormonal steroids. Furthermore, according to unpublished results from our laboratory, all tissues express detectable but variable amounts of the androgen receptor gene and thus constitute potential targets for the androgens. Since the purpose of this review is to inform the reader about toxicologic rather than physiologic aspects of androgen action, we will focus our discussion on the cellular and molecular effects of these steroids primarily in nonreproductive tissues such as the liver and muscle.

The central role of the liver in steroid metabolism has already been mentioned. In addition to its role in steroid inactivation, the liver also serves as an important target for the androgenic steroids (36). In fact, many of the pathologic conditions

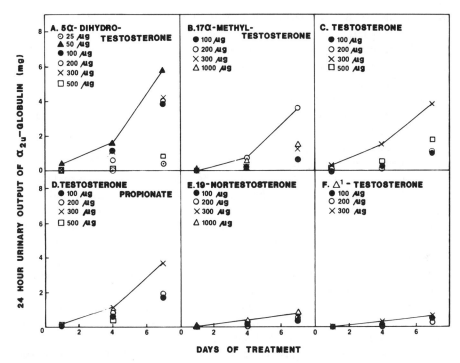

FIG 3. Comparative effects of androgenic and anabolic steroids on the hepatic induction of α_{2u}-globulin in the rat. Various doses of testosterone and testosterone derivatives (μg/100 g body wt) were administered daily as subcutaneous injections to ovariectomized female rats, and the daily urinary output of α_{2u}-globulin was determined by specific immunoassay. Each point is an average of values from four experimental animals. The points representing the optimum doses are joined together. Based on this assay, the potencies of various androgenic steroids are as follows (A–F): 5α-dihydrotestosterone > 17α-methyl testosterone > testosterone > testosterone propionate > 19-nortestosterone >Δ+1-testosterone. (From ref. 38, with permission.)

associated with prolonged use of the androgenic-anabolic steroids emanate from the adverse effects of these steroids on hepatic gene expression. Earlier reports from our laboratory have described detailed analyses of the androgenic regulation of α_{2u}-globulin in the rat liver (38). α_{2u}-Globulin is a male pheromone-binding protein and is the major secretory protein produced by the liver of male rats. α_{2u}-Globulin is almost quantitatively filtered through the kidneys into the urine, providing a convenient noninvasive method to monitor its daily output. The liver also expresses a high level of 5α-reductase (40), and thus it is likely that both testosterone and nortestosterone are mostly converted to DHT and DHN in the liver before they interact with the androgen receptor. Results presented in Fig. 3 show that the synthetic anabolic steroid nortestosterone is a very weak inducer of α_{2u}-globulin. Compared with DHT, nortestosterone is about 40-fold less effective in stimulating α_{2u}-globulin production. These results indicate that the receptor-binding data, suggesting about 16-fold lower affinity of DHN than DHT for the androgen receptor (45), may be an overestimation of nortestosterone function. Furthermore, 17α-methyl testosterone functions considerably better than testosterone in the stimulation of α_{2u}-globulin synthesis. The latter observation is in accord with the expectation that because of its 17α-alkylation, methyl testosterone is a poor substrate for the hepatic steroid-inactivating enzymes. Thus, lower receptor affinity of methyl testosterone is more than compensated by its ability to withstand hepatic catabolism.

The skeletal muscle represent about one third of the total body mass, and it also happens to be an important target for androgenic steroids (29). Soon after the chemical characterization of androgens, both animal experiments and human studies showed that these hormonal steroids cause nitrogen retention and an increase in body weight (22,23). Subsequent studies revealed that the increase in body weight is due to a corresponding increase in muscle mass. It was also established that castration or androgen supplementation does not change the number of myofibrils but rather alters the protein content of the individual myofibrils (24,25). Such a myotropic effect of the androgen has raised two major scientific enigmas: (1) the possible existence of a purely anabolic steroid acting through a nonandrogen receptor mechanism, and (2) the mechanism of the myotropic action of the hormone in the young adult male, where physiologic levels of androgens are sufficient to saturate all of the available androgen receptor.

As mentioned earlier, a massive amount of effort has gone into the synthesis and testing of androgen analogs, with the hope of identifying a purely anabolic steroid. These studies have not produced adequate success, and results obtained so far can be explained on the basis of tissue-specific differences in enzymatic alterations of these androgen analogs, followed by their action through the mediation of the androgen receptor (8). These issues have already been discussed (see "Androgenic vs. Anabolic Actions of the Male Sex Hormone" above) and will not be repeated here, save to mention that we have noted a relatively high level of androgen receptor gene expression in the skeletal muscle. In our laboratory, we have developed a highly sensitive and reproducible reverse transcriptase/polymerase chain reaction–based assay for the androgen receptor mRNA (44). Results presented in Fig. 4 show that the level of the androgen receptor in the skeletal muscle is almost as high as that in the kidney, a well accepted androgen target, and is about 2-fold higher than in the liver. Although the high level of the androgen receptor has already been documented in the levator ani muscle (3), critics have argued that this particular muscle is a reproductive tissue and the presence of the androgen receptor in the levator ani is not reflective of a receptor-based action of anabolic steroids in the skeletal muscle. However, our results clearly establish that, based on the receptor mRNA content, the skeletal muscle can indeed be considered an important target for the androgenic steroids.

It is generally accepted that the circulating levels of androgens in the normal male are several-fold higher than the dissociation constant (K_d) of the androgen receptor for its ligands (8). In this situation, almost all of the receptors in the

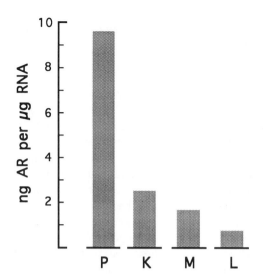

FIG 4. Comparative levels of the androgen receptor mRNA in the skeletal muscle, prostate, kidney and liver in young adult (3-month-old) male rats. Androgen receptor (AR) mRNA was assayed by the competitive reverse transcriptase/polymerase chain reaction (44). Steady-state levels of AR mRNAs per μg total RNA in the prostate (P), kidney (K), skeletal muscle from the hind leg (M), and liver (L) are shown.

target tissues of young adult males will be saturated with androgenic steroids. If the myotropic action of the androgens is mediated via the androgen receptor system, as appears to be the case, then the stimulatory effect of pharmacologic doses of androgens on muscle mass in the male becomes a regulatory paradox. A number of authors have suggested that androgens in pharmacologic doses can function as glucocorticoid antagonists and this may be the mechanism for its myotropic action in the young adult male (26,28). This argument is based on the fact that glucocorticoids are known to induce protein catabolism. The antiglucocorticoid effect of high levels of androgens may therefore prevent protein catabolism in the muscles without any change in protein synthesis and thereby increase muscle mass. One problem with this explanation is that it invokes two separate mechanisms for the myotropic action of androgens, ie, one for the male mediated through glucocorticoid receptor and another for the female mediated via androgen receptor. In the light of a recent report showing differential stability of the androgen receptor after its binding to different hormonal ligands (51), it is very plausible that pharmacologic doses of anabolic steroids promote an androgen receptor–mediated increase in muscle protein synthesis both in the male and female by reducing the normal rate of receptor turnover.

PATHOLOGIC MANIFESTATIONS OF
CHRONIC ANDROGEN TREATMENT

A chronically high level of circulating androgens causes virilization in women and a marked decrease of gonadotropin secretion in men (49). In young adult women, pharmacologic doses of androgens cause hirsutism, acne, alopecia, clitorimegaly, amenorrhea, and other virilizing symptoms. In men, low levels of gonadotropins can result in the shrinkage of the testes and azoospermia. Conversion of a small percentage of the androgens to estrogenic steroids in the adipose tissue can also lead to gynecomastia. Many of these reproductive abnormalities are reversible after discontinuation of the androgen treatment. In addition to these reproductive abnormalities, high doses of androgens can also cause toxic effects in both sexes. A number of reports have described serious liver pathology associated with the chronic use of androgenic steroids (5,10,13,16,47). Since androgens promote erythropoiesis through increased erythropoietin production, patients suffering from Fanconi's anemia are often treated with androgenic steroids. These patients frequently develop liver pathology involving generalized hyperplasia, hyperplastic nodules, and benign hepatomas. Protracted androgen treatment also results in the development of blood-filled cysts in the liver known as peliosis hepatitis (5,10). Dysfunctions of bile metabolism leading to jaundice are also frequently seen in healthy adults taking high doses of androgenic steroids (43). Similar to the reproductive abnormalities, many of these liver pathologies are generally reversed after discontinuation of the androgen treatment (49).

We have already mentioned that the liver is an important target for androgenic steroids and produces a number of secretory proteins with important transport functions (38). Hepatic synthesis of some of these proteins is under the regulation of sex hormones, and supraphysiologic levels of androgens can adversely affect their homeostasis. For example, hepatic production of apolipoproteins is regulated by sex hormones, and supraphysiologic doses of androgens simultaneously increase the circulating levels of low density lipoproteins and decrease the high density lipoproteins, thus adversely affecting cholesterol homeostasis and predisposing the androgen-treated subject to atherosclerosis (18,41). In addition to these functional abnormalities and tumorigenesis, ultrastructural changes in the parenchymal cells of the liver after both short- and long-term treatment with androgenic steroids have also been reported (14).

SUMMARY AND CONCLUSIONS

With the discovery of two apparently distinct effects of the male sex hormones, one androgenic primarily influencing reproductive functions, and the other anabolic increasing the skeletal muscle mass, it has been suggested that these hormones may act on target organs by two different mechanisms. Biochemical and molecular biological studies have shown, however, that all androgens act through a single steroid hormone receptor, the androgen receptor. This protein is encoded by a single gene localized on the X chromosome. On binding of the hormone ligand, the conformationally altered receptor protein is transported to the cell nucleus, where it seeks out and interacts with specific DNA sequence elements (androgen response elements) in the promoters of target genes. Through protein–protein contacts with the basal transcriptional machinery, either directly or through intermediaries, the transcription rate of the target gene is enhanced, giving rise to higher levels of the gene product. Given that the androgen receptor is present in all tissues examined, every tissue in the body is a potential target for androgen action. Differences in the levels of the androgen receptor in various tissues may play some role in the degree of the effect of the androgens on physiologic responses. Perhaps the major contributor to differential androgen response is the various means by which the ligand can be enzymatically modified. These modifications include sulfurylation, glucuronidation, oxido-reduction and aromatization, which decrease, increase, or alter the ability of the ligand to activate the receptor protein, respectively. Herein probably lies the mechanism for the observed differences in the anabolic versus androgenic activities of the various male sex hormones, both natural and synthetic. For example, male reproductive tissues, unlike the skeletal muscle, contain high levels of 5α-reductase, which converts testosterone to DHT, a compound ten times better able to activate the androgen receptor. In reproductive tissues, anabolic steroids such as 19-nortestosterone are also acted on by 5α-reductase. The 5α-reduced nortestosterone has a markedly lower affinity for the receptor than the parent steroid. Thus, nortestosterone rapidly loses its receptor-binding ability in the reproductive tissues, while maintaining its full potency in the muscle. The abuse of anabolic steroids among athletes leads to numerous detrimental side effects in the reproductive organs, as well as in nonreproductive targets, especially in the liver of both males and females. Given the limited knowledge of the numbers and types of liver genes stimulated or repressed by the androgen receptor, it is difficult to pinpoint the exact mechanism by which altered androgen action gives rise to these pathologies. Continued study of the genes regulated by the androgen receptor under normal and pathologic conditions will begin to provide a mechanistic understanding of these side effects.

ACKNOWLEDGMENTS

Supported by NIH grant R-37 DK 14744.
We thank Ms. Katrine Krueger for her excellent secretarial assistance.

REFERENCES

1. Akerblom IE, Slater EP, Beato M, Baxter JD, Mellon PL. Negative regulation by glucocorticoids through interference with a cAMP response enhancer. *Science.* 1988;241:350–353.
2. Anderson KM, Liao S. Selective retention of dihydrotestosterone by prostatic nuclei. *Nature.* 1968;219:277–279.
3. Bartsch W, Krieg M, Voigt KD. Quantification of endogenous testosterone, 5α-dihydrotestosterone and 5α-androstane-3α-, 17β-diol in subcellular fractions of the prostate, bulbocabernosus/levator ani muscle, skeletal muscle and heart muscle of the rat. *J Steroid Biochem.* 1980;13:259–264.
4. Beato M. Gene regulation by steroid hormones. *Cell.* 1989;56:335–344.
5. Boyd PR, Mark GL. Multiple hepatic adenomas and a hepatocellular carcinoma in a man on oral methyl testosterone for eleven years. *Cancer.* 1977;40:1765–1770.
6. Brown CJ, Goss SJ, Lubahn DB, et al. Androgen receptor locus on the human X chromosome: regional localization to Xq11-12 and description of a DNA polymorphism. *Am J Hum Genet.* 1989;44:264–269.
7. Bruchovsky N, Wilson JD. The conversion of testosterone to 5α-androstan-17β-ol-3-one by rat prostate in vivo and in vitro. *J Biol Chem.* 1968;243:2012–2021.
8. Celotti F, Cesi PN. Anabolic steroids: a review of their effects on the muscles, of their possible mechanisms of action and their use in athletics. *J Steroid Biochem Mol Biol.* 1992;43:469–477.

9. Chang CS, Kokontis J, Liao ST. Structural analysis of complementary DNA and amino acid sequences of human and rat androgen receptors. *Proc Natl Acad Sci U S A.* 1988;85:7211–7215.

10. Coombes GB, Reiser J, Paradinas EJ, Burr I. An androgen associated hepatic adenoma in a transsexual. *Br J Surg.* 1978;65:869–870.

11. Evans RM. The steroid and thyroid hormone receptor superfamily. *Science.* 1988;240:889–895.

12. Faber PW, van Rooij HC, van der Korput HA, *et al.* Characterization of the human androgen receptor transcription unit. *J Biol Chem.* 1991;266:10743–10749.

13. Falk H, Thomas LB, Popper H, Ishak KG. Hepatic angiosarcoma associated with androgenic-anabolic steroids. *Lancet.* 1979;2:1120–1123.

14. Gragera R, Saborido A, Molano F, Jimenez L, Muniz E, Megias A. Ultrastructural changes induced by anabolic steroids in liver of trained rats. *Histol Histopathol.* 1993;8:49–55.

15. Gurpide E. Enzymatic modulation of hormonal action at the target tissue. *J Toxicol Environ Health.* 1978;4:249–268.

16. Hickson RC, Ball KL, Falduto MT. Adverse effects of anabolic steroids. *Med Toxicol Adverse Drug Exp.* 1989;4:254–271.

17. Hoberman JM, Yesalis CE. The history of synthetic testosterone. *Sci Am.* 1995;272:76–81.

18. Hurley BF, Seals DR, Hagberg JM, *et al.* High-density-lipoprotein cholesterol in bodybuilders and powerlifters. Negative effects of androgen use. *JAMA.* 1984;252:507–513.

19. Hutchison KA, Dittmar KD, Pratt WB. All of the factors required for assembly of the glucocorticoid receptor into a functional heterocomplex with heat shock protein 90 are preassociated in a self-sufficient protein folding structure, a "foldosome." *J Biol Chem.* 1994;269:27894–27899.

20. Jenster G, van der Korput HA, van Vroonhoven C, van der Kwast TH, Trapman J, Brinkmann AO. Domains of the human androgen receptor involved in steroid binding, transcriptional activation, and subcellular localization. *Mol Endocrinol.* 1991;5:1396–1404.

21. Junkmann K. Long-acting steroids in reproduction. *Recent Prog Horm Res.* 1957;13:389–428.

22. Kenyon AT, Sandiford I, Bryan AH, Knowlton K, Koch FC. The effect of testosterone propionate on nitrogen, electrolyte, water and energy metabolism in eunuchoidism. *Endocrinology.* 1938;23:135–153.

23. Kochakian CD. Effect of male hormone on protein metabolism of castrate dogs. *Proc Soc Exp Biol Med.* 1935;32:1064–1065.

24. Kochakian CD, Tillotson C. Influence of several steroids on the growth of individual muscles of the guinea pig. *Endocrinology.* 1957;60:607–618.

25. Kochakian CD, Tillotson C, Austin J, Dougherty A, Haage V, Coalson R. The effect of castration on the weight and composition of the muscles of the guinea pig. *Endocrinology.* 1956;58:315–326.

26. Konagaya M, Max SR. A possible role for endogenous glucocorticoid in orchiectomy-induced atrophy of the rat levator ani muscle: studies with RU38486, a potent glucocorticoid agonist. *J Steroid Biochem.* 1986;25:305–308.

27. Luke MC, Coffey DS. Human androgen receptor binding to the androgen response element of prostate specific antigen. *J Androl.* 1994;15:41–51.

28. Mayer M, Rosen F. Interaction of glucocorticoids and androgens with skeletal muscle. *Metabolism.* 1977;26:937–962.

29. Mooradian AD, Morley JE, Korenman SG. Biological actions of androgens. *Endocr Rev.* 1987;8:1–28.

30. Nardulli AM, Shapiro DJ. DNA bending by nuclear receptors. *Receptor.* 1993;3:247–255.

31. Pearce D, Yamamoto KR. Mineralocorticoid and glucocorticoid receptor activities distinguished by nonreceptor factors at a composite response element. *Science.* 1993;259:1161–1165.

32. Rennie PS, Bruchovsky N, Leco KJ, *et al.* Characterization of two cis-acting DNA elements involved in the androgen regulation of the probasin gene. *Mol Endocrinol.* 1993;7:23–36.

33. Richard-Foy H, Hager GL. Sequence-specific positioning of nucleosomes over the steroid-inducible MMTV promoter. *EMBO J.* 1987;6:2321–2328.

34. Riegman PHJ, Vlietstra RJ, van der Korput JAGM, Brinkmann AO, Trapman J. The promoter of the prostate-specific antigen gene contains a functional androgen responsive element. *Mol Endocrinol.* 1991;5:1921–1930.

35. Roy AK. Regulation of hormone action in target cells by specific hormone inactivating enzymes. *Proc Soc Exp Biol Med.* 1992;199:265–272.

36. Roy AK, Chatterjee B. Sexual dimorphism in the liver. *Annu Rev Physiol.* 1983;45:37–50.

37. Roy AK, Chatterjee B. Androgen action. *Crit Rev Eukaryot Gene Expr.* 1995;5:157–177.

38. Roy AK, Chatterjee B, Demyan WF, Milin BS, Motwani NM, Nath T, Schiop MJ. Hormone and age-dependent regulation of α_{2u} globulin gene expression. *Recent Prog Horm Res.* 1983;39:425–461.

39. Rundlett SE, Wu X, Miesfeld RL. Functional characterization of the androgen receptor confirms that the molecular basis of androgen action is transcriptional regulation. *Mol Endocrinol.* 1990;4:708–714.

40. Russell DW, Wilson JD. Steroid 5α-reductase: two genes/two enzymes. *Annu Rev Biochem.* 1994;63:26–61.
41. Semmens J, Rouse I, Beilin LJ, Masarei JRL. Relationship of plasma HDL cholesterol to testosterone, estradiol and sex hormone binding globulin levels in men and in women. *Metabolism.* 1983;32:428–432.
42. Simental JA, Sar M, Lane MV, French FS, Wilson EM. Transcriptional activation and nuclear targeting signals of the human androgen receptor. *J Biol Chem.* 1991;266:510–518.
43. Slater SD, Davidson JF, Patrick RS. Jaundice induced by stanozolol hypersensitivity. *Postgrad Med J.* 1976;52:229–232.
44. Supakar PC, Song CS, Jung MH, *et al.* A novel regulatory element associated with age-dependent expression of the rat androgen receptor gene. *J Biol Chem.* 1993;268:26400–26408.
45. Toth M, Zakar T. Relative binding affinities of testosterone, 19-nortestosterone and their 5α-reduced derivatives to the androgen receptor and to other androgen-binding proteins: a suggested role of 5α-reductive steroid metabolism in the dissociation of "myotropic" and "androgenic" activities of 19-nortestosterone. *J Steroid Biochem.* 1982;17:653–660.
46. Tsai MJ, O'Malley BW. Molecular mechanisms of action of steroid/thyroid receptor superfamily members. *Annu Rev Biochem.* 1994;63:451–486.
47. Turani H, Levi J, Zevin D, Kessler E. Hepatic lesions in patients on anabolic androgenic therapy. *Isr J Med Sci.* 1983;19:332–337.
48. Umesono K, Evans RM. Determinants of target gene specificity for steroid/thyroid hormone receptor. *Cell.* 1989;57:1139–1146.
49. Wilson JD. Androgen abuse by athletes. *Endocr Rev.* 1988;9:181–199.
50. Wilson JD, Gloyna RE. Intranuclear metabolism of testosterone in the accessory organs of male reproduction. *Recent Prog Horm Res.* 1970;26:309–336.
51. Zhou Z, Lane MV, Kemppainen JA, French FS, Wilson EM. Specificity of ligand-dependent androgen receptor stabilization: receptor domain interactions influence ligand dissociation and receptor stability. *Mol Endocrinol.* 1995;9:208–218.

Endocrine Toxicology, 2nd ed.,
Edited by J. A. Thomas and H. D. Colby
Copyright © 1997 Taylor & Francis

9

Role of Cadmium in the Etiology of Cancer of the Prostate

Michael P. Waalkes, *Sabine Rehm, †Timothy P. Coogan, and ‡Jerrold M. Ward

*Inorganic Carcinogenesis Section, and ‡Office of Laboratory Animal Sciences National Cancer Institute, Frederick Cancer Research and Development Center, Frederick, Maryland 21702-1201; *Department of Toxicology, Smithkline Beecham Pharmaceuticals, King of Prussia, Pennsylvania 19406; †Robert Wood Johnson Pharmaceutical Research Institute, Spring House, Pennsylvania 19477*

CADMIUM AND PROSTATIC DISEASE

Prostate cancer in humans is a common and often lethal neoplastic disease. In many countries, including the United States, the incidence and mortality rate of prostate cancer continue to rise. Prostate cancer has a complex etiologic basis making linkage to a single factor difficult to detect. Cadmium is a metallic toxin of continuing environmental and occupational concern. Epidemiologic studies indicate that exposure to cadmium is occasionally associated with human malignant prostatic disease. Studies also indicate that cadmium levels in the human prostate positively correlate with neoplasia. The association between cadmium and human prostate cancer remains controversial, and until recently there was a lack of relevant evidence in animals. However, over the last few years several rodent studies have indicated that cadmium can induce prostate tumors in the rat. Some of these chronic studies indicate a possible hormonal dependence of cadmium-induced prostatic carcinogenesis. Other supportive work includes the finding of malignant transformation of rat prostatic epithelial cells with cadmium exposure *in vitro*. Additionally, one of the primary cellular tolerance systems for detoxication of cadmium, specifically the metallothionein gene, appears to be poorly active in the region of the rat prostate that is sensitive to cadmium carcinogenicity. Development of prostate cancer in rats after exposure to cadmium supports but does not conclusively establish a possible role for this toxic metal in the etiology of human prostate cancer. Additional effort is required to define the precise role of cadmium in this important human malignancy.

Exposure to cadmium, a very toxic metal, continues to be a substantial environmental and occupational concern. Cadmium has several diverse acute and chronic toxic effects (29,30), including carcinogenicity (47,98,101). Cadmium was recently accepted by the International Agency for Research on Cancer as a human carcinogen (47), primarily based on activity as a pulmonary carcinogen (82). Cadmium is also an effective and potent rodent carcinogen and has been associated with tumors of the lung, testes, and hematopoietic system among other possible sites (47,96,98,101).

Prostate cancer is a common and potentially lethal malignant disease in humans. Of recent concern is the observation that both the incidence and mortality rate of prostate cancer continue to rise in the United States (83). Prostate cancer has a very complex etiology, being dependent on a variety of, as yet, only poorly defined elements. This multifactorial etiology makes linkage to a single factor, such as cadmium exposure, difficult to establish (63). Though genetic makeup probably plays an important role in dictating general sensitivity, incidence rates in immigrant populations indicate that environmental factors are also important in the development of prostate cancer.

Exposure to cadmium has been linked with human prostate cancer in several but not all epidemiologic studies. This association has been controversial, in part because of a previous lack of applicable animal data. In the last several years, experimental data supporting a possible role of cadmium in the etiology of prostate cancer have accumulated, including results of chronic carcinogenicity testing in rats. This chapter will discuss the epidemiologic and experimental data that support a potential role for cadmium as an etiologic component in the development of prostate cancer.

ASPECTS OF PROSTATE ANATOMY AND PHYSIOLOGY RELEVANT TO CANCER

A primary experimental model for human prostate cancer has been the rat. The rat prostate is arranged in multiple, discrete bilateral lobes including the ventral lobes, dorsolateral lobes, and the dorsocranial lobes (39). The dorsocranial lobes are located on the concave aspect of the seminal vesicles and often are referred to as coagulation gland. Embryologically, the prostate epithelium in the rat is derived from the endoderm, while the seminal vesicle epithelium stems from the mesoderm (37). Precisely how the prostatic lobes of the rat compare to the very different anatomic organization of the human prostate is not absolutely defined. The human prostate is a compact organ, in which three different, distinct anatomic zones have been identified, including a large peripheral zone, a central zone, and a small transition zone. Most human prostate cancers (70%) arise in the peripheral zone, while 25% or more of all cancers are found in the transition zone; the remainder are located in the central zone (57). It has been proposed that the ventral prostate of the rat embryologically has no human homologue (70), and therefore tumors arising in this lobe would not be a relevant model for human cancer (9). However, it is not currently clear whether an embryologic homology is equivalent to a functional or pathologic homology, and how these various aspects will contribute to the understanding of prostate tumor etiology and pathogenesis remains to be defined. As there is certainly no perfect animal model for prostate cancer (13)—and given the importance of the disease for humans—any study that may indicate possible etiologic factors should be considered of value. Because of the anatomic, physiologic, and pathologic differences between the prostate gland in the human and rat, it is very difficult to draw valid comparisons; however, it seems premature to disqualify lesions arising in the ventral prostate of the rat as irrelevant for prostatic disease in humans.

Spontaneous tumor development in the rat is common in the ventral lobes but rarely occurs in the dorsolateral lobes (8). In contrast, chemically induced prostate carcinomas typically occur in the dorsolateral prostate (11,45,60,75). Several chemical compounds, often in conjunction with supplementary hormonal treatment, induce invasive carcinomas indiscriminately in seminal vesicles and dorsocranial prostate in rats, which, like most human prostate cancers, exhibit a glandular pattern, readily invade, form scirrhous components, and metastasize to the lung (87). However, these tumors do not show the complete histologic range of malignancies seen in the human prostate. Tumors arising in the rat ventral lobe frequently do not extend beyond the confinements of the organ, do not metastasize, and do not show significant scirrhous components (68,74,103,104).

Tumors arising in the rat ventral prostate do, however, exhibit a cribriform growth pattern and may form squamous cell carcinomas (68,74,103,104), and though these histologic variants do not occur in tumors arising from the dorsolateral or dorsocranial lobe, they are not infrequently observed in human prostate cancers (58,108).

Furthermore, invasive carcinomas in the seminal vesicles are frequently induced in experimental models with rats (15,87), and unless studied histologically at early stages of tumor development, they may be mistaken for prostatic neoplasms arising from the dorsolateral prostate. For instance, in a system intended as a model for prostate cancer, a high incidence of prostate carcinomas is reported after *N*-nitrosomethylurea and testosterone implants in Lobund Wistar rats (64–66). However, these tumors were frequently measured only as palpable masses and not histologically, or otherwise analyzed at a late stage in tumor progression. When studied at an early stage, this model has been found actually to result in more than a 70% incidence of carcinomas of the seminal vesicles that are highly malignant, show early invasion, grow quickly into large palpable masses, and metastasize to the peritoneal cavity and lung (15,87). Few carcinomas of the other accessory sex glands are found with this system, and almost none become large palpable masses that metastasize (15,87). Despite the assertion to the contrary (64), a grossly visible tumor 0.5–1.5 cm in diameter should probably not be considered as an early manifestation specifically of a prostate tumor, particularly considering the invasive nature of these seminal vesicle neoplasms and the close proximity of the accessory sex glands in the male rat. Although comparative studies in the rat may help resolve some of these issues, selection of a single rodent model for prostate cancer may not be a realistic choice because the human disease is highly variable and clearly multifaceted in nature (13).

The structural maintenance and proper functioning of the male accessory sex tissues, including the prostate, depends on androgens (14). Castration or estrogen treatment can result in severe prostatic atrophy (14,20,28). Prostate tumors are likewise frequently androgen-dependent in the early stages of development and can show regression with castration or estrogen therapy (14,20,28). Androgens can also be effective alone or in combined treatments as promoters of prostatic carcinogenesis in rodent models (12,60,68,77). Elevated levels of circulating androgen have been associated in some studies with human prostate cancer (10).

Cadmium, at sufficient doses, can rapidly induce severe necrosis of the rodent testes, resulting subsequently in chronic testicular degeneration and atrophy (31,103). This causes a loss of testicular function, including a marked decline in androgen secretion (31). Doses of cadmium below the level required for induction of overt testicular necrosis can also adversely affect testicular androgen production (54). Consequently, accessory sex tissue regression and atrophy can occur (30), a factor that may have direct bearing on the ability of cadmium to induce prostatic carcinogenesis in rodents. In addition to this effect, cadmium exposure can also cause testicular proliferative lesions or tumors in rats, mice, and hamsters (103–105).

CADMIUM AND PROSTATE CANCER IN HUMANS

Epidemiologic Studies-Occupational Exposure

The human epidemiology of cadmium and cancer has recently been reviewed (47). With regard to cancer of the prostate, Potts (67) reported an association between cadmium exposure and prostate cancer in workers from two nickel-cadmium battery plants in the United Kingdom who had been exposed for at least 20 years. Three deaths from prostate cancer were identified in a total of 74 workers (67). Kipling and Waterhouse (50), using a larger group of men from the same plants who had been exposed to cadmium for 1 or more years (248 total workers), found an additional case of death from prostate cancer. The total of four cases in these workers constituted a significantly elevated incidence in comparison with regional death rates from prostate cancer (50). In a further study of workers in these same two nickel-cadmium battery plants, eight prostate cancer deaths in 458 workers who had been employed for at least 1 year in jobs involving high cadmium exposure were detected, a significant elevation over the expected rates (eight observed, 1.99 expected) (81).

In a Swedish cadmium plant, Kjellström *et al.* (51) found a significant elevation of prostate cancer in 94 cadmium-exposed workers when compared with a unexposed group of 328 men. This elevation was not, however, statistically significant when compared with the prevailing regional rates (51).

Lemen et al. (55), investigating a group of 292 white males in a United States plant with 2 or more years of cadmium exposure, found four cases of prostate cancer death, a nonsignificant 3.5-fold increase over expected rates (1.15 cases). Prostate cancer mortality, however, was significantly increased in workers with 20 or more years latency from the original onset of exposure to cadmium (four observed, 0.88 expected). When Thun et al. (91) expanded this study group to 602, one of the previously identified cases of prostate cancer death was not considered because the individual was thought to have only indirect exposure to cadmium and, though relative risk for prostate cancer was still greater than 1 (2.13), the statistical significance of this association was lost. The omission of this case was stated by the authors to be, to a certain extent, arbitrary (91).

Using a combined cohort consisting of the data from several previous reports from the United States, United Kingdom, and Sweden, Elinder et al. (23) concluded that there was a significant association between cadmium exposure and death from prostate cancer in this pooled group. The validity of this technique of combining data from different geographic and exposure settings could well be questioned.

Prostate cancer was elevated in three occupational categories, including welders, that were stated as having potential exposure to cadmium in a study of cancer mortality patterns in Massachusetts (22). In a similar study of data from over 3000 counties throughout the United States, a significant association between prostate cancer in white males and occupation in the primary metal products or fabricated metal products industries was observed (7), though no direct cadmium exposure data were available.

Many other studies have failed to find a significant association between an increased risk of prostate cancer and occupational cadmium exposure (3,43,44,47–49,52,72), including studies following up on populations in which positive correlations had previously been detected. However, Elinder et al. (23) noted that for studies available before 1985, most indicated that the association of prostate cancer and occupational exposure to cadmium had a relative risk greater than 1, a pattern that has generally held during subsequent years (see ref. 47 for review).

Epidemiologic Studies—Environmental Exposure

In a study of environmental cadmium exposure, prostate cancer rates were compared to cadmium concentrations measured in water, waste, soil, and food stocks in geographic regions of Alberta, Canada (4). The area with the highest rate of prostate cancer had consistently higher environmental cadmium levels, while the area with the lowest rate showed the lowest cadmium levels (4). More recently, in a study of white males from urban areas in Utah, high intake of cadmium in the diet was associated with prostate tumors (1). A combination of high dietary cadmium, occupational cadmium exposure, and smoking (a good source of cadmium) (29) was associated with increased risk of aggressive (metastatic, or localized but undifferentiated) prostate cancers (1). Likewise, in another study of Utah men, in the 68–74-year-old age group, a high dietary intake of cadmium (>61 µg per day) significantly increased risk of prostatic malignancy in comparison with categorically matched controls (109).

Comments on Human Epidemiologic Data

The available epidemiologic studies concerning cadmium and prostate cancer have at least two major limitations. First, only a very few exposure groups have been studied. Second, studies have almost exclusively used populations of European origin, and there are clear population-based differences in rates for cancer of the prostate based on ethnicity (10). The fact that most studies are limited to fatal cancers is a further limitation. The reason for this is that prostate cancer is unusual as a potentially fatal human malignancy because there is a large discrepancy between the rate of histologically recognizable tumors and the much lower incidence of clinically recognized cancer (73). Many cases would be inadvertently missed when death alone is used as the endpoint for incidence of prostate malignancy. The fact that survival has progressively improved with early detection (73) may also be of importance in a population that might be alerted or sensitized to the potential risk. Potential cofactors in prostate carcinogenesis have not been analyzed, although rodent studies indicate several factors, including zinc, androgens, and estrogens, may modify tumor incidence (10,100,104). For environmental exposure, the correlation of regional environmental levels of a toxin with the regional prevailing rate of a particular disease is fraught with difficulties in interpretation, including the appropriate control of a number of inherent additional variables.

CADMIUM LEVELS IN HUMAN PROSTATE TISSUE

Some studies have presumably detected an association between cadmium exposure and malignant prostatic disease by measurement of prostatic tissue levels of cadmium. Cadmium levels can, in fact, be elevated in cases of prostatic carcinoma (24–27,35,62). For instance, in Nigerian black men, prostatic cadmium levels were eight times higher in cases of prostate cancer than in normal prostate tissue (62). Likewise in a study performed in United Kingdom, cadmium levels in resected prostates from patients with prostatic carcinoma were 25-fold higher than in normal prostate tissue taken at autopsy (35). A series of studies in Germany (24–27) showed elevated prostatic cadmium levels in a variety of prostate tumor types-adenocarcinoma, scirrhous carcinoma, and solid carcinoma. Cadmium levels were higher in the epithelium of the tumors, with the highest levels in the nuclear fraction of poorly differentiated carcinomas (24–26). In many of these studies, zinc levels were reduced in neoplastic prostate tissue, in conjunction with the elevations in tissue cadmium (27,35,62). Lahtonen (53) found no significant differences in cadmium concentrations between malignant or normal prostate tissue in Finnish men.

Interpretation of these findings should be done with caution. The regional levels of cadmium in normal prostate tissue vary widely with anatomic location (56), and thus sampling may be a major source of variability. Furthermore, with tumor progression, cellular proliferation could dilute cellular concentrations of metals such as cadmium. The level of cadmium present in a given tissue probably represents a combination of both recent exposure and chronic accumulation. The very long biological half-life of cadmium (25 years in humans) indicates that tissue levels probably reflect past exposure, at least in part. The depression of prostatic zinc levels concurrent with elevated cadmium in malignant prostates is intriguing, given the capacity of zinc to antagonize cadmium carcinogenesis at many sites in rodents (32,33). Defining whether elevated cadmium levels in samples from cancerous prostates are etiologic or circumstantial will require further study.

CADMIUM AND PROSTATE CANCER IN CHRONIC RODENT STUDIES

Cadmium was established as a potent metallic carcinogen in rodents over 30 years ago (38). Cadmium produces sarcomas at the site of intramuscular or subcutaneous injection and testicular interstitial cell tumors or proliferations (32,33,36,38,46,47,71). Early efforts showed the ability of zinc to prevent or reduce the necrotizing and carcinogenic effects of cadmium within the testes (32,33). The carcinogenic potential of inhaled cadmium is definitively established in rats (86), a finding in clear support of the metal's potential as a human pulmonary carcinogen (47). Several recent studies have shown that cadmium, given by various routes, can induce tumors of the rat prostate (Table 1). The dose dependency of cadmium-induction of prostate tumors is complex and depends on effects of the metal on other tissues, in particular the testes (101).

Direct injection of cadmium into the rat prostate has produced malignant prostatic carcinomas (40,41). When rats were injected with 0.44 mg Cd/rat into the right lobe of the ventral prostate and observed for the next 9 months, the first case of invasive prostatic carcinoma was detected only 56 days after cadmium injection (40,41). A total of five cases of invasive carcinoma eventually occurred in 100 cadmium-injected rats, while cadmium also induced 11 cases of carcinoma in situ, 29 cases of atypical hyperplasia, and 38 cases of simple hyperplasia. In the control rats, five (25%) had simple hyperplasia and one rat (5%) had atypical hyperplasia (40,41). Subsequent work showed that repeated intraprostatic injections of cadmium produced prostatic carcinomas in a dose-related fashion at a incidence of up to 60% over the 9 months after cadmium injections (42). At

TABLE 1. *Evidence for an Association Between Cadmium Exposure and Prostatic Cancer in Rats.*

Exposure route	Results[a]	Reference
Intraprostatic injection	Adenocarcinomas[b]	40–42
Oral	Adenomas	100
Subcutaneous	Adenomas/adenocarcinomas	103,104
Intramuscular	Adenomas/adenocarcinomas	76[c],104

[a]Tumors originate exclusively within the ventral lobe of the prostate.
[b]Potentially metastatic.
[c]In combination with 3,2'-dimethyl-4-aminobiphenyl.

least one case of metastases was detected from these cadmium-induced tumors (42). Gunn et al. (34) gave rats cadmium by direct injection into the ventral lobe of the prostate, but no prostate tumors developed over the next 16 months, although the dosage used was much lower than that of Hoffmann et al. (40–42).

The injection of a single subcutaneous dose of cadmium in rats (1–40 μmol/kg) resulted in an approximately 3-fold increase in prostate tumor incidence as compared with control rates over the subsequent 2 years (103). However, prostate tumors were only elevated at doses of cadmium below the threshold (<5.0 μmol/kg) for testicular toxicity. At these lower cadmium doses, a clear dose-related increase in prostate tumors occurred (103). The tumors were mainly adenomas and were exclusively located within the ventral lobe. Multiplicity of tumorous foci in the prostate also showed a dose relationship at doses of cadmium of at least 2.5 μmol/kg (103). In contrast, multiplicity of preneoplastic foci (ie, hyperplasia) increased with cadmium dose throughout most of the entire dosage range, indicating that cadmium induced initiating events but promotional factors (ie, testosterone) were likely not present at sufficient levels to encourage tumor development at doses exceeding the threshold for overt cadmium-induced testicular toxicity. In rats, testosterone is a promoter in two stage systems of prostatic carcinogenesis (10,12,68,77). Testicular androgen production is essential for the appropriate growth and maintenance of the prostate, while prostate tumors can often be testosterone-dependent (10). Thus, the testicular effects of cadmium could account for a lack of prostatic tumorigenicity at cadmium doses causing severe testicular dysfunction (103).

Zinc is an effective inhibitor of the testicular effects of cadmium (31,101). Another study showing potential for cadmium as a prostatic carcinogen examined the effects of zinc treatments (0–3000 μmol/kg, subcutaneously) on cadmium (30 μmol/kg, subcutaneously) carcinogenicity in rats over a 2-year period (104). When zinc treatment was given at doses sufficient to prevent cadmium-induced chronic testicular degeneration, the incidence of prostate tumors was elevated 4-fold over controls (104). Rats receiving doses of zinc that were not effective in preventing the testicular toxicity of cadmium did not show an elevated incidence of prostate tumors (104). Likewise, cadmium, when given intramuscularly at doses not resulting in chronic degenerative effects in the testes, induced a marked elevation in prostate tumor incidence (104). This again implicates a dependence of tumor formation on unimpaired testicular function. These tumors again were exclusively located within the ventral lobe of the prostate (104).

Cadmium treatment will also potentially enhance the formation of prostate tumors induced by organic carcinogens in rats (76). Combined 3,2'-dimethyl-4-aminobiphenyl and cadmium given to rats acted synergistically to induce carcinomas of the prostate (76). Again, the prostate carcinomas developed only in the ventral lobes (76), reinforcing the evidence for the lobe-specific nature of the carcinogenic or co-carcinogenic effects of cadmium.

Evidence from chronic studies in rats also indicates that oral cadmium exposure can induce proliferative lesions of the ventral prostate (100). When rats were given dietary cadmium (25, 50, 100 and 200 ppm) combined with diets either adequate (60 ppm) or marginally deficient (7 ppm) in zinc over an 18-month period, an increase in the overall incidence of prostatic proliferative lesions (combined focal atypical hyperplasia and adenomas of the ventral prostate) was associated with cadmium exposure (100). The highest incidence of prostatic proliferative lesions occurred at 50 ppm cadmium in zinc-adequate groups, reaching 23% of the total; this was significantly increased over the 2% incidence seen in control rats (100). Prostatic proliferative lesions occurred at a significantly lower incidence with zinc-deficient diets, which were associated with an increase in the incidence of prostatic atrophy, indicating inadequate androgen support of accessory sex tissue (100). Dietary zinc deficiency can be suppressive of testicular function and reduce androgen support of sex accessory tissues, such as the prostate (69).

Chronic studies in rats indicate that the rat ventral prostate is a potential target site for cadmium-induced neoplasia. This occurs whether cadmium is given orally, parenterally, or by direct injection. Cadmium induces the full spectrum of prostatic proliferative lesions, including invasive, potentially metastatic adenocarcinomas. These data are generally supportive of a potential role for cadmium in the etiology of human prostate neoplasia.

STUDIES RELATED TO CADMIUM AS A PROSTATIC CARCINOGEN IN RODENTS OR HUMANS

Other, indirect evidence for an association between cadmium exposure and prostate cancer also exists (Table 2). In a study of relatively short duration, oral exposure to cadmium produced prostatic hypertrophy in a dose-related fashion as reflected in increased prostate tissue weights when assessed over a 6-month exposure period (95). Histologic changes in the prostates were not assessed (95). However, no ultrastructural changes occurred in the prostates of rats treated for up to 10 months with cadmium in the drinking water (6).

TABLE 2. *Studies Related to the Prostatic Carcinogenesis of Cadmium in Rodents or Humans.*

Cadmium exposure	Results	Reference
In vivo	Prostatic hypertrophy in rats	95
In vivo	Testosterone-dependent cadmium accumulation in rats	102
In vitro	Malignant transformation of rat prostatic epithelium	88,89
In vitro	Growth stimulation of human prostatic epithelium	106,107
In vitro	Stimulation of 5α-reductase in human prostatic homogenates	79

In vivo testosterone treatment will effect the distribution and retention of cadmium by the rat prostate (102). With the use of constant-release testosterone implants after castration, androgen replacement was found to approximately double prostatic cadmium accumulation and prolonged the residence time of the metal in this tissue (102). These data correlate with chronic rat studies indicating that testicular androgen support is potentially important for cadmium induction of prostate tumors.

Studies by Terracio and Nachtigal (88,89) have demonstrated the ability of cadmium to induce transformation of prostatic epithelial cells. Primary cultures of rat ventral prostatic epithelial cells underwent transformation in vitro after exposure to cadmium, and these cadmium-transformed cells produced malignant tumors when injected into newborn rats, whereas untreated prostate cells did not (88,89). This indicates the carcinogenic effects in the prostate are due to direct interactions of cadmium with prostatic epithelial cells. These findings are also consistent with long-term studies in rats that consistently show that the ventral prostate is a target site for cadmium induction of prostate tumors (40–42, 76,100,103,104).

Using cultured human prostatic epithelium, Webber (106,107) has shown cadmium to be a growth stimulant. Selenium prevents cadmium-induced growth stimulation, a finding attributed to the anticarcinogenic effects of the metalloid (106,107).

Cadmium when added in vitro to homogenates of human prostate tissue stimulated 5a-reductase activity, as indicated by increases in 5a-reduced testosterone metabolites (79). Cadmium exposure also reduced the breakdown of 5a-reduced testosterone metabolites, suggesting the metal could result in a higher than normal concentration or half-life of the biologically active form of testosterone, 5a-dihydrotestosterone (DHT) and thereby stimulate growth in hormone-dependent prostatic neoplasia (79).

Cadmium is also effective in in vitro inhibition of specific binding of DHT to cytosolic proteins isolated from mouse prostate (21,90). Inhibition of these protein-binding interactions could block androgen action and inhibit cellular growth in the prostate and may be partially responsible in vivo for cadmium-induction of prostatic atrophy at high doses (90).

SENSITIVITY FACTORS TO CADMIUM IN THE PROSTATE

There are several factors that no doubt contribute to determining a target site in metal carcinogenesis. Metals such as cadmium, as toxins or carcinogens, tend to be highly tissue-specific (96). Tissue proximity to locally high concentrations of metal or otherwise direct exposure of a cell population to a metal compound probably contributes in many cases of disease. For instance, in the lung after inhalation of cadmium-containing particulate matter, high local concentrations of the metal could occur. Likewise, proximity to locally high concentrations of cadmium clearly occurs at repository-type injection sites. At these sites, biological reactions to an irritating deposit could further dissolve and release metal. The direct injection of cadmium into the prostate probably has at least an element of these factors involved. However, tumors occurring in juxtaposition to high local metal concentrations very often are sarcomas (34,96) and do not arise from the epithelial components of the local tissue, as do the cadmium-induced adenocarcinomas of the prostate (40–42).

Specific disposition of the carcinogenic metals within a tissue may also be a general factor in determining the target cell (96). However, within the rat prostate, the accumulation of cadmium does not explain the lobe specificity of cadmium carcinogenicity (19). In fact, the dorsolateral lobe of the rat prostate actually accumulates much more cadmium than the ventral lobe (19), indicating that toxicokinetics is not the basis of sensitivity. Other target sites of cadmium carcinogenesis in rodents also accumulate very little of the metal, including the testes (96). Thus specific disposition is not likely a primary factor in dictating target site in cadmium-induced prostate carcinogenesis.

Specific sensitivity factors probably help dictate target tissues in metal carcinogenesis, and absence or suppression of normal defense mechanisms against the particular metal may contribute to a unique sensitivity (96). Though the precise carcinogenic mechanism of action of cadmium remains unidentified (96), the level of metallothionein (MT) gene expression may play a role in determining susceptibility to cadmium-induced tumors. MT is clearly a key element in endogenous or acquired cellular tolerance to cadmium toxicity. MT is a high affinity metal-binding protein, which is found in many tissues and is highly inducible by several metals, including cadmium and zinc (97). Of the amino acids in MT, approximately 30% are cysteine residues. This high content of cysteinyl thiol groups probably accounts for the high affinity of cadmium for MT, and detoxication is believed to occur through high-affinity sequestration. MT levels may play a critical role in determining the sensitivity or resistance of a given tissue or cell to various aspects of cadmium toxicity, including carcinogenicity (101). For instance, cell lines in which the MT gene appears to be quiescent can be quite sensitive to cadmium-induced genotoxicity (78), whereas in cell lines with an active MT gene stimulation of MT expression before exposure to cadmium markedly reduces the genotoxic effects of cadmium (16,18). Cadmium can activate certain proto-oncogenes (80), and this activation can be prevented or reduced in some cases by enhancement of cellular MT levels (2).

In this regard, MT may be only poorly expressed in the ventral lobe of the rat prostate, and the MT gene in this particular lobe appears generally unresponsive to metal stimuli (17,19,93,102). Basal levels of MT mRNA are at or below detection limits in the rat ventral prostate, as measured by recombinant or in situ hybridization techniques (17,19,93,102). Likewise, basal MT protein levels, when measured by a variety of techniques, are also very low in the ventral prostate, again often at or near detection limits (17,19,85,92,93,102). MT gene expression is not stimulated by cadmium in the ventral prostate (17,19,102), despite cadmium concentrations in this lobe in excess of those that activate the gene in other tissues, such as the liver (17,19). MT protein accumulation has been detected in the ventral prostate, but only when cadmium is given concurrently with testosterone (85), and testosterone itself may be a primary inducer of MT gene expression (93).

In contrast to the ventral lobe, high basal MT mRNA levels are found in the dorsolateral lobe of the rat prostate (17,19,93,102). In fact, the dorsolateral lobe of the rat prostate actually accumulates much more cadmium than the ventral lobe (19), an observation indicating that disposition of the metal in the prostate is not a primary factor dictating sensitivity.

Cadmium induction of prostate tumors in the rat has only been detected thus far within the ventral lobe, and not in the dorsolateral lobe. The poor basal expression and the lack of metal-induced stimulation of the MT gene in the ventral lobe of the rat prostate thus correlate with the lobe-specific sensitivity to cadmium carcinogenicity. A deficiency in responsiveness of this primary cellular defense system against cadmium toxicity may be a major aspect determining sensitivity to cadmium carcinogenesis within the rat prostate. In a similar fashion, it appears that the species-based differences in the sensitivity to pulmonary carcinogenicity of inhaled cadmium are founded in the relative expression of MT in the lungs of rats and mice (61).

Immunohistochemically, there is little evidence that MT occurs within the ventral lobe of the rat prostate, although the dorsal prostate shows significant concentrations and levels in the ventral lobe are often not modified by metal treatments (59,85,93,94). The results of immunohistochemical studies of MT in the rat prostate can be variable and dependent on the precise technique used (5); however, overall they indicate that MT may be poorly expressed in the ventral lobe of the rat prostate. Immunohistochemical localization of MT in the human prostate varies extensively with zonal locale, but large portions of the gland show very weak staining (84).

The one study designed to determine the biochemical nature of the cadmium-binding proteins in the rat prostate failed to isolate authentic MT from either the dorsolateral or ventral lobes of the rat prostate (99). A cadmium-binding protein of similar molecular weight to MT was isolated from both lobes of the rat prostate by standard techniques for MT purification; however, when analyzed for amino acid content, these proteins proved to be quite distinct from MT (99). Definition of the exact nature of these low molecular weight metal-binding proteins in the prostate will require further study.

SUMMARY

Cancer of the prostate is an important and potentially deadly form of human cancer. The complex etiology of prostate cancer makes linkage to a single factor such as cadmium exposure difficult. Epidemiologic reports occasionally link occupational or environmental cadmium exposure to prostate cancer in human populations. The International Association for Research on Cancer, in its first evaluation of the carcinogenicity of cadmium (46), mentioned the prostate as a possible human target site for carcinogenesis, and this was not excluded as a possibility in the most recent evaluation (47). Several studies show cadmium levels in the human prostate to correlate with incidence of malignant disease, although causation cannot necessarily be presumed with such ex post facto measurements. Several chronic studies show cadmium can produce the full cascade of proliferative lesions within the rat prostate, including invasive adenocarcinoma. A complex dose-response relationship between cadmium and prostate tumors in the rat implies that the effects of cadmium in an entirely different tissue (eg, the testes) may modify prostatic response. A similar nonlinear dose relationship in humans, if it did exist, would confuse the issue of causation. The observation of malignant transformation of rat prostatic epithelial cells after cadmium exposure in vitro is sound supportive evidence of carcinogenic potential. MT, a protein associated with tolerance to cadmium genotoxicity, appears to be poorly expressed and unresponsive in the rat ventral lobe, the portion of the prostate that is sensitive to cadmium carcinogenicity.

Just as in studies of pulmonary malignancies in rodents following inhalation of cadmium, studies observing prostate cancer in rodents support the postulate that cadmium could be a possible factor in human prostatic carcinogenesis. However, it cannot be assumed that all, or even many, human prostate cancers are associated with cadmium exposure, and rodent data do not allow a conclusive connection. Commonality of target sites between human and rodents is a frequent observation with human carcinogens, despite large species-specific pathophysiologic differences (110). Further research is necessary to define more adequately the risks of prostate cancer associated with human exposure to cadmium.

REFERENCES

1. Abd Elghany N, Schumacher MC, Slattery ML, West DW, Lee JS. Occupation, cadmium exposure and prostate cancer. *Epidemiology.* 1990;1:107–115.
2. Abshire MK, Buzard GS, Shiraishi N, Waalkes MP. Induction of proto-oncogene expression in rat L6 myoblasts by cadmium is inhibited by zinc preinduction of the metallothionein gene. *J Toxicol Environ Health.* In press.
3. Andersson K, Elinder C-G, Hogstedt C, Kjellström T, Spang G. Mortality among cadmium and nickel exposed workers in a Swedish battery factory. *Toxicol Environ Chem.* 1984;9:53–62.
4. Bako G, Smith ESO, Hanson J, Dewar R. The geographical distribution of high cadmium concentrations in the environment and prostate cancer in Alberta. *Can J Public Health.* 1982;73:92–96.
5. Bataineh ZM, Heidger Jr PM, Thompson SA, Timms BG. Immunocytochemical localization of metallothionein in the rat prostate gland. *Prostate.* 1986;9:397–410.

6. Battersby S, Chandler JA, Morton MS. The effect of orally administered cadmium on the ultrastructure of the rat prostate. *Urol Res.* 1982;10:123–130.

7. Blair A, Fraumeni JF. Geographic patterns of prostate cancer in the United States. *J Natl Cancer Inst.* 1978;61:1379–1384.

8. Bosland MC. Adenocarcinoma, prostate, rat. In: Jones TC, Mohr U, Hunt RD, eds. *Genital System.* New York, NY: Springer-Verlag; 1987:252–260.

9. Bosland MC. Animal models for the study of prostate carcinogenesis. *J Cell Biol.* 1992;16H:89–98.

10. Bosland MC. Male reproductive system. In: Waalkes MP, Ward JM, eds. *Carcinogenesis: Target Organ Toxicology Series.* New York, NY: Raven Press; 1987:339–402.

11. Bosland MC, Prinsen MK. Induction of dorsolateral prostate adenocarcinomas and other accessory sex gland lesions in male Wistar rats by a single administration of *N*-methyl-*N*-nitrosourea, 7,12-dimethylbenz(a)anthracene, and 3,2'-dimethyl-4-aminobiphenyl after sequential treatment with cyproterone acetate and testosterone propionate. *Cancer Res.* 1990;50:691–699.

12. Bosland MC, Prinsen MK, Kroes R. Adenocarcinomas of the prostate induced by *N*-nitroso-*N*-methylurea in rats pretreated with cyproterone acetate and testosterone. *Cancer Lett.* 1983;18:69–78.

13. Coffey DS, Isaacs JT. Requirements for an idealized animal model of prostatic cancer. In: *Model for Prostate Cancer.* New York, NY: Alan R. Liss; 1980:379–391.

14. Coffey DS, Isaacs JT. Control of prostate growth. *Urology.* 1981;3:*(Suppl)* 17–24.

15. Cohen MB, Heidger PM, Lubaroff DM. Gross and microscopic pathology of induced prostatic complex tumors arising in Lobund-Wistar rats. *Cancer Res.* 1994;54:626–628.

16. Coogan TP, Bare RM, Waalkes MP. Cadmium-induced DNA damage: effects of zinc pretreatment. *Toxicol Appl Pharmacol.* 1992;113:227–233.

17. Coogan TP, Shiraishi N, Waalkes MP. Apparent quiescence of the metallothionein gene in the rat ventral prostate: association with cadmium-induced prostate tumors in rats. *Environ Health Perspect.* 1994;102: 37–40.

18. Coogan TP, Bare RM, Bjornson EJ, Waalkes MP. Enhanced metallothionein gene expression protects against cadmium-induced genotoxicity in cultured rat liver cells. *J Toxicol Environ Health.* 1994;41:129–141.

19. Coogan TP, Shiraishi N, Waalkes MP. Minimal basal activity and lack of metal-induced activation of the metallothionein gene correlates with lobe-specific sensitivity to the carcinogenic effects of cadmium in the rat prostate. *Toxicol Appl Pharmacol.* 1995;103:164–173.

20. DeVita VT, Hellman S, Rosenberg SA, eds. *Cancer: Principles and Practice of Oncology.* Philadelphia, Pa: JB JLippincott; 1982.

21. Donovan MP, Schein LG, Thomas JA. Inhibition of androgen-receptor interaction in mouse prostate gland cytosol by divalent metal ions. *Mol Pharmacol.* 1980;17:156–162.

22. Dubrow R, Wegman DH. Cancer and occupation in Massachusetts: a death certificate study. *Am J Ind Med.* 1984;6:207–230.

23. Elinder G-C, Kjellström T, Hogstedt C, Andersson K, Spang G. Cancer mortality of cadmium workers. *Br J Ind Med.* 1985;42:651–655.

24. Feustel A, Wennrich R. Determination of the distribution of zinc and cadmium in cellular fractions of BPH, normal prostate and prostatic cancers of different histologies by atomic and laser absorption spectrometry in tissue slices. *Urol Res.* 1984;12:253–256.

25. Feustel A, Wennrich R. Zinc and cadmium in cell fractions of prostatic cancer tissues of different histological grading in comparison to BPH and normal prostate. *Urol Res.* 1984;12:147–150.

26. Feustel A, Wennrich R, Dittrich H. Zinc, cadmium and selenium concentrations in separated epithelium and stroma from prostatic tissues of different histology. *Urol Res.* 1987;15:161–163.

27. Feustel A, Wennrich R, Steiniger D, Klauss P. Zinc and cadmium concentration in prostatic carcinoma of difference histological grading in comparison to normal prostate tissue and adenofibromyomatosis (BPH). *Urol Res.* 1982;10:301–303.

28. Flanders WD. Review: prostate cancer epidemiology. *Prostate.* 1984;5:621–629.

29. Friberg L, Elinder C-G, Kjellström T, Nordberg GF, eds. *Cadmium and Health: A Toxicological and Epidemiological Appraisal.* Boca Raton, Fla: CRC Press; 1986;2 vol.

30. Goering PL, Waalkes MP, Klaassen CD. Cadmium toxicity. In: Goyer RA, Cherian MG. eds. *Handbook of Experimental Pharmacology; Toxicology of Metals, Biochemical Effects.* New York, NY: Springer-Verlag; 1994:189–214.

31. Gunn SA, Gould TC. Cadmium and other mineral elements. In: Johnson AD, Gomes WR, Vandemark NL. eds. *The Testis, Volume III: Influencing Factors.* New York, NY: Academic Press; 1970;3:377–427.

32. Gunn SA, Gould TC, Anderson WAD. Cadmium-induced interstitial-cell tumors in rats and mice and their prevention by zinc. *J Natl Cancer Inst*. 1963;31:745–753.

33. Gunn SA, Gould TC, Anderson WAD. Effect of zinc on cancerogenesis by cadmium. *Proc Soc Exp Biol Med*. 1964;115:653–657.

34. Gunn SA, Gould TC, Anderson WAD. Specific response of mesenchymal tissue to cancerogenesis by cadmium. *Arch Pathol*. 1967;83:493–499.

35. Habib FK, Hammond GL, Lee IR, et al. Metal-androgen interrelationships in carcinoma and hyperplasia of the human prostate. *J Endocrinol*. 1976;71:133–141.

36. Haddow A, Roe FJC, Dukes CE, Mitchley BCV. Cadmium neoplasia: sarcomata at the site of injection of cadmium sulphate in rats and mice. *Br J Cancer*. 1964;18:667–673.

37. Hayashi N, Sugimura Y, Kawamura J, Donjacour AA, Cunha GR. Morphological and functional heterogeneity in the rat prostatic gland. *Biol Reprod*. 1991;45:308–321.

38. Heath JC, Daniel IR, Dingle JT, Webb M. Cadmium as a carcinogen. *Nature*. 1962;193:592–593.

39. Hebel R, Stromberg MW. Accessory genital glands. In: Hebel R, Stromberg MW, eds. *Anatomy of the Laboratory Rat*. Baltimore, Md: Williams & Wilkins; 1976:70–71.

40. Hoffmann L, Putzke H-P, Kampehl H-J, et al. Carcinogenic effects of cadmium on the prostate of the rat. *J Cancer Res Clin Oncol*. 1985;109:193–199.

41. Hoffmann L, Putzke H-P, Simonn C, et al. Spielt Kadmium eine Rolle in der Ätiologie und Pathogenese des Prostatakarzinoms. *Z Ges Hyg* 1985;31:224–227.

42. Hoffman L, Putzke H-P, Bendel L, Erdmann T, Huckstorf C. Electron microscopic results on the ventral prostate of the rat after CdCl$_2$ administration. A contribution towards etiology of the cancer of the prostate. *J Cancer Res Clin Oncol*. 1988;114:273–278.

43. Holden H. A mortality study of workers exposed to cadmium fumes. In: *Proceedings of 2nd International Cadmium Conference*. London, UK: Cadmium Association; 1979:211–216.

44. Holden H. Further mortality studies on workers exposed to cadmium fumes. In: *Seminar on Occupational Exposure to Cadmium*. London, UK: Cadmium Association; 1980:23–24.

45. Hoover DM, Best KL, McKenney BK, Tamura RM, Neubauer BL. Experimental induction of neoplasia in the accessory sex organs of male Lobund-Wistar rats. *Cancer Res*. 1990;50:142–146.

46. *International Agency for Research on Cancer Monographs: Volume 11, Cadmium, nickel, some epoxides, miscellaneous industrial chemicals and general considerations on volatile anesthetics*. Lyon, France: IARC; 1976:39–74.

47. *International Agency for Research on Cancer Monographs: Volume 58, Beryllium, cadmium, mercury, and exposures in the glass manufacturing industry*. Lyon, France: IARC; 1993:119–238.

48. Kazantzis G, Blanks RG. A mortality study of cadmium exposed workers. In: Cook ME, Hiscock SA, Morrow H, Volpe RA, eds. *7th International Cadmium Conference*. London, UK: Cadmium Association; 1992:150–157.

49. Kazantzis G, Lam T-H, Sullivan KR. The mortality of cadmium-exposed workers: a five-year update. *Scand J Environ Health*. 1988;14:220–223.

50. Kipling MD, Waterhouse JAH. Cadmium and prostatic carcinoma. *Lancet*. 1967;i:730–731.

51. Kjellström T, Friberg L, Rahnster B. Mortality and cancer morbidity among cadmium-exposed workers. *Environ Health Perspect*. 1979;28:199–204.

52. Kolonel L, Winkelstein Jr W. Cadmium and prostatic carcinoma. *Lancet*. 1977;10:566–567.

53. Lahtonen R. Zinc and cadmium concentrations in whole tissue and in separated epithelium and stroma from human benign prostatic hypertropic glands. *Prostate*. 1985;6:177–183.

54. Laskey JW, Rehnberg GL, Laws SC, Hein JF. Reproductive effects of low acute doses of cadmium chloride in adult male rats. *Toxicol Appl Pharmacol*. 1984;73:250–255.

55. Lemen RA, Lee JS, Wagoner JK, Blejer HP. Cancer mortality among cadmium production workers. *Ann N Y Acad Sci*. 1976;271:273–279.

56. Lindegaard PM, Hansen SO, Christensen JEJ, Anderson BB, Andersen, O. The distribution of cadmium within the human prostate. *Biol Trace Elem Res*. 1990;25:97–104.

57. McNeal JE. Prostatic microcarcinomas in relations to cancer origin and the evolution to clinical cancer. *Cancer*. 1993;71(suppl):984–991.

58. McNeal JE, Reese JH, Redwine EA, Freiha FS, Stamey TA. Cribriform adenocarcinoma of the prostate. *Cancer*. 1986;58:1714–1719.

59. Nishimura H, Nishimura N, Tohyama C. Localization of metallothionein in the genital organs of the male rat. *J Histochem Cytochem*. 1990;38:927–933.

60. Nobel RL. The development of prostatic adenocarcinoma in Nb rats following prolonged sex hormone administration. *Cancer Res*. 1977;37:1929–1933.

61. Oberdörster G, Cherian MG, Baggs RB. Correlation between cadmium-induced pulmonary carcinogenicity, metallothionein expression, and inflammatory processes: a species comparison. *Environ Health Perspect.* 1994;102:257–264.
62. Ogunlewe JO, Osegbe DN. Zinc and cadmium concentrations in indigenous blacks with normal, hypertrophic, and malignant prostate. *Cancer.* 1989;63:1388–1392.
63. Piscator M. Role of cadmium in carcinogenesis with special reference to cancer of the prostate. *Environ Health Perspect.* 1981;40:107–120.
64. Pollard M, Luckert PH. Early manifestations of induced prostate tumors in Lobund-Wistar rats. *Cancer Lett.* 1992;67:113–116.
65. Pollard M, Luckert PH, Snyder D. Prevention and treatment of experimental prostate cancer in Lobund-Wistar rats, I: effects of estradiol, dihydrotestosterone and castration. *Prostate.* 1989;15:95–103.
66. Pollard M, Luckert PH, Sporn MB. Prevention of primary prostate cancer in Lobund-Wistar rats by *N*-(4-hydroxyphenyl)retinamide. *Cancer Res.* 1991;51:3610–3611.
67. Potts CL. Cadmium proteinuria—the health of battery workers exposed to cadmium oxide dust. *Ann Occup Hyg.* 1965;8:55–61.
68. Pour PP, Stepan K. Induction of prostatic carcinomas and lower urinary tract neoplasms by combined treatment of intact and castrated rats with testosterone propionate and *N*-nitrosobis(2-oxopropyl)amine. *Cancer Res, ed.* 1987;47:5699–5706.
69. Prasad AS. Clinical and biochemical spectrum on zinc deficiency in human subjects. In: *Clinical, Biochemical, and Nutritional Aspects of Trace Elements.* New York, NY: Alan R. Liss; 1982:3–62.
70. Price D. Comparative aspects of development and structure in the prostate. *Monogr Natl Cancer Inst.* 1963;12:1–25.
71. Roe FJC, Dukes CE, Cameron KI, Pugh RCB, Mitchley BCV. Cadmium neoplasia: testicular atrophy and Leydig cell hyperplasia and neoplasia in rats and mice following subcutaneous injection of cadmium salts. *Br J Cancer.* 1964;18:674–681.
72. Ross RK, Shimizu H, Paganini-Hill A, Honda G, Henderson BE. Case-control studies of prostate cancer in blacks and whites in southern California. *J Natl Cancer Inst.* 1987;78:869–874.
73. Scardino PT, Weaver R, Huson MA. Early detection of prostate cancer. *Hum Pathol.* 1992;23:211–222.
74. Shirai T, Fukushima S, Ikawa E, Tagawa Y, Ito N. Induction of prostate carcinoma in situ at high incidence in F344 rats by a combination of 3,2'-dimethyl-4-aminobiphenyl and ethinyl estradiol. *Cancer Res.* 1986;46:6423–6426.
75. Shirai T, Imaida K, Iwasaki S, Mori T, Tada M, Ito N. Sequential observation of rat prostate lesion development induced by 3,2'-dimethyl-4-aminobiphenyl and testosterone. *Jpn J Cancer Res.* 1993;84:20–25.
76. Shirai T, Iwasaki S, Masui T, Mori T, Kato T, Ito N. Enhancing effect of cadmium on rat ventral prostate carcinogenesis induced by 3,2'-dimethyl-4-aminobiphenyl. *Jpn J Cancer Res.* 1993;84:1023–1030.
77. Shirai T, Tagawa Y, Taguchi O, et al. Low tumorigenic response to 3,2'-dimethyl-4-aminobiphenyl administration in the prostate of rats castrated at birth. *Jpn J Cancer Res.* 1988;79:1293–1296.
78. Shiraishi N, Hochadel JF, Coogan TP, Koropatnick J, Waalkes MP. Sensitivity to cadmium-induced genotoxicity in rat testicular cells is associated with minimal expression of the metallothionein gene. *Toxicol Appl Pharmacol.* 1995;130:229–236.
79. Sinquin G, Morfin RF, Floch HH. Testosterone metabolism by homogenates of human prostates with benign hyperplasia: effects of zinc, cadmium and other bivalent cations. *J Steroid Biochem.* 1984;20:773–780.
80. Smith JB, Smith L, Pijuan V, Zhuang Y, Chen Y-C. Transmembrane signals and prootoncogene induction evoked by carcinogenic metals and prevented by zinc. *Environ Health Perspect.* 1994;102:181–190.
81. Sorahan T, Waterhouse JAH. Cancer of the prostate among nickel-cadmium battery workers. *Lancet.* 1985;i:459. Letter.
82. Stayner L, Smith R, Thun M, Schorr T, Lemen R. A dose-response analysis and quantitative assessment of lung cancer risk and occupational cadmium exposure. *Ann Epidemiol.* 1992;2:177–194.
83. Stephens T. A mixed bag of cancer trends. *J Natl Inst Health Res.* 1991;3:71–72.
84. Suzuki T, Umeyama T, Ohma C, et al. Immunohistochemical study of metallothionein in normal and benign prostatic hyperplasia of human prostate. *Prostate.* 1991;19:35–42.
85. Suzuki T, Yamanaka H, Nakajima K, et al. Induction of metallothionein by $CdCl_2$ administration in rat prostate. *Prostate.* 1993;22:163–170.
86. Takenaka S, Oldiges H, König H, Hochrainer D, Oberdörster G. Carcinogenicity of cadmium chloride aerosols in Wistar rats. *J Natl Cancer Inst.* 1983;70:367–373.

87. Tamano S, Rehm S, Waalkes MP, Ward JM. High incidence of seminal vesicle adenocarcinoma in a Lobund-Wistar rat model of prostatic cancer using *N*-nitrosomethylurea and testosterone. *Vet Path.* In press.

88. Terracio L, Nachtigal M. Transformation of prostatic epithelial cells and fibroblasts with cadmium chloride in vitro. *Arch Toxicol.* 1986;58:141–151.

89. Terracio L, Nachtigal M. Oncogenicity of rat prostate cells transformed in vitro with cadmium chloride. *Arch Toxicol.* 1988;61:450–456.

90. Thomas JA, Donovan MP, Waalkes MP, Curto KA. Some protein-heavy metal interactions in the rodent prostate cell. In: Murphy GP, Sandberg AA, Karr JP, eds. *The Prostatic Cell.* New York, NY: Alan R. Liss; 1981:459–474.

91. Thun MJ, Schnorr TM, Smith AB, Halperin WE, Lemen RA. Mortality among a cohort of US cadmium production workers—an update. *J Natl Cancer Inst.* 1985;74:325–333.

92. Timms BG, Hagen JA. Immunohistochemical localization of metallothionein in the rat prostate gland during postnatal development. *Prostate.* 1989;14:367–382.

93. Tohyama C, Suzuki JS, Homma N, Nishimura N, Nishimura H. Regulation of metallothionein biosynthesis in genital organs of male rats. In: Suzuki KT, Imura N, Kimura M, eds. *Metallothionein III.* Basel, Switzerland: Birkhäuser Verlag: 1993:443–457.

94. Umeyama T, Saruki K, Imai K, et al. Immunohistochemical demonstration of metallothionein in the rat prostate. *Prostate.* 1987;10:257–264.

95. Visser AJ, Deklerk JN. The effect of dietary cadmium on prostate growth. *Trans Am Assoc Genito-Urinary Surgeons.* 1979;70:66–68.

96. Waalkes MP. Metal Carcinogenesis. In: Goyer RA, Waalkes MP, Klaassen CD, eds. *Organ Specific Toxicity to Heavy Metals.* San Diego, Calif: Academic Press; 1994:5:47–69.

97. Waalkes MP, Goering PL. Metallothionein and other cadmium-binding proteins: Recent developments. *Chem Res Toxicol.* 1990; 3:281–288.

98. Waalkes MP, Oberd´rster G. Cadmium carcinogenesis. In: Foulkes EC, ed. *Biological Effects of Heavy Metals. Vol II: Metal Carcinogenesis.* Boca Raton, Fla: CRC Press; 1990:129–157.

99. Waalkes MP, Perantoni A. Apparent deficiency of metallothionein in the Wistar rat prostate. *Toxicol Appl Pharmacol.* 1989;101:83–94.

100. Waalkes MP, Rehm S. Carcinogenicity of oral cadmium in the male Wistar (WF/NCr) rat: effect of chronic dietary zinc deficiency. *Fundam Appl Toxicol.* 1992;19:512–520.

101. Waalkes MP, Coogan TP, Barter RA. Toxicological principles of metal carcinogenesis with special emphasis on cadmium. *Crit Rev Toxicol.* 1992;22:175–201.

102. Waalkes MP, Rehm S, Perantoni A, Coogan TP. Cadmium exposure in rats and tumors of the prostate. In: Nordberg GF, Alessio L, Herber RFM, eds. *Cadmium in the Human Environment: Toxicity and Carcinogenicity.* Lyon, France: IARC; 1992;390–400.

103. Waalkes MP, Rehm S, Riggs CW, et al. Cadmium carcinogenesis in the male Wistar [Crl:(WI)BR] rats: dose-response analysis of tumor induction in the prostate and testes and at the injection site. *Cancer Res.* 1988;48:4656–4663.

104. Waalkes MP, Rehm S, Riggs CW, et al. Cadmium carcinogenesis in the male Wistar [Crl:(WI)BR] rats: dose-response analysis of effects of zinc on tumor induction in the prostate and in the testes and at the injection site. *Cancer Res.* 1989;49:4282–4288.

105. Waalkes MP, Rehm S, Sass B, Kovatch R, Ward JM. Chronic carcinogenesis and toxic effects of a single subcutaneous dose of cadmium in male NFS and C57 mice and male Syrian hamsters. *Toxic Subst J.* 1994;13:15–28.

106. Webber MM. Selenium prevents the growth stimulatory effects of cadmium on human prostatic epithelium. *Biochem Biophys Res Comm.* 1985;127:871–877.

107. Webber MM. Normal, benign and malignant human prostatic epithelium: in vitro cell models for studies on the etiology, treatment, and prevention of benign and malignant human prostatic neoplasia. In: Webber MM, Sekely LI, eds. *In Vitro Models for Cancer Research: Carcinoma of the Prostate and Testis.* Boca Raton, Fla: CRC Press; 1985:25–41.

108. Wernert N, Goebbels R, Bonkhoff H, Dhom G. Squamous cell carcinoma of the prostate. *Histopathology.* 1990;17:339–344.

109. West DW, Slattery ML, Robison LM, French TK, Mahoney AW. Adult dietary intake and prostate cancer risk in Utah: a case-control study with special emphasis on aggressive tumors. *Cancer Causes Control.* 1991;2:85–94.

110. Wilbourn J, Haroun L, Heseltine E, Kaldor J, Partensky C, Vainio H. Response of experimental animals to human carcinogens: an analysis based upon the IARC Monographs programme. *Carcinogenesis.* 1986;7:1853–1863.

Endocrine Toxicology, 2nd ed.,
Edited by J. A. Thomas and H. D. Colby
Copyright © 1997 Taylor & Francis

10

Actions of Chemicals and Other Factors on Leydig Cell Growth and Proliferation

John A. Thomas

*Department of Academic Services,
University of Texas Health Sciences Center, San Antonio, Texas 78284-7722*

INTRODUCTION

The incidence of testicular tumors in man is considerably different from that in nonhuman species. Testicular tumors in man are rare relative to testicular tumors in rodents. Furthermore, the type of testicular tumor in men is most frequently of germ cell or Sertoli cell origin. In rats (and some strains of mice), the cell type of the gonadal tumor is most often the Leydig cell. Leydig cell tumors in rats are quite restrictive and are found more frequently in the Fischer (35) and the Wistar strains (74).

Despite species differences with regard to cell types of testicular neoplasms, certain gonadal disease profiles in the human testis, as in rodents, can be associated with occupational and chemical exposures. In humans, testicular tumors of nongerm cell origin represent 5–10% of all testicular neoplasms (22). The nongerm cell tumors represent a heterogeneous group of relatively rare neoplasms, both malignant and benign. Sex cord–gonadal stromal tumors constitute a large portion of this small group, with the majority being either Leydig cell or Sertoli cell in origin. Jacobsen (39) has recently reviewed the status of malignant Sertoli cell tumors of the testis and indicated that they are very rare in man. The majority of male germ cell tumors are gonadal (11,14). Table 1 shows the classification of human testicular tumors (52).

Carcinoma *in situ* of the testes was first described by Wilms in the late nineteenth century as a condition of atypical intratubular cells adjacent to an invasive tumor (62). Cancer of the testes is most often a precursor of invasive germ cell tumor. Testicular cancer is perhaps the most common cancer in men 20–35 years of age. Prior to the mid-1970s, the mortality rate for testicular cancer was very high. Nowadays, there are several effective chemotherapeutic agents, alone or in

TABLE 1. *Classification of Human Testicular Tumors.* *

Type	Occurrence–All ages (%)
Germ cell tumors	95
Seminoma	40
Embryonal carcinoma	24
Teratocarcinoma	25
Teratoma	5
Choriocarcinoma	1
Yolk sac tumor	<1
Nongerm cell tumors	5
Sex cord–stromal tumor	3
Leydig cell tumor	2
Sertoli cell tumor (androblastoma)	
Granulosa cell tumor	
Other sex cord–stromal tumors	
Adnexal tumors	<2
Rete testis carcinoma	
Mesothelioma	
Other adnexal tumors	

*(Adapted from ref. 52.)

combination, that can be used in the treatment regimen. Cisplatin, vinblastine, and bleomycin have produced cure rates nearing 90% (59). Treatment for testicular cancer has dramatically improved in the last decade (44). The highest incidence of testicular cancer is recorded in Denmark; northern Europe has higher than southern Europe. The incidence is low in non-Caucasians and lower in black than in white Americans (40,57). Cryptorchidism appears to be an established nonchemical risk factor, although there may be a hereditary component (29). Other nonchemical risk factors including prenatal radiation, mumps, and testicular temperature have been suggested (45,70). Premature birth is associated with a greater risk for testicular cancer (31).

A few risk factors for cancer of the testes have been consistently discovered (7). While cryptorchidism has most consistently been found to be a risk factor for testicular cancer, inconsistent or contradictory risk factors have included urban-rural settings, familial aggregation, genetic predisposition, mumps-orchitis, testicular trauma, inguinal hernia, and religion (56,65). Vasectomy does not seem to affect testicular cancer risk (32).

There is evidence that certain occupations and chemical exposures are associated with an increased risk of testicular tumors (3). Table 2 reveals occupational/industrial settings that have been associated with an increased risk of testicular neoplasms. Ducatman (23) reported an association between testicular germ cell tumors and aircraft repairmen. Dimethylformamide was linked to developing testicular cancer. Mills et al. (50) linked crude petroleum and natural gas extraction industries with an increased risk of testicular cancer (ie, germ cell). A survey of testicular cancer among U.S. Navy personnel who were working as avi-

TABLE 2. *Occupations or Industrial Settings Linked to Testicular Neoplasms.*[a]

Agriculture
Aircraft repairman[b]
Aviation technicians, engine men, mechanics
Leather tanners
Natural gas and petroleum workers[b]
Sawmill and wood workers

[a]See refs. 3,23.
[b]Reported as germ cell tumors.

ation support technicians, engine men, and mechanics revealed a higher rate of gonadal cancer, after adjustment for age with that of the United States popula- tion (30). Diethylstilbestrol (DES), given prenatally, failed to show an increased risk of testicular cancer (31). The development of Leydig cell tumors has been associated with clomiphene treatment for oligozoospermia (10).

Advancing age, as a variable in the incidence of testicular cancers in mammals, is not an apparent risk factor in men. Conversely, the aging male rodent, partic- ularly certain strains, is closely linked to the occurrence of spontaneous testicu- lar tumors, as well as relative ease in producing chemically induced neoplasms.

MORPHOLOGIC PERSPECTIVE—HYPERPLASIA/NEOPLASIA

The use of various morphologic descriptive terms to describe the histologic progression of events in the neoplastic process has not always been precise or without controversy or differing interpretations. Cancer development proceeds, through sequential or contemporaneous morphologic changes, from normal, pre- neoplastic, and premalignant to highly malignant neoplasms (26). Definitions that seek to establish concepts and provide reasonable uniformity for classifying neoplasms are important in cell biology and carcinogenesis. An often-held no- tion is that proliferative lesions (ie, abnormalities of tissue growth) can be clear- ly and unambiguously categorized as so-called nonneoplastic, benign neoplasia (ie, hyperplasia or dysplasia) or malignant neoplasia. Historically, convenient clinical categorization of morphologic terminology has not been synchronized or necessarily correlated with descriptive terminology of modern cell biology. Ac- cording to Eustis (26), the earliest lesions to emerge have been termed preneo- plastic. Such lesions are considered to be precursors of neoplasia. Lesions can be grouped as hyperplasia or dysplasia. The term hyperplasia is defined morpho- logically as an increase in the number of normal cells in normal arrangement within any particular tissue. Hyperplasia can occur as a regenerative or repara- tive response to cellular degeneration and necrosis. Hyperplasia can also occur with hormonal stimulation.

Loehrer (44) has remarked on the myriad nongerm-cell histologic subtypes used to describe human teratomas. These many and varied classifications of testicular tumors have also created some confusion. Despite some of the limitations of morphologic techniques in defining various stages in the progression of cellular changes, it is assumed, for purposes of this review, that Leydig cell hyperplasia can proceed to neoplasia. Further, and in an effort to classify such events strictly, the term hyperplasia/neoplasia has been adopted. This dilemma in distinguishing Leydig cell hyperplasia from Leydig cell neoplasia has been previously encountered, particularly in describing chemical-induced testicular lesion (27).

Mori and Christensen (51) have presented an excellent morphometric analysis of Leydig cells in the normal rat. The Leydig cell is a key structure of the testes. It is a highly differentiated cell containing abundant darkly stained cytoplasm, polyhedral shape, and prominent mitochondria with extensive cristae and peroxisomes (8,25,72). Quantitative information about normal rat Leydig cells and their organelles provides valuable insight into biochemical and physiologic processes. A knowledge of the normal growth and development of Leydig cells is necessary in order to better understand chemically induced or hormonally perturbated internal environments.

In the whole rat testes, the Leydig cells represent only about 3%. While the embryonic source of the Leydig cells is unknown, there has been significant progress in understanding the development of Leydig cells in the rat from birth to adulthood (21). Each cubic centimeter (about 1 g) of rat testes contains about 22 million Leydig cells (51). An average Leydig cell has a volume of about 1200 μm^3 and a plasma membrane surface area of about 1500 μm^2. Adult rat Leydig cell number increases from approximately 250,000 to about 25 million per testis between birth and 90 days of age (27).

The smooth endoplasmic reticulum (SER), the most prominent organelle in the Leydig cell and the major site of steroidogenic enzymes, has a surface area nearly seven times that of the plasma membrane. The SER represents well over half the total membrane area of the Leydig cell. The nuclei of Leydig cells occupy about 0.3% of the testicular volume. It should be noted, however, that the comparative abundance of SER membranes in Leydig cells varies from species to species (15). Quantitation of the cell biology of the Leydig cell may shed insight into pathologic changes associated with the events of hyperplasia/neoplasia.

REGULATION OF THE TESTICULAR LEYDIG CELLS

Several comprehensive reviews have described the mammalian Leydig cell life history, structure, function, and regulation (21,24,87). Ewing (27) has also provided an excellent synopsis of the physiology of the Leydig cell and chemicals that alter its function.

The physiologic activity of the testes is modulated by follicle-stimulating hormone (FSH) and luteinizing hormone (LH), which is also known as interstitial cell–stimulating hormone (ICSH) in the male. These two pituitary gonadotropic hormones are closely related and appear to be secreted by a single class of pituitary cells. FSH acts on the germinal epithelium and modulates the process of spermatogenesis, while LH acts on the Leydig cells to stimulate testosterone production.

The principal role of the Leydig cell is the biosynthesis and secretion of the male sex hormone testosterone in response to stimulation by LH. Located on the surface of the Leydig cell are specific glycoprotein receptors that, when activated by LH, lead to an initial cascade of cellular events involving cyclic adenosine monophosphate (cAMP). It has been estimated that there are about 20,000 LH receptors per Leydig cell (15). These receptors undergo developmental changes (66), and the sensitivity to LH or human chorionic gonadotropin (hCG) may be affected (53). The synthesis of testosterone occurs through a series of biochemical reactions. The rate-limiting step in the biosynthesis of testicular steroids is the conversion of cholesterol to pregnenolone. LH is the primary regulator of testosterone biosynthesis, but FSH may play a primary role by enhancing Leydig cell receptivity to LH stimulation.

While FSH and LH exert modulating effects on the testes mediated through the adenohypophysis, testicular cells are also regulated by factors produced locally in the testes (46). These local regulatory factors include peptide growth factors, pro-opiomelanocortin (POMC) derivatives, neuropeptides and steroids. Several growth factors have also been isolated from the testes (Table 3). Locally produced growth factors may play a putative mitogenic role in the testis. Several peptide growth factors originate from different cell types and are produced at different phases during testicular development. Most of the growth factors isolated from the testis have been identified in other nongonadal organs and tissues.

Insulin-like growth factor I (IGF-I) and transforming growth factor β (TGF-β) may play a nonmitogenic paracrine role in testicular function (2,4). IGF-I stimulates Leydig cells, leading to an increased production of androgen (4). Testicular macrophages stimulate testosterone production when added to Leydig cells in vitro (86). Interleukin-1β also stimulates the production of steroids by isolated Leydig cells (81). It has also been suggested that the cytokines may contribute to maintaining the blood–testis barrier (80). To what extent these cytokines can influence Leydig cell hyperplasia/neoplasia is not fully understood.

Noncytokines can also provide local regulation of the testis. Local biosynthesis of vasopressin can occur in Leydig cells in vitro (37). Vasopressin has both a stimulatory and an inhibitory effect on testosterone production by Leydig cells (67). Vasopressin receptors (ie, V1) have been characterized on primary Leydig cells, as well as on Leydig tumor cells (1,48,73).

The Leydig cell has been described as a diffuse neuroendocrine system (18). It is evident that steroidogenesis is not the sole function of the Leydig cell. In addition to the Leydig cell's containing binding sites for hormones, growth factors, and neuroactive substances, these cells also have markers for neuronal and neuroendocrine cells (eg, neuron-specific enolase, or NSE). The detection of testicular NSE, along with tachykinins, substance P, neurokinin A, and others, provides evidence for the neuroendocrine nature of the Leydig cell (18).

TABLE 3. *Growth Factors Isolated from the Testis.*[a]

Growth factor[b]	Testicular origin	Proposed mitogenic target in testis
IGF-I	Sertoli cells	NI
IGF-II	Germ cells	NI
TGF-fl	Sertoli cells	NI
	Peritubular cells	
Inhibin	Sertoli cells	NI
SGF	Sertoli cells	Sertoli cells?
bFGF	NI	NI
TGF-α	Sertoli cells	NI
	Peritubular cells	
SCSGF (=TGF-α?)	Sertoli cells	Germ cells?
EGF		
RTFGF	Rete testis fluid	NI
tIL-1	Sertoli cells	Germ cells
NFG-β	Germ cells	NI

[a]See refs. 46,68.

[b]Key: IFG-I and-II, insulin-like growth factor I and II; TGF-α and -fl, transforming growth factor α and fl; SGF, seminiferous growth factor; bFGF, basic fibroblast growth factor; SCSGF, Sertoli cell–secreted growth factor; EGF, epidermal growth factor; RTFGF, rete testis fluid–derived growth factor; tIL-1, testicular interleukin-1-like factor; NGF-β, nerve growth factor β, NI, no information available.

FACTORS AFFECTING LEYDIG CELL HYPERPLASIA

Spontaneous Leydig cell tumors in humans–and even in most strains of rat–are rare. Malignancy of such tumors occurs with even less frequency. Certain strains of rat, such as Fischer 344 (F344) rats, however, represent an exception to this otherwise rare occurrence. The exact etiology of Leydig tumor formation in F344 rats is not known, but several factors have been implicated (Table 4). A variety of hormonal manipulations, either directly or indirectly, can produce Leydig cell hyperplasia (12). Prolactin stimulation, whether provoked by drugs or prolactin-secreting tumors, can stimulate the Leydig cell. Aging has long been associated with hyperplasia of several endocrine tissues, notably the prostate gland. Cryptorchidism is a risk factor in human testicular cancers, but its effect differs between mice and rats. Ordinarily, experimental cryptorchidism produces a loss or impairment of Leydig cells in rats. In mice, the administration of prenatal estrogen increases the incidence of cryptorchidism and hence causes the development of testicular tumors (64). Cadmium injection and vascular ligation can produce interstitial cell tumors of the testes (34,83). Testicular necrosis, whether induced by cadmium or vascular ligation, may contribute to a preneoplastic condition. Presumably, a parabiotic experimental design involving a castrate and a normal partner produces an excess of pituitary LH release in the former causing LH-induced hyperplasia in the normal partner. Other nongonadotropic pituitary hormones, usually in combination with estrogens and/or androgen, may produce hormonal synergism leading to tissue hyperplasia.

TABLE 4. *Factors Affecting Leydig Cell Hyperplasia.*[a]

Long-term stimulation by luteinizing hormone or human chorionic gonadotropin
Increased secretion of prolactin
Aging
Surgically induced cryptorchidism (mice only?)
Cadmium administration (vascular ligation)
Parabiosis (castrate/normal pairing)
Intrasplenic grafts at testicular tissue
Prenatal estrogen or estrogen-like hormones
Other trophic hormones (growth hormone, adrenocorticotropic hormone, thyroid-stimulating hormone, etc)

[a]Most demonstrable effects are seen in rodents, particularly F344 strains.

While the high incidence of Leydig cell tumors is most often strain-specific, the phenomenon of aging is interrelated. The background tumor incidence in a 2-year National Toxicology Program (NTP) study revealed that the most commonly occurring tumor in untreated male F344 rats was in the Leydig cell (88 1/8) (35). Around the age of 24 months, approximately 95% of the F344 rats exhibit some degree of interstitial neoplasia (12,13,33,38,69,79,85).

In Wistar rats (substrain U), 78% developed spontaneous Leydig cell tumors (74). The first signs of tumor development were apparent in 1-month-old U-rats. Conversely, Walsh and Poteracki (84) reported recently that testicular interstitial cell tumors were not common in Wistar rats; only 4% were observed to have Leydig cell tumors. A similar low incidence in Wistar rats was reported by Kroes et al. (43) and by Bomhard et al. (5). Maekawa and co-workers (47) reported a 93% incidence in Leydig cell tumors in 98 Slc: Wistar rats. The Han-Wistar strain exhibited an 18% incidence (49), while the Wistar-Imamichi strain reportedly had a 23% incidence in Leydig cell tumors (20). Based on these varying incidences of Leydig cell tumors, it is evident that genetics plays an important role in the genesis of hyperplasia.

CHEMICALS/DRUGS AFFECTING LEYDIG CELL PROLIFERATION

Ewing (27) has recently reviewed those compounds that impair or kill Leydig cells, and the focus in this section will be to emphasize those agents or factors that cause Leydig cell hyperplasia/neoplasia. Certainly, there is a list of agents that impair or kill Leydig cells, including ethanol, drugs, industrial chemicals, different heavy metals, and xenoestrogens (75–77). These are also useful in vitro models to study acute toxicity on Leydig cells (9). The induction of testicular tumors in rodents, usually Leydig cell tumors, has been reviewed by several investigators (6,42,54,55). Several chemicals have been reported to cause testicular tumors in rodent bioassays (36,71). Table 5 reveals a list of chemicals and drugs capable of producing Leydig cell hyperplasia/neoplasia. Generally, the mechanism(s) of tumors produced in the rat interstitial cell is not known. Drugs and chemicals that

TABLE 5. *Chemicals and Drugs Causing Leydig Cell Hyperplasia/Neoplasia in Rodents.*[a]

Agent/chemical/drug	Agent class or biologic activity
Cadmium	Heavy metal
Estrogen	Hormone
Guanadrel	Adrenergic blocker
Linuron	Herbicide
S0Z-200-110, isradine, isadipine, felodipine	Calcium channel blocker
Flutamide	Antiandrogen
Gemfibrozil, clofibrate	Hypolipidemic agent
Finasteride	5α-reductase inhibitor
Cimetidine	Histamine (H$_2$) receptor blocker
Hydralazine, reserpine	Antihypertensive agent
Carbamazepine	Anticonvulsant/analgesic
Vidarabine	Antiviral agent
Mesulergine	Dopamine (D$_2$) agonist/antagonist
Clomiphene	Treatment of infertility
Perfluorooctanoate	Industrial ingredient (plasticizers, lubricant/wetting agents)
Dimethylformide	Industrial use (tannery and leather goods, metal dyes)
Diethylstilbestrol	Synthetic hormone
Nafarelin	Luteinizing hormone–releasing hormone analog
Nitrosamine	Industrial uses
Methoxychlor	Pesticide with estrogen properties
Oxolinic acid	Antimicrobial agent
Spironolactone	Diuretic
Metronidazole	Antiprotozoal
Cyclophosphamide	Antineoplastic
Methylcholanthrene	Experimental carcinogen
Procymidone	Systemic fungicide

[a]See refs. 7,19,27,58,61.

cause increases in endogeneous LH (eg, clomiphene) often lead to Leydig cell hyperplasia/neoplasia. Mesulergine, which acts as an antagonist-agonist at dopamine (D$_2$) receptors, may induce Leydig tumors in rats by pertubating circulating prolactin and affecting Leydig cell LH receptors (61). Prenatal estrogen treatment (eg, with DES) can increase the frequency of cryptorchidism, which in turn can lead to a greater than normal incidence of Leydig cell tumors. It is apparent that these chemicals and drugs have a wide diversity of chemical structures and biologic activity. The chemicals include biological activity associated both with and without inherent estrogenicity. Cadmium-induced testicular tumors have been reviewed by Waalkes and Oberdorst (82). The testicular tumorigenicity of cadmium does not differ markedly among rat strains with a low spontaneous incidence of these neoplasms. The majority of cadmium-induced Leydig cells are benign, but high doses can cause malignant neoplasms. Chemicals and drugs that cause peroxisome proliferation show a propensity to cause Leydig cell hyperplasia/neoplasia. Gemfibrozil, a hypolipidemic agent, causes interstitial cell tumors (28). Phthalate acid esters, also known to cause peroxisomal proliferation (78) exert a direct effect on Leydig cell structure and function (41).

Cook and co-workers (16,17) have investigated the mechanisms for Leydig cell tumorigenesis. Linuron, a herbicide with structural similarities to the antiandrogen flutamide, appears to induce Leydig cell tumors by causing a sustained hypersecretion of LH (16). Thus, linuron, a less potent antiandrogen than flutamide, produces Leydig cell tumors via an antiandrogenic mechanism involving sustained hypersecretion of LH. Still another possible mechanism of chemical-induced Leydig cell tumors is that caused by ammonium perfluorooctanoate (C-8) (17). C-8 produces an increased incidence of Leydig cell adenomas by a mechanism that appears to involve an increase in serum estradiol levels. Thus C-8, like linuron, appears to involve endocrine-mediated mechanism(s) yet by different hormones.

The possible mechanism(s) of finasteride-induced Leydig cell hyperplasia is also associated with increased serum levels of LH (60). Finasteride, a selective inhibitor of 5α-reductase, decreases the conversion of testosterone to dihydrotestosterone. The actions of finasteride on Leydig cells appear to be secondary to increased serum LH, and they occur only at very high doses.

Certain calcium channel blockers also induce Leydig cell tumors (63). While increases in serum gonadotropins were noted, there also appeared to be a reduction in testicular LH receptors. A 20% decrease in testicular LH receptors indicated a modest down-regulation in response to what might have also involved an increase in steroidogenesis (63).

Although chemical-and drug-induced Leydig cell tumors are frequently associated with sustained released of LH, there are still a large number of agents whose mechanism is unknown or at least does not seem to involve this gonadotropin. Further, there are factors that appear to make this process of tumorigenesis quite species-specific to the rat.

REFERENCES

1. Ascoli M, Pignataro OP, Segaloff DL. Vasopressin biosynthesis in rodent Leydig cells. *J Biol Chem.* 1989;264:6674–6681.
2. Avallet O, Vigier M, Perrard-Sapori MH, Saez JM. Transforming growth factor-β inhibits Leydig cell functions. *Biochem Biophys Res Commun.* 1987;146:575–581.
3. Barsano CP, Thomas JA. Endocrine disorders of occupationaland environmental origin. *Occup Med.* 1992;7:479–502.
4. Benahmed M, Morera AM, Chauvin MC, de Perettiet E. Somatomedin C/insulin-like growth factor I as a possible intratesticular regulator of Leydig cell activity. *Mol Cell Endocrinol.* 1987;50:69–77.
5. Bomhard E, Karbe E, Loeser E. Spontaneous tumors of 2000 Wistar TN/W.70 rats in two-year carcinogenicity studies. *J Environ Pathol Toxicol Oncol.* 1986;7:35–52.
6. Boorman GA, Rehm S, Waalkes MP, et al. Seminoma, testis, rat. In: Jones TC, Mohr U, Hunt RD, eds. *Genital system.* Berlin: Springer-Verlag; 1987:192–195.
7. Waalkes MP, Ward JM, eds. *Carcinogenesis.* New York, NY: Raven Press; 1994.
8. Browne ES, Flasch MV, Sohal GS, Bhalla VK. Gonadotropin receptor occupancy and stimulation of cAMP and testosterone production by purified Leydig cells: critical dependence on cell concentration. *Mol Cell Endocrino.* 1990;70:49–63.
9. Brun HP, Leonard JF, Moronvalle V, Caillaud JM, Melcion C, Cordier A. Pig Leydig cell culture: a useful in vitro test for evaluating the testicular toxicity of compounds. *Toxicol Appl Pharmacol.* 1991;108:307–320.

10. Bujan L, Mieusset R, DeZong Z, Mansat A, Pontonnier F. Development of Leydig cell tumour in association with clomiphene treatment for oligozoospermia. *Br J Urol.* 1992;69:659–660.

11. Chaganti RSK, Rodriguez E, Mathew S. Origin of adult male mediastinal germ-cell tumours. *Lancet* 1994;343:1130–1132.

12. Christensen AK, Peacock KC. Increase in Leydig cell number in the testes of adult rats treated chronically with an excess of human chorionic gonadotropin. *Biol Reprod.* 1980;22:383–391.

13. Coleman GL, Barthold SW, Osbaldiston GW, Foster SJ, Jonas AM. Pathological changes during aging in barrier-reared Fischer 344 male rat. *J Gerontol.* 1977;32:258–278.

14. Collins DH, Pugh RCB. Classification and frequency of testicular tumours. *Br J Urol.* 1964;36:1–11.

15. Conn PM, Tsuruhara T, Dufau M, Catt KJ. Isolation of highly purified Leydig cells by density gradient centrifugation. *Endocrinology.* 1977;101:639–642.

16. Cook JC, Mullin LS, Frame SR, Biegel LB. Investigation of a mechanism for Leydig cell tumorigenesis by Linuron in rats. *Toxicol Appl Pharmacol.* 1993;119:195–204.

17. Cook JC, Murray SM, Frame SR, Hurtt ME. Induction of Leydig cell adenomas by ammonium perfluorooctanoate: a possible endocrine-related mechanism. *Toxicol Appl Pharmacol.* 1992;113:209–217.

18. Davidoff MS, Schulze W, Middendorff R, Holstein AF. The Leydig cell of the human testisóa new member of the diffuse neuroendocrine system. *Cell Tissue Res.* 1993;271:429–439.

19. Davies TS, Monro A. Marketed human pharmaceuticals reported to be tumorigenic in rodents. *J Am Coll Toxicol.* 1995;14:90–107.

20. Deerberg F, Rapp KG, Rehn S. Mortality and pathology of Han:Wist rats depending on age and genetics. *Exp Biol Med.* 1982;7:63–71.

21. de Kretser DM, Kerr JB. The cytology of the testis. In: Knobil E, Neill J, et al., eds. *The Physiology of Reproduction.* New York, NY: Raven Press; 1988;837.

22. Dilworth JP, Farrow GM, Oesterling JE. Non-Germ cell tumors of testis. *Urology.* 1991;37:399–417.

23. Ducatman AM, Conwill DE, Crawl J. Germ cell tumors of the testicle among aircraft repairmen. *J Urol.* 1986;136:834–836.

24. Dufau ML, Pock R, Newbauer A, Catt KJ. In vitro bioassay of LH in human serum: the rat interstitial cell testosterone (RICT) assay. *J Clin Endocrinol Metab.* 1988;42:958–976.

25. Eik-Nes KB. Biosynthesis and secretion of testicular steroids. In: Greep RO, Astwood EB, Hamilton DW, Geiger S, eds. *Handbook of Physiology.* Washington, DC: American Physiological Society; 1975:95–115.

26. Eustis SL. The sequential development of cancer: a morphological perspective. *Toxicol Lett.* 1989;49:267–281.

27. Ewing LL. The Leydig cell. In: Scialli AR, Clegg ED, ed. *Reversibility in Testicular Toxicity Assessment.* Boca Raton, Fla: CRC Press; 1992:89–125.

28. Fitzgerald JE, Sanyer JL, Schardein JL. Carcinogen bioassay and mutagenicity studies with the hypolipidemic agent gemfibrozil. *J Natl Cancer Inst.* 1981;67:1105–1112.

29. Forman D, Gallagher R, Moller H, Swerdlow TJ. Aetiology and epidemiology of testicular cancer: report of a consensus group. *EORTC Genitourinary Group Monograph 7: Prostate Cancer Testicular Cancer.* New York, NY: Wiley-Liss; 1990:245–253.

30. Garland FC, Gorham ED, Garland CF, Ducatman AM. Testicular cancer in US Navy personnel. *Am J Epidemiol.* 1988;127:411–414.

31. Gershman ST, Stolley PD. A case-control study of testicular cancer using Connecticut tumour registry data. *Int J Epidemiol.* 1988;17:735–742.

32. Giovannucci E, Tosteson TD, Speizer FE. A long-term study of mortality in men who have undergone vasectomy. *N Engl J Med.* 1992;326:1392–1398.

33. Goodman DG, Ward JM, Squire RA, Chu KC, Linhart MS. Neoplastic and nonneoplastic lesions in aging F344 rats. *Toxicol Appl Pharmacol.* 1979;48:237–248.

34. Gunn SA, Gould TC, Anderson WAD. Comparative study of interstitial cell tumors of rat testis induced by cadmium injection and vascular ligation. *J Natl Cancer Inst.* 1965;35:329–337.

35. Haseman JK, Arnold J, Eustis SL. Tumor incidences in Fischer 344 rats: NTP historical data. *Pathology of the Fischer Rat* Reference C and Atlas. New York, NY: Academic Press; 1990;555–564.

36. Huff J, Cirvello J, Haseman J. Chemicals associated with site-specific neoplasia in 1934 long-term carcinogenesis experiments in laboratory rodents. *Environ Health Perspect.* 1991;93:247–270.

37. Ivell R, Hunt N, Hardy M, Nicholson H, Pickering B. Vasopressin biosynthesis in rodent Leydig cells. *Mol Cell Endocrinol.* 1992;89:59–66.

38. Jacobs BB, Huseby RA. Transplantable Leydig cell tumors in Fischer rats: hormone responsivity and hormone production. *J Natl Cancer Inst.* 1967;41:1141–1153.

39. Jacobsen GK. Malignant Sertoli cell tumors of the testis. *J Urol Path.* 1993;1:233–255.
40. Jensen OM, Esteve J, Moller H, Renard H. Cancer in the European Community and its member states. *Eur J Cancer.* 1990;26:1167–1256.
41. Jones HB, Garside DA, Liu R, Roberts JC. The influence of phthalate esters on Leydig cell structure and function in vitro and in vivo. *Exp Mol Pathol.* 1993;58:179–193.
42. Kirkman H, Kempson RL. Tumours of the testis and accessory male sex gland. In: Turusov VS, ed. *Pathology of Tumours in Laboratory Animals. Vol 3: Tumours of the Hamster.* Lyon, France: International Agency for Research on Cancer; 1982;34;175–190.
43. Kroes R, Garbis-Berkvens JM, deVries T, Van Nesselrooy HJ. Histopathological profile of a Wistar rat stock including a survey of the literature. *J Gertontol.* 1981;36:259–279.
44. Loehrer Sr PJ, Williams SD, Einhorn LH. Testicular cancer: the quest continues. *J Natl Cancer Inst.* 1988;80:1373–1382.
45. Loughlin JE, Robboy SJ, Morrison AS. Risk factors for cancer of the testis. *N Engl J Med.* 1980;303:112–113.
46. Maddocks S, Parvinen M, Soder O, Punnonen J, Pollanen P Regulation of the testis. *J Reprod Immunol.* 1990;46:33–50.
47. Maekawa A, Onodera H, Tanigawa H, et al. Neoplastic and non-neoplastic lesions in aging Slc:Wistar rats. *J Toxicol Sci.* 1983;8:279–290.
48. Maggi M, Morris PL, Kassis S, Radbard D. Identification and characterization of arginine vasopressin receptors in the clonal murine Leydig-derived TM_3 cell line. *Int J Androl.* 1989;12:65–71.
49. Maita K, Matsunuma N, Masuda H, Suzuki Y. The age-related tumor incidence in Wistar-Imamichi rat. *Exp Anim* 1979;28:555–560.
50. Mills PK, Newell GR, Johnson DE. Testicular cancer associated with employment in agriculture and oil and natural gas extraction. *Lancet* 1984;1:207–209.
51. Mori H, Christensen K. Morphometric analysis of Leydig cells in the normal rat testis. *J Cell Biol.* 1980;84:340–354.
52. Morse MJ, Witmore WF. Neoplasms of the testis. In: Walsh PC, Gittes F, Perlmutter AD, eds. *Campbell's Urology.* Philadelphia, PA: Saunders; 1986;2:1535–1583.
53. Misro MM, Ganguly A, Das RP. Is testosterone essential for maintenance of normal morphology in immature rat Leydig cells? *Int J Androl.* 1993;16:221–226.
54. Mostofi FK, Bresler VM. Tumours of the testis. In: Turusov VS, ed. *Pathology of Tumours in Laboratory Animals. Vol 1: Tumours of the Rat.* Lyon, France: International Agency for Research on Cancer; 1979:399–407.
55. Mostofi FK, Sesterhenn IA, Bresler VM. Tumors of the testis. In: Turusov VS, Mohr U, eds. *Pathology of Tumours in Laboratory Animals. Vol 1: Tumours of the Rat.* Lyon, France: International Agency for Research on Cancer; 1990:399–407.
56. Muir CS, Nectoux J. Epidemiology of cancer of the testis and penis. *Natl Cancer Inst Monogr.* 1979;53:157–164.
57. Muir C, Waterhouse J, Mack T, et al. Cancer incidence in five continents. *IARC Sci Publ* 5. 1987;88.
58. Murakami M, Hosokawa S, Yamada T, et al. Species-specific mechanism in rat Leydig cell tumorigenesis by procymidone. *Toxicol Appl Pharmacol.* 1995;131:244–252.
59. Peckham M. Testicular cancer. *Rev Oncol* 1 1988;439–453.
60. Prahalada S, Majka JA, Soper KA, et al. Leydig cell hyperplasia and adenomas in mice treated with finasteride, a 5α-reductase inhibitor: a possible mechanism. *Fundam Appl Toxicol.* 1994;22:211–219.
61. Prentice DE, Siegel RA, Donatsch P, Qureshi S, Ettlin RA. Mesulergine induced Leydig cell tumours, a syndrome involving the pituitary-testicular axis of the rat. *Arch Toxicol.* 1992;15:197–204.
62. Reinberg Y, Manivel JC, Fraley EE. Carcinoma *in situ* of the testis. *J Urol.* 1989;142:243–247.
63. Roberts SA, Nett TM, Hartman HA, Adams TE, Stoll RE. SDZ 200-110 induces Leydig cell tumors by increasing gonadotropins in rats. *J Am Coll Toxicol.* 1989;8:487–504.
64. Sato B, Spomer W, Huseby RA. The testicular estrogen receptor system in two strains of mice differing in susceptibility to estrogen-induced Leydig cell tumors. *Endocrinology.* 1979;104:822–831.
65. Schottenfeld D, Warshauer ME, Sherlock S. The epidemiology of testicular cancer in young adults. *Am J Epidemiol.* 1980;112:232–246.
66. Shan LX, Hardy MP. Developmental changes in the levels of luteinizing hormone receptor and androgen receptor in rat Leydig cells. *Endocrinology.* 1992;131:498–508.
67. Sharpe RM, Cooper RM. Vasopressin biosynthesis in rodent Leydig cells. *J Endocrinol.* 1987;113:89–96.

68. Soder O, Pollanen P, Syed V, et al. Mitogenic factors in the testis. *Serono Symp Publ Series*. 1989;53:215–225.
69. Solleveld HA, Haseman JK, McConnell EE. Natural history of body weight gain, survival, and neoplasia in the F344 rat. *J Natl Cancer Inst*. 1984;72:929–940.
70. Strader CH, Weiss NS, Daling JR. Vasectomy and the incidence of testicular cancer. *Am J Epidemiol*. 1988;128:56–63.
71. Swirsky GL, Slone TH, Manley NB. Target organs in chronic bioassays of 533 chemical carcinogens. *Environ Health Perspect*. 1991;93:233–246.
72. Tahka KM. Current aspects of Leydig cells function and its regulation. *J Reprod Fertil*. 1986;78:367–380.
73. Tahri-Joutei A, Pointis G. AVP receptors of mouse Leydig cells are regulated by LM and E2 and influenced by experimental cryptorchidism. *FEBS Lett*. 1989;254:189–193.
74. Teerds KJ, De Rooij DG, De Jong FH, Rommerts FFG. Rapid development of Leydig cell tumors in a Wistar rat substrain. *J Androl*. 1991;12:171–179.
75. Thomas JA. in Casarett & Doull's Toxic Responses of the Reproductive System. Toxicology, the Basic Science of Poisons, 4th ed. Pergamon Press; 1991.
76. Thomas JA. Gonadal-specific metal toxicology. In: Goyer RA, Waalkes MP, Klassen CD, eds. *Metal Toxicology*. San Diego, CA: Academic Press; 1995:413–446.
77. Thomas JA, Barsano CP. Occupational reproductive risks. In: *Encyclopedia of Environmental Control Technology*. Houston, TX: Gulf Publishing Co.; 1994;7:195–215.
78. Thomas JA, Thomas MJ. Biological effects of DI-(2-ethylhexyl) phthalate and other phthalic acid esters. *CRC Crit Rev Toxicol*. 1984;13:283–317.
79. Thompson SW, Huseby RA, Fox MA, Davis CL, Hunt RD. Spontaneous tumors in the Sprague-Dawley rat. *J Natl Cancer Inst*. 1961;27:1037–1057.
80. Verhoeven G, Cailleau J. Stimulatory effects of epidermal growth factor on steroidogenesis in Leydig cells. *Mol Cell Endocrinol*. 1986;47:57–68.
81. Verhoeven G, Cailleau J, Van Damme J, Billiau A. Interleukin-1 stimulates steroidogenesis in cultured rat Leydig cells. *Mol Cell Endocrinol*. 1988;57:51–60.
82. Waalkes MP, Oberdorst G. Biological effects of heavy metals. In: Foulkes ED, ed. *Metal Carcinogenesis*. Boca Raton, FL: CRC Press; 1990;129–158.
83. Waalkes MP, Rehm S, Riggs CW. Cadmium carcinogenesis inmale Wistar {Crl: (WI)BR: rats} dose-response analysis of tumor induction in the prostate and testes and at the injection site. *Cancer Res*. 1988;48:4656–4663.
84. Walsh KM, Poteracki J. Spontaneous neoplasms in control Wistar rats. *Fundam Appl Toxicol*. 1994;22:65–72.
85. Walsh PC. The endocrinology of testicular tumors. *Recent Results Cancer Res*. 1979;60:196–201.
86. Yee JB, Hutson JC. Effects of testicular macrophage-conditioned medium on Leydig cells in culture. *Endocrinology*. 1985;116:2682–2684.
87. Zirkin BR, Ewing LL. Leydig cell differentiation during maturation of the rat testis: a stereological study of cell number and ultrastructure. *Anat Rec*. 1987;219:157–169.

Endocrine Toxicology, 2nd ed.,
Edited by J. A. Thomas and H. D. Colby
Copyright © 1997 Taylor & Francis

11

Toxic Effects of Cyproheptadine and Its Analogs in Insulin-Producing Cells

Lawrence J. Fischer

*Institute for Environmental Toxicology
Michigan State University, East Lansing, Michigan 48824*

INTRODUCTION

A small group of synthetic chemicals having diverse chemical structures are known to have selective actions that disrupt the functions of the insulin-producing β-cells of the endocrine pancreas. Exposure to these chemicals can lead to a temporary or permanent diabetic state characterized by a loss of glycemic control. The involvement of environmental factors, including chemical exposures, in the etiology of human diabetes has been considered for many years. A genetic predisposition for the disease is well accepted, but the triggers for the disease, which may be diverse in nature, remain elusive. It is reasonable to investigate chemicals for their ability to produce deleterious effects in the β-cells of the islets of Langerhans because human exposure to certain chemicals has yielded diabetic conditions characterized by hypoinsulinemia (1).

The islets of Langerhans in the pancreas of mammalian species contain four types of cells, each secreting a different polypeptide hormone. The β-cells secrete insulin, while the α-cells secrete glucagon, which has actions opposing those of insulin. The δ-cells secrete somatostatin, and the PP-cells secrete pancreatic polypeptide. The hypoglycemic and hyperglycemic actions of insulin and glucagon, respectively, are major factors in controlling blood glucose. Somatostatin may play a secondary role by attenuating, in a paracrine fashion, the secretion of glucagon and perhaps insulin. The action of pancreatic polypeptide remains to be fully elucidated, but it has little effect on glucose homeostasis. In most species, the hormone-secreting cells of the islets of Langerhans cells are located within a particular architecture in the pancreatic islet, and the biological significance of this cellular arrangement merits continuing investigation. From studies carried on to date, it is the insulin-producing cells, located in the central core of each pancreatic islet, that are most susceptible to chemical-induced damage. Chemical agents that specifically damage α-cells or PP-secreting cells are not known. Thus, this report will focus on insulin cell damage.

The majority of the chemicals known to selectively damage the insulin-secreting cells produce necrosis, cell death, and a permanent diabetic state. Typical of these agents are streptozotocin and alloxan, which have been widely used to produce experimental diabetes in many species of laboratory animals. These agents produce cytotoxicity through generation of reactive chemical species that react with critical cell components, including DNA (60). Evidence exists to suggest that loss of nicotinamide adenine dinucleotide (NAD) due to excessive poly-ADP-ribosylation triggered by massive DNA damage may be involved in the cytotoxic action of each of these agents. Pyriminil (Vacor), a rodenticide, produces a permanent diabetic state in humans surviving the severe peripheral neuropathy that occurs after ingestion of the chemical (34). Evidence for selective destruction of β-cells by pyriminil has been obtained from histologic examination of postmortem tissues. Pentamidine, a drug used to treat schistosomal infections, produces a diabetic state in a fraction of the treated patients (44). This diabetogenic effect is due to a selective destruction of β-cells (4). Because insulin-producing cells appear to be particularly sensitive to the cytotoxic effects of these chemicals, it has become accepted that among the hormone-producing cells of the endocrine pancreas, the β-cells are particularly vulnerable to chemical insult (38).

Among the chemicals known to produce adverse effects in insulin-producing cells is the antihistamine-antiserotonin drug cyproheptadine (CPH). This agent and a group of structurally related analogs produce a reversible inhibition of insulin synthesis and release. CPH and its analogs have a unique and specific action in the endocrine pancreas. This laboratory and several others have investigated the toxicology, metabolism, and mechanism of action of CPH over a 20-year period. The results provide a fascinating example of target organ toxicity selective for an important endocrine organ. It is the purpose of this chapter to integrate published reports and some unpublished information into a cohesive description of the toxic action of an interesting group of diabetogenic chemicals.

CHARACTERISTICS OF β-CELL TOXICITY OF CYPROHEPTADINE

Morphologic Measurements

Light microscopy provided the initial evidence of CPH-induced selective damage to the endocrine pancreas (59), whereas specific damage to organelles in the insulin-producing cells was obtained using electron microscopy (Fig. 1). The earliest morphologic change resulting from CPH is a reduction in the number of insulin-secretion granules, which occurs about 15 hours after a single oral dose of 45 mg/kg of the drug in rats (37). Abnormalities in the endoplasmic reticulum can also be observed within 24 hours after a single dose. Subsequent daily oral doses result in a progressive dilation of the intercisternal space followed by vesic-

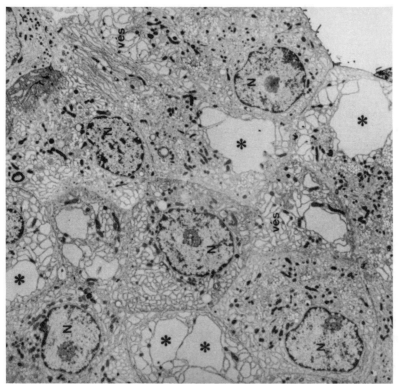

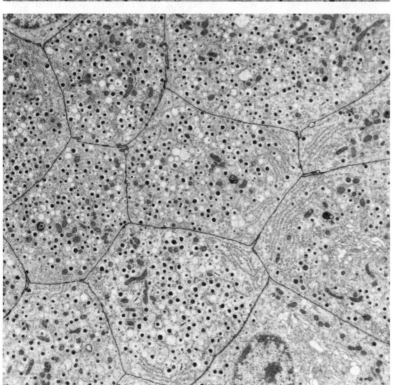

FIG. 1. Electronmicrographs of pancreatic β-cells from control (left) and CPH-treated (right) rats. Treatment occurred over 14 days using an oral daily dose of 45 mg/kg. Cells in control animals contain numerous insulin-secretion granules, while very few are found in cells from treated animals. Treatment also produces intense vesiculation (ves) of the rough endoplasmic reticulum and cytoplasmic vacuole formation (denoted by an asterisks). N, nucleus.

ulation of the endoplasmic reticulum. Loss of insulin-secretion granules is nearly complete after four daily doses of CPH. Small vesicles of endoplasmic reticulum appear to coalesce, eventually forming large cytoplasmic vacuoles that are visible after four daily doses. Cytoplasmic vacuole formation progresses by increasing vacuole size and the number of involved cells. It reaches a maximum at approximately 2 weeks of daily doses. No abnormalities in mitochondria, nucleus, Golgi apparatus, or other cell organelles were observed during CPH treatment.

Ultrastructural alterations in the islets of Langerhans caused by oral doses of CPH are dose-dependent and specific for insulin-producing β-cells. Glucagon-secreting α-cells and somatostatin-secreting δ-cells appear normal after 2 weeks of treatment. No histologic or ultrastructural changes in the acinar cells of the exocrine pancreas have been observed after daily CPH treatment for up to 2 weeks. Normal numbers of zymogen granules and normal-appearing rough endoplasmic reticulum are observed in pancreatic acinar cells after CPH treatment (37).

The morphologic changes observed in pancreatic β-cells from CPH-treated rats can be reproduced when isolated pancreatic islets are cultured for 8 days with the drug (49). These results indicate that the structural abnormalities observed in intact animals are a result of a direct action within the endocrine pancreas. The culture of isolated rat pancreatic islets with higher concentrations (50 μmol/L) of CPH for 6 days indicated a loss of insulin and a somewhat smaller reduction in glucagon. A loss of glucagon has not been observed with CPH treatment in vivo, and its occurrence in tissue culture was probably due to cell death from the high concentration of the drug applied (24). The presence of intense lysosomal activity also observed in the cultured islet cells signals a possible stress phenomenon that is not observed in intact animals treated with the drug.

The genesis of the changes observed in the endoplasmic reticulum in CPH-treated rats is not entirely understood. After initiation of treatment, there is dilation in the intercisternal space of the endoplasmic reticulum, which could be caused by accumulation of protein products at the site of synthesis. This alters the normal architecture of that organelle and leads to the formation of small vesicular structures that coalesce to form large vacuoles containing material that has a proteinaceous appearance in electron micrographs. An ultrastructural-immunocytochemical analysis produced no evidence of insulin-like material in the vacuoles, suggesting that an accumulation of pre-proinsulin or other insulin precursors was apparently not a part of the vacuolation process (52). The identity of the material in the vesicles and resulting vacuoles observed after CPH treatment remains unknown. The appearance of the vacuoles, however, is not characteristic of glycogen deposition or hydropic degeneration (37).

A report by Richardson indicated that cytoplasmic vacuoles could not be found in hypophysectomized CPH-treated rats (48). This result, indicating an intact pituitary was necessary for CPH-induced vacuole formation, was confirmed by Hintze et al. (28). However, the later report showed that a loss of pancreatic insulin and vesiculation of the rough endoplasmic reticulum did occur in hypophysectomized rats. The pituitary apparently plays a role in vacuole formation but does not alter the ability of CPH to cause changes in the endoplasmic reticulum and produce a loss of pancreatic insulin.

A hallmark characteristic of the toxic effects produced by CPH in the endocrine pancreas is that they are reversible. An exception to this is alterations resulting from exposure during fetal development (these will be discussed later). As previously mentioned, very few insulin-secretion granules can be observed in β-cells after several days of CPH treatment, but on withdrawal of the drug, increased numbers can be observed within 24 hours (51). The large cytoplasmic vacuoles are slow to disappear and can be found in recovering cells 8 days after CPH withdrawal. At that time, cells are well granulated with secretion granules, in spite of the presence of large cytoplasmic vacuoles.

Biochemical Measurements

Results from measurements of glucose tolerance, pancreatic and serum insulin, and in vitro insulin synthesis and secretion support and extend the morphologic evidence obtained in CPH-treated animals. Loss of pancreatic insulin reaches a maximum after two daily oral doses of 45 mg/kg and remains at 25% of control over the remainder of a 2-week treatment schedule as shown in Fig. 2 (51). This loss of insulin is accompanied by hyperglycemia and glucose intolerance (37). Plasma insulin levels in CPH-treated animals remain within normal limits in spite of the hyperglycemia. The absence of normal blood insulin in the presence of hyperglycemia is indicative of a possible secretion deficiency. Abnormal insulin secretion in vivo is more easily observed when insulin release is challenged with an acute stimulus such as that used in a glucose tolerance test.

Consistent with morphologic evidence indicating a return of insulin-secretion granules on withdrawal of CPH treatment, pancreatic levels of proinsulin and insulin also increase after treatment (51). Within 24 hours, pancreatic insulin levels are normal and continue to rise before eventually returning to control levels over a 2-week period. The overshoot in pancreatic insulin that occurs after withdrawal of CPH is probably due to stimulated insulin synthesis resulting from treatment-related hyperglycemia. The mild hyperglycemia that may be seen during treatment reverses slowly, ie, within 10 days. Serum levels of insulin remain within normal limits during treatment but appear to exhibit short excursions on initiation and withdrawal of treatment.

An ability of CPH to alter insulin secretion has been observed using perfused rat pancreas segments in vitro (50). Pancreas tissue taken from animals treated with a single 45 mg/kg oral dose of CPH or with eight daily doses exhibits a deficiency in insulin release on challenge using a variety of stimulants such as glucose, leucine, dibutyryl cyclic adenosine monophosphate (cAMP), and tolbutamide. A reduction in stimulated insulin release observed at 3 and 24 hours after completion of drug treatment returns to normal by 48 hours. This indicates that CPH-induced inhibition of insulin release is also reversible.

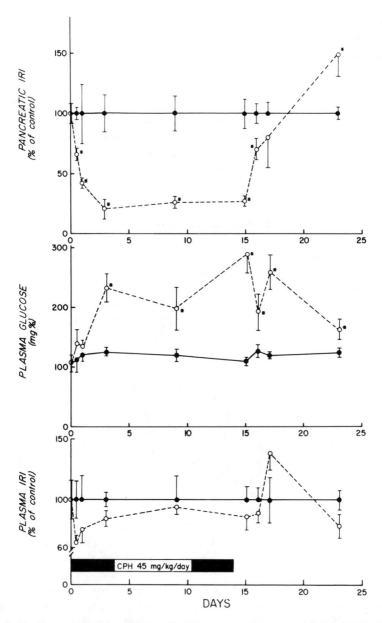

FIG. 2. Pancreatic immunoreactive insulin (IRI), plasma glucose, and plasma IRI in rats during and after daily treatment with CPH (45 mg/kg) given orally for a 2-week period. ●—●, Water-treated controls; ○—○, CPH-treated animals. Asterisks (*) indicate a significant difference from control (P<0.05). (From ref 51, with permission.)

The deficiency of stimulated insulin secretion from pancreas tissue obtained from treated animals may be attributed to the pancreatic insulin depletion produced by CPH, or it could result from a direct effect of CPH on the insulin-release mechanism. A direct effect of CPH on insulin secretion was demonstrated by treating pancreas tissue segments or isolated pancreatic islets from untreated rats with CPH in vitro and observing decreased hormone release in response to a glucose stimulus (14,33,50). The mechanism for this direct inhibition by CPH of insulin release appears to be an inhibition by the drug of the depolarization-induced uptake of extracellular Ca^{++} into insulin-secreting cells (14). Because glucose metabolism is required for insulin secretion, it is possible that CPH acts as an inhibitor by altering the catabolism of glucose. This possibility was eliminated by finding no effect of the drug on glucose metabolism in isolated rat pancreatic islets (33).

An increase in intracellular free Ca^{++} is the ultimate trigger for exocytosis of insulin-secretion granules from β-cells (39), and therefore direct inhibition of calcium uptake by CPH can explain the CPH-induced inhibition of insulin secretion observed in vitro and in vivo. Undoubtedly, the reduction of pancreatic insulin content in CPH-treated animals that occurs 12–24 hours after a dose and persists with repeated treatment contributes to abnormal insulin release. It is important to note that the ability of CPH to block calcium uptake into cells may explain why the drug inhibits the secretion of a variety of peptide hormones including glucagon (33), prolactin, growth hormone (31), thyroid-stimulating hormone (TSH) (15), and adrenocorticotropic hormone (ACTH) (36).

An inhibitory effect of CPH on the synthesis of insulin in β-cells appears to be a likely cause for the decline of pancreatic levels of the hormone. Using isolated pancreatic islets from untreated rats, CPH was found to inhibit the incorporation of ^{3}H-leucine into proinsulin and insulin in a concentration-dependent manner (27). At a concentration of 16 μmol/L, a 70% inhibition of synthesis of the proinsulin occurs, with no inhibition of the synthesis of other proteins in the islets. These results show CPH has a selective action for inhibition of insulin precursor synthesis. An inhibition of proinsulin synthesis in vivo should result in a decline in the pancreatic levels of the prohormone followed by a decline in levels of insulin. This pattern is observed when levels of proinsulin and insulin are measured after a single oral dose of CPH to rats. Proinsulin decline reaches a maximum about 6 hours after the dose, whereas insulin loss from the pancreas is first observed at 24 hours (27).

While the loss of pancreatic insulin in CPH-treated rats can be explained by inhibition of proinsulin synthesis, a drug-induced inhibition of the conversion of proinsulin to insulin might also contribute to insulin depletion. Pulse-chase experiments in the presence and absence of CPH show that incorporation of ^{3}H-leucine into proinsulin was inhibited during a 30-minute pulse and that a commensurate reduction in labeled insulin occurred during a 120-minute chase period (27). In separate experiments, addition of 10 μmol/L CPH only during the chase period did not alter the production of labeled insulin from labeled proinsulin (unpublished results from this laboratory). Monensin (10 µmol/L), known to inhibit the conversion of proinsulin to insulin (22) and used as a positive control in the experiment, was found to slow the formation of labeled insulin when added during the chase period. These data indicate that the primary reason CPH depletes pancreatic insulin is its inhibition of proinsulin synthesis.

It is now well established that the effect of CPH to inhibit insulin synthesis is reversible. This was first detected by finding that islets isolated from CPH-treated animals, although depleted of cellular stores of insulin, were capable of synthesizing insulin at a high rate (27). During the islet isolation procedure, CPH is removed from the tissue allowing the islets to resume synthesis of the hormone. The rapid recovery of pancreatic insulin after stopping CPH treatment of animals is consistent with this view.

Structure–Activity Relationships

Assessment of the ability of various chemicals to produce CPH-like effects in the endocrine pancreas permits identification of an active chemical structure, or toxicophore, responsible for the insulin-depleting action of CPH. Early studies utilized histologic evidence of cytoplasmic vacuole formation as evidence of islet cell toxicity (18). It became evident that several drugs and other synthetic chemicals possess the ability to produce cytoplasmic vacuolation in β-cells of the islets of Langerhans. Structural features of active compounds indicated that the tricyclic ring structure of CPH is not required, but a 4-substituted piperidine or piperazine ring was a necessity. Substitution of the nitrogen atom of the heterocyclic ring is not a requirement for activity because the *N*-desmethyl cyproheptadine metabolite of CPH (DMCPH) produces insulin depletion and disruption of the endoplasmic reticulum of pancreatic β-cells.

Structure–activity relationships also indicate that the antihistaminic or antiserotonin actions of CPH are not involved in producing β-cell alterations. Chemicals such as DMCPH that do not possess these pharmacologic activities (16) are active in producing toxicity in β-cells (18). However, some other known antihistamines, including cyclizine do cause β-cell toxicity because they possess the correct structure for CPH-like activity in the endocrine pancreas (30). A basic structure having potent activity for producing alterations in β-cell structure and function typical of CPH is 4-diphenylmethylpiperidine (4-DPMP). The structural isomers 2-DPMP and 3-DPMP possess no toxic activity in the endocrine pancreas, demonstrating the specific structural requirements for this activity (26). The structures of CPH, 4-DPMP, and 2-DPMP are shown in Fig. 3.

All of the chemicals exhibiting CPH-like effects have structural similarities to 4-DPMP, except for one, hexamethylmelamine, an antitumorigenic compound. Rats treated at least 4 weeks with the drug exhibit characteristic morphologic changes in the pancreatic β-cells (43). These include a loss of insulin-secretion granules, disruption of the endoplasmic reticulum, and large cytoplasmic vac-

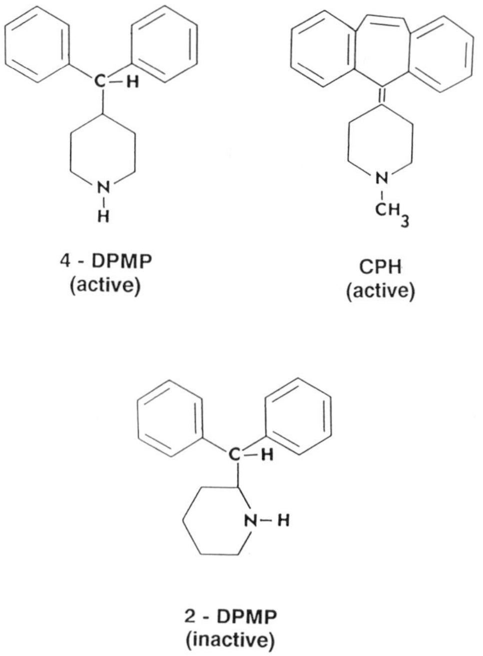

4 - DPMP
(active)

CPH
(active)

2 - DPMP
(inactive)

FIG. 3. Chemical structures of active and inactive diphenylmethylpiperidine (DPMP) analogs of CPH.

uoles. The structure of hexamethylmelamine is very different from 4-DPMP, and should this compound be found also to exhibit inhibition of insulin biosynthesis, the current structure–activity relationships thought to be involved in CPH-like pancreatic toxicity will require revision. Further studies of hexamethylmelamine action are warranted.

Species Differences and Toxicity in Humans

The rat is very susceptible to the toxic effects of CPH and its analogs in the endocrine pancreas. A systematic study of species differences has not been carried out, but early work indicated that mice, hamsters, and rabbits did not exhibit cytoplasmic vacuolization in β-cells after repeated daily doses of CPH (59). Beliles (2) reported that EX10-542A, a morphanthridine analog of CPH, produced vacuoles in rat pancreatic islets but was inactive in dogs.

Histologic evidence of CPH-like toxicity is insufficient to detect the more subtle morphologic effects and the corresponding functional changes found in pancreatic β-cells. This laboratory has examined mice treated with daily oral doses of 45 mg/kg for 8 days. With the use of methods identical to those used for rats (51), reversible hyperglycemia and loss of pancreatic insulin were found in treated mice (Fig. 4). These data and electron microscopic evidence indicate that the mouse is fully susceptible to the effects of CPH but the ultrastructural lesions in β-cells do not progress to the formation of large cytoplasmic vacuoles. The reason for this is not clear, but longer treatment than 8–14 days may be necessary in mice.

The inhibitory effects of CPH on insulin secretion and synthesis observed in rodents have not been studied in larger animals or primate species used in the laboratory. However, studies in humans provide evidence that the drug has inhibitory effects on insulin secretion. CPH has been used clinically to stimulate appetite, particularly in children, and a study of its potential mechanism of action for this effect included glucose tolerance tests and serum insulin measurements. A dose of 4 mg/day for 4 weeks to eight pediatric patients resulted in a serum insulin response to intravenous glucose that was blunted (21). This indicated a possible effect of the drug on insulin secretion and/or synthesis.

Results from several human studies using short-term treatment with CPH failed to indicate an alteration in glucose tolerance or show a decreased insulin response to a glucose challenge (3,55). However, it may be difficult to exhibit the inhibitory effects of CPH on insulin secretion using clinical doses of the drug because high-

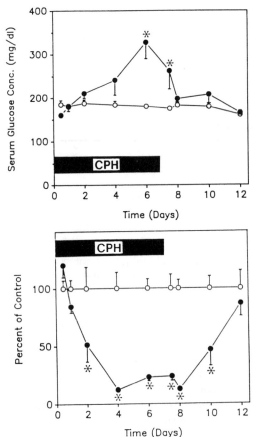

FIG. 4. Pancreatic insulin content (left) and serum glucose concentrations (right) in Swiss Webster mice given eight daily oral doses of CPH (45 mg/kg). ●——●, CPH-treated; ○——○, water-treated controls. Immunoreactive insulin in pancreas is expressed as a percentage of control at each time point. Each point is the mean ± SE (N=5). Asterisks (*) denote values significantly different from control.

er doses than those exhibiting its therapeutic effects are usually required in laboratory animal studies.

Direct evidence that CPH can inhibit the synthesis and release of human insulin has been reported by Jahr et al. (32) from studies using pancreatic islets isolated from human pancreas. The addition of 0.5–100 μmol/L CPH directly to human islets decreased, in a concentration-dependent manner, glucose-stimulated insulin release and incorporation of ^{3}H-leucine into insulin. These data, derived using the same in vitro methodology as laboratory animal experiments, provide evidence that the inhibitory effects of CPH are likely to be observed in humans after sufficiently high doses of the drug.

Susceptibility of Fetal, Newborn, and Young Animals

Development of the insulin-producing cells in the rat pancreas occurs relatively late in gestation, and the response of those cells to glucose does not occur until after birth (12,54). Immaturity of the endocrine pancreas is also associated with greater susceptibility to the toxic effects of CPH and its analogs. Administration of usual insulin-depleting doses of CPH (eg, 45 mg/kg) to pregnant rats produces fetal death and structural abnormalities in the offspring (13,56). However, lower maternal doses of 5–11 mg/kg CPH or DMCPH given daily for the last 8 days of gestation produces a dose-dependent loss of insulin in fetal animals obtained by cesarean section just before birth (8). This effect is specific for insulin, as fetal glucagon and somatostatin levels are normal. These doses of CPH do not alter fetal body weight or pancreas weight measured just before birth. Importantly, no loss of pancreatic insulin in maternal animals occurs with these lower doses of CPH (8). This result dramatically demonstrates the higher susceptibility of the fetal animal to the effects of CPH.

Results from drug disposition studies (described later) indicate CPH and its metabolites can reach the fetal animal, suggesting a direct effect of the drug in fetal tissue. Experiments using isolated pancreatic islets obtained at day 21 of gestation from fetal rats indicates that CPH inhibits proinsulin biosynthesis at lower concentrations (5 μmol/L) than those found to be inhibitory (16 μmol/L) using adult islets (8). Stimulated insulin release from fetal pancreas is also directly inhibited by CPH. These functional deficits, when considered with evidence of morphologic changes in the endoplasmic reticulum of fetal pancreatic β-cells, indicate that CPH produces toxic effects in the developing pancreas that are qualitatively the same as those produced in adult animals. However, quantitatively the fetal pancreatic tissue appears to be more sensitive because it contains levels of CPH and its metabolites equal to or less than those found to be incapable of depleting insulin from maternal pancreas after daily treatment of pregnant rats with the drug (9).

The effects of CPH in the fetal animal appear to have long-lasting consequences of a type that have not been observed in adult rats. Newborn rats from CPH-treated mothers have 50% less pancreatic insulin when compared with appropriate control animals (8). The low insulin levels in the neonate exposed to CPH *in utero* return to normal by 3 days after birth. This rate of recovery from chemical-induced insulin depletion in the neonatal rat is similar to that observed in adult animals treated with CPH (51). However, the offspring exposed *in utero* to CPH during the last 8 days of gestation continue to accumulate insulin in the pancreas (7). By 50 days of age, they have twice the levels of pancreatic insulin compared with appropriate control animals (Table 1). Similar abnormalities are not observed in levels of pancreatic glucagon or somatostatin in the offspring from CPH-treated pregnant rats, indicating specificity for insulin cells. Cross-fostering studies show that this unusual defect in the endocrine pancreas is due to exposure of the fetal animal, and not due to differences in the postnatal maternal environment in animals treated during pregnancy. The long-lasting nature of this unusual effect was verified by also observing a 2-fold higher level of insulin at 100 days of age. Measurements in older animals have not been conducted.

The functional status of the endocrine pancreas containing excessive insulin in the 50-day-old offspring of CPH-treated pregnant rats may be abnormal, because oral glucose tolerance is deficient, as shown in Fig. 5. These results could arise from a deficiency in insulin release and/or insulin action. The ability of these animals to metabolize glucose and to respond to exogenous insulin remains to be investigated.

The action of CPH in the developing endocrine pancreas is a critical area for further research. The results obtained represent a unique demonstration of a chemical-induced alteration in the fetus that results in abnormal functioning of the endocrine pancreas in adulthood. Even though details of the events that lead to an uncontrolled increase in levels of pancreatic insulin remain to be elucidated, the results are indicative of the vulnerability of developing β-cells and show that a diabetic-like condition can result in adulthood from chemical exposures in the fetal animal.

The higher susceptibility of fetal rats to the insulin-depleting action of CPH prompted an investigation of the age at which an adult-like sensitivity to the toxic effects of the drug could be observed. Two oral daily doses of 5 mg/kg CPH will produce a reduction of pancreatic and serum insulin in 10- and 15-day-old ani-

TABLE 1. *Effects of Cyprohepatadine (CPH) on Pancreatic and Serum Insulin and Serum Glucose in 50-Day-Old Offspring from Dams Treated During Pregnancy with Either CPH or Water.[a]*

Maternal treatment	CPH[b]	H$_2$O
Pancreatic insulin (ng/mg)	115 ± 3	219[c] ± 12
Serum insulin (ng/mL)	2.7 ± 0.2	2.6 ± 0.3
Serum glucose (mg/dL)	146 ± 4	142 ± 2

[a]Each value represents a mean ± SE for 12–18 animals from five different litters.

[b]CPH, 11 mg/kg, was given by gastric intubation once daily during the last 8 days of gestation. Body weights and pancreas weights of 50-day-old animals exposed to CPH in utero were not different from control.

[c]Significant difference (P<0.05) from water-treated controls. No significant difference was found in serum insulin or glucose.

(From ref. 7, with permission.)

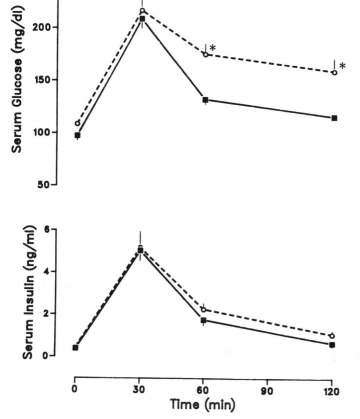

FIG. 5. Oral glucose tolerance (top) and corresponding serum insulin levels (bottom) in 50-day-old male offspring from pregnant rats treated with water (■—■) or 11 mg/kg CPH (O—O) orally for the last 8 days of gestation. Each value is the mean ± SE (N=5 litters). Asterisks (*) indicate a significant difference from control. (From ref. 9, with permission.)

mals, whereas no effects from this dose can be observed in 25- and 50-day-old rats (6). Comparison of dose–response relationships in rats of different ages show that by age 25 days (weaning on day 22), an adult-like susceptibility to the pancreatic effects of CPH occurs. The relationship between this decreasing susceptibility with age and the development of an adult pattern for metabolism of the drug will be presented in the next section.

A higher susceptibility in young rats to CPH-like insulin-depleting activity may be a common characteristic for diabetogenic chemicals. The CPH analog 4-DPMP exhibits greater potency for depletion of pancreatic insulin in 9-day-old rats when compared with doses required for insulin depletion in 21-day-old animals (5). It is not known whether younger rats are more susceptible to the insulin-depleting action of 4-DPMP because of an observed slower elimination of the chemical or because of the inherently greater sensitivity of the immature pancreas to the action of the chemical. Further investigations of the metabolism and toxicity of this chemical are required.

RELATIONSHIPS BETWEEN DRUG DISPOSITION AND TOXICITY

The metabolic fate of CPH in the rat and other laboratory animals was initially studied as part of an effort to understand differences among species for exhibiting pancreatic islet cell vacuolization after repeated treatment with the drug. Later studies using biochemical measurements of CPH action in the endocrine pancreas indicated that species differences in toxicity were less prominent than originally indicated using histologic evidence. However, significant age-related differences in susceptibility to the effects of CPH were observed, and drug disposition studies were performed to explore a possible pharmacokinetic basis for the greater sensitivity of young animals to the insulin-depleting effects of the drug. A suspicion that drug metabolites may contribute to CPH toxicity was fueled by knowledge that the *N*-demethylated product desmethyl-CPH (DMCPH) could be found in pancreatic tissue of CPH-treated rats (58) and that this product could produce cytoplasmic vacuoles in the islets of Langerhans when given in repeated oral doses to rats (18).

Metabolism and Excretion

Results from studies of the biotransformation of CPH in various species show the drug to be extensively metabolized (17,23,29,35,45). A number of different metabolites and a small fraction of unchanged drug are excreted in urine. Differences among species in the pattern of metabolites produced from a chemical are not unusual, and this is the case for the biotransformation of CPH in rats, mice, dogs, cats, and humans. A variety of *N*-demethylated and hydroxylated metabolites are produced in these species. Metabolites in the rat are of particular interest because of the relatively large amount of toxicity data available in that species. The pathways of CPH metabolism in the rat are shown in Fig. 6.

The rat and other species demethylate CPH to form the DMCPH. The rat is unusual, however, in also forming the 10,11-epoxide of DMCPH, which appears as a major metabolite in the urine (23,29). Rats also excrete a small amount of CPH-epoxide in urine (see Fig. 6), and this undemethylated epoxide may be an intermediate in the formation of DMCPH-epoxide. Other species excrete hydroxylated and conjugated metabolites of CPH and DMCPH in the urine (23). Humans also metabolize CPH in a pattern dissimilar to that of the rat, and undetectable amounts of DMCPH-epoxide are found in human urine (29).

The tricyclic epoxide metabolites formed from CPH, CPH-epoxide and DMCPH-epoxide, do not have the chemical reactivity typical of arene oxides. These epoxides are stable in urine, and hydrolysis to dihydrodiols is slow or does not occur. They also appear to be poor substrates for epoxide hydrolase, an enzyme that converts reactive and unreactive epoxides to dihydrodiols. Stable epoxides of CPH and other drugs can be found intact in tissues, where they may exhibit pharmacologic activity via interaction with receptors. An example is the

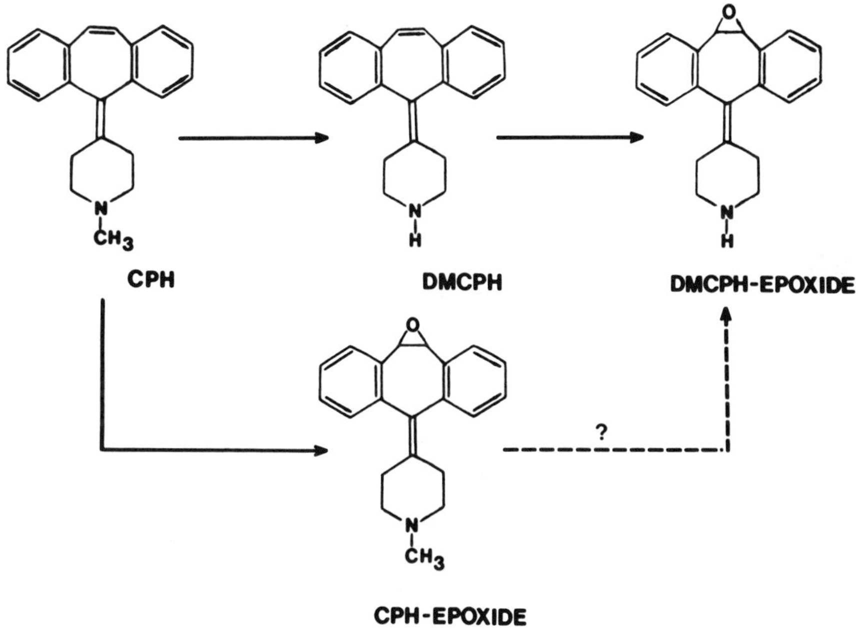

FIG. 6. Pathways of CPH metabolism in the rat. (From ref. 7, with permission.)

pharmacologically active, stable epoxide metabolite of the tricyclic anticonvulsant drug carbamazepine (47).

Activities of Cyproheptadine Metabolites in Pancreatic Tissue

The possible importance of drug metabolites in the toxicity of CPH to the endocrine pancreas was demonstrated by studies in which metabolism and toxicity of the drug were assessed in animals pretreated with known inhibitors of drug metabolism. Pretreatment of rats with the inhibitors SKF-525A and DDEP increases CPH tissue levels, decreases tissue levels of drug metabolites, and *reduces* the depletion of pancreatic insulin after a dose of CPH (11). It was clear from the results of these experiments that pancreatic insulin depletion closely follows tissue levels of DMCPH-epoxide, indicating that this metabolite may be of particular toxicologic importance.

The biological activities of CPH metabolites in rat tissues have been directly assessed using in vitro systems (10). All of the metabolites—DMCPH, DMCPH-epoxide, and CPH-epoxide—have higher potency than the parent compound for inhibiting proinsulin synthesis (^{3}H-leucine incorporation) in pancreatic islets isolated from adult rats. The concentration response curves in Fig. 7 show that DMCPH-epoxide has the highest potency followed by CPH-epoxide > DMCPH

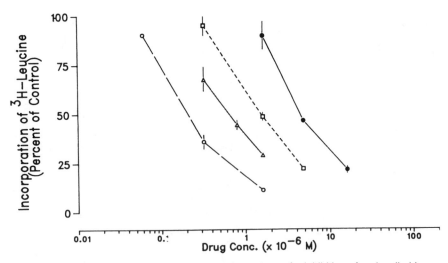

FIG. 7. Concentration response curves comparing potency for inhibition of proinsulin biosynthesis by CPH and its metabolites in pancreatic islets from adult rats. ●——●, CPH; □——□, CPH-epoxide; △——△, DMCPH; ○——○, DMCPH-epoxide. Values are reported as percentage of control (nontreated) islets. Values are the mean ± SE (N=5). (From ref. 10, with permission.)

> CPH. DMCPH-epoxide, the major rat metabolite isolated and purified from urine, is 20 times more potent than CPH. All of the metabolites show selectivity for inhibition of proinsulin synthesis, as they have little or no effect on the synthesis of other islet cell proteins. In contrast, the potency with which metabolites inhibit glucose-stimulated insulin secretion is lower than that for CPH. Fig. 8 shows that the order of potency for inhibiting hormone secretion is CPH > DMCPH > CPH-epoxide > DMCPH-epoxide.

The potencies with which CPH and its metabolites inhibit insulin synthesis and secretion have been determined using in vitro systems such as isolated rat pancreatic islets. The relevance of these values to potency in vivo can be questioned, and comparisons of concentrations effective in vitro with those found in rat pancreas tissue after effective doses in vivo are informative. Alterations of insulin cell function by CPH and its metabolites in vitro occur at media concentrations between 0.1 μmol/L and 15 μmol/L (10). Pancreas tissue levels of CPH and its active metabolites after doses of the drug that produce alteration in insulin cell function in vivo are within the same concentration range (6,9,58). Therefore, it seems reasonable to apply potency values obtained in vitro to estimate the biological effects that may occur in vivo. This approach will be described in the next section, which addresses age-related differences in toxicity.

The rank order potencies of CPH and its metabolites for inhibiting insulin synthesis and secretion contributes to an understanding of the diabetogenic action of the drug. Because the comparative potencies are different—in fact, opposite— for inhibition of insulin synthesis and for inhibition of secretion, the mechanisms

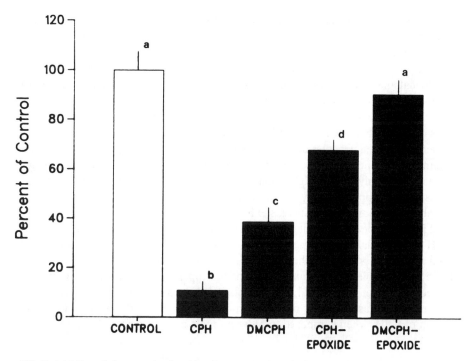

FIG. 8. Inhibition of glucose-stimulated insulin secretion from isolated pancreatic islets by equimolar concentrations (1.6 µmol/L) CPH and its metabolites. Values are expressed as percentage of secretion in nontreated control islets. Values are the mean ± SE (N=5). Values represented by bars having the same letters are not significantly different. (From ref. 10, with permission.)

for these effects must be different. This is consistent with results from mechanistic studies conducted to date. An inhibition of Ca^{++} uptake by CPH and metabolites appears to be involved with effects on secretion, while effects on synthesis (discussed later) may involve specific steps in the transcription and translation of the insulin gene. Further, knowledge of the relative potencies of metabolites is helpful in discerning the role that biotransformation plays in age-related differences in susceptibility to the effects of CPH.

Age-Related Differences in Metabolism and Toxicity

The previously described high susceptibility of the fetal rat to the insulin-depleting action of CPH is due, at least in part, to toxic concentrations of the drug and its active metabolites in fetal pancreatic tissue. After an oral dose, the unchanged drug and all of its metabolites are found in both maternal and fetal tissues (9). Generally, unchanged CPH and the metabolites DMCPH and DMCPH-epoxide are found in 3–8 times higher concentrations in maternal tissues when compared with corresponding fetal tissues. The pancreas, however is the only tissue in which the potent, active metabolite DMCPH-epoxide is found in the fetus at concentrations equal to those present in maternal tissue (Fig. 9). With knowledge of the relative potencies of CPH and its metabolites for inhibition of insulin biosynthesis (10), it can be calculated from tissue concentrations that the relative biological activity of drug-related material in the fetal pancreas at 6 hours after stopping CPH treatment are CPH = 1, DMCPH = 18, and DMCPH-epoxide = 66. This indicates that metabolites, particularly DMCPH-epoxide, are contributing most of the insulin-inhibitory activity in fetal pancreas during daily treatment of the pregnant rat. Considering the maternal pancreas levels of CPH and metabolites, the calculated total biological activity is only slightly higher than in the fetus. Because maternal and fetal pancreas contain approximately the same total biological activity from CPH and its metabolites but only fetal pancreas exhibits a drug-related reduction in insulin (8), fetal β-cells appear to exhibit a higher sensitivity to the insulin-depleting action of CPH and its metabolites. This analysis assumes that concentrations in maternal and fetal pancreas tissue reflect those in β-cells of the islets of Langerhans. This seems to be a reasonable assumption because of the apparent ease with which CPH and metabolites enter all tissues; however, specific data to support it are not available.

The higher susceptibility of newborn and young rats to the insulin-depleting action of CPH, when compared to older animals can be attributed in part to tox-

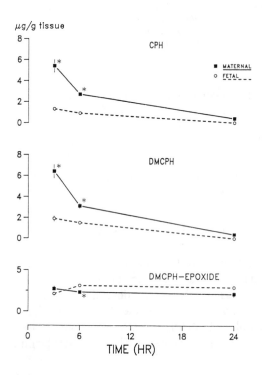

FIG. 9. Fetal and maternal levels of CPH and its active metabolites DMCPH and DMCPH-epoxide in the pancreas after completion of eight daily oral doses of CPH (11 mg/kg) to pregnant rats. An asterisk (*) denotes a statistically significant maternal–fetal difference. (From ref. 11, with permission.)

icokinetic differences. A study of tissue levels of the drug and its metabolites after oral administration to 10-, 15-, 25- and 50-day-old rats showed that the potent insulin-synthesis inhibitor DMCPH-epoxide reached higher and more prolonged levels in younger animals when compared with adults (ie, 50-day-old) animals (6). With the use of the area under tissue-level curves for 10- and 50-day-old rats and calculation of the total biological activity in the tissue based on the relative potencies of CPH and its individual metabolites, it can be seen from the results in Table 2 that younger animals are exposed to higher activity levels than adults. This may account for some but probably not all of the increased susceptibility of young animals to the diabetogenic effects of CPH. It is likely that the relative immaturity of the endocrine pancreas in young rats also contributes in some way to the increased susceptibility observed in young rats. Studies investigating this possibility have not been conducted to date.

In summary, studies of the metabolism of CPH have provided valuable information regarding its diabetogenic action. The fact that all of the metabolites found in rat tissues after CPH treatment are more active as inhibitors of insulin synthesis than the parent compound explains why the rat is among the most susceptible species. Humans, not converting CPH to DMCPH-epoxide, may be among the less sensitive species. All of the active metabolites possess chemical structures with the necessary requirements for insulin-depleting activity, as presented earlier. This lends verification to the previously described structure–activity relationships. Finally, the high sensitivity of fetal and newborn rats to the effects of CPH may be due in part to the production and accumulation of higher levels of

TABLE 2. *Comparison of Activity Indices Derived from Pancreatic Levels of CPH and Its Metabolites in 10- and 50-Day-Old Rats.*

	Product in tissue	Area under tissue level curve (μg h/g)	Potency ratio[a]	Activity index[b]
10-Day-old rats	CPH	41.6 ± 1.4	1.0	41.6 ± 1.4+*
	DMCPH	2.5 ± 0.2	9.0	22.8 ± 2.1
	CPH-epoxide	9.9 ± 0.3	3.4	33.8 ± 1.0+*
	DMCPH-epoxide	58.0 ± 2.3	22.1	1281.8 ± 51.5+*
	Total			1375,5 ± 48.1+*
50-Day-old rats	CPH	2.1 ± 0.1	1.0	2.1 ± 0.1
	DMCPH	2.3 ± 0.2	9.0	18.3 ± 1.5
	CPH-epoxide	0	3.4	0
	DMCPH-epoxide	38.5 ± 2.6	22.1	850.8 ± 57.1
	Total			873.9 ± 57.1

[a]Potency ratio was based on the IC_{50} values of CPH and its metabolites [6] for inhibition of proinsulin synthesis in pancreatic islets isolated from 50-day-old rats.
[b]Activity index is the area under the curve times the potency ratio. Each value is the mean ± SEM for three experiments.
(From ref. 6, with permission.)

DMCPH-epoxide. This potent metabolite, while contributing in large measure to the diabetogenic effects of CPH in rats, will be useful in future experiments to determine the molecular mechanism of action whereby CPH-like compounds reversibly inhibit insulin biosynthesis.

BIOCHEMICAL MECHANISMS OF TOXICITY

Declines in pancreatic and serum insulin after treatment with CPH are the result of inhibition of insulin synthesis and secretion by the drug and its metabolites. As previously described, the mechanisms for inhibition of synthesis and secretion appear to be different, based on results from structure–activity relationship studies. Evidence for the calcium channel–blocking action of CPH appears to be adequate for explaining the ability of CPH to inhibit insulin secretion. Inhibition of synthesis occurs by a mechanism that is now under investigation in this laboratory. A description of results from experiments exploring the mechanistic aspects of CPH-induced inhibition of proinsulin and insulin biosynthesis follows.

Clonal Insulin-Producing Cells as Models

Cellular systems used as appropriate models for intact organ systems are valuable tools for use in studies of mechanisms of toxicity. Results obtained using isolated pancreatic islets showed that CPH and its metabolites had direct actions in the endocrine pancreas. When isolated islets are used, the amount of tissue available is limited; isolation damage can be confounding, and the isolation procedure is tedious and time-consuming. Thus, isolated islets have distinct disadvantages that often offset the advantage of using primary cells. Cell culture systems lessen these disadvantages, but their usefulness can often be limited by abnormalities in the function of immortalized cells.

The use of the clonal insulin-secreting cell lines RINm5F and HIT-T15 as possible model systems for CPH actions in vivo was explored. Both of these cell lines have been used extensively in studies of insulin cell function in connection with diabetes research. The HIT cell line is derived from SV40-transformed hamster pancreatic islet cells, while RINm5F cells originate from a radiation-induced rat insulinoma (19,53). HIT cells retain an ability to secrete insulin in response to glucose, while RINm5F cells are unresponsive to glucose stimulation (25,46). However, in RINm5F cells other stimulants such as high potassium, glyceraldehyde and amino acids can provoke insulin release (46).

Exposure of these cell lines to CPH for 48 hours produces a concentration-dependent decline in cellular and media insulin, with a maximum loss of approximately 70% using 10 μmol/L of the drug (40). Typical of effects observed in isolated islets and in intact animals, recovery of insulin levels occurs within a 48-hour period. The CPH-induced loss of cellular insulin can be attributed to a concentration-related, specific inhibition of proinsulin synthesis (^{3}H-leucine incorporation), similar to that observed with isolated pancreatic islets. In addition to alterations in insulin synthesis, insulin secretion is inhibited in response to appropriate stimuli in each cell line, with maximal effects occurring at 10 μmol/L CPH. If RINm5F cells are to be considered an adequate model system for the insulin-depleting effects of CPH and analogs in vivo, the structure–activity relationships determined using intact animals should be the same as those determined in the clonal cell system. This appears to be the case because the active analog 4-DPMP, but not the inactive 2-DPMP, produces a loss of cellular insulin from RINm5F cells in culture (42). In addition, the CPH metabolite DMCPH-epoxide, known to be more potent than its parent compound as an inhibitor of insulin biosynthesis in rat pancreatic islets, is more potent than CPH for producing a decline in cellular insulin in RINm5F cells (42). These results indicate that RINm5F cells and probably the less well-tested HIT cells are adequate models for the actions of CPH in pancreatic β-cells. In addition to establishing their adequacy as model systems, the observation of identical actions for CPH and its analogs in each cell line shows that glucose responsiveness, a characteristic of HIT but not RINm5F cells, is not required for the chemicals to inhibit insulin synthesis and secretion.

Levels of Insulin mRNA

The major events occurring in the biosynthesis of insulin are schematically presented in Fig. 10. A reduction by CPH and its analogs of the level of pre-proinsulin mRNA (PPImRNA) for insulin synthesis would result in a loss of pre-proinsulin, proinsulin, and insulin from pancreatic β-cells. The time course for the decline of insulin and its precursors in rats after a single dose of CPH indicates that effects on both transcription and translation may be involved in the insulin-depleting effects of the drug (41). Measurements of PPImRNA, proinsulin, and insulin in the pancreas after a single oral dose of CPH show the time-dependent changes depicted in Fig. 11. The data indicate that a decline of PPImRNA occurs after a dose of CPH, and consistent with this effect are declines in proinsulin and insulin concentrations in pancreatic tissue. Pre-proinsulin could not be measured because of its very rapid conversion to proinsulin. The early time course of decline is informative because proinsulin loss occurs somewhat more rapidly than the loss of PPImRNA. This suggests that it may be possible for CPH to inhibit the production of proinsulin and insulin without producing a loss of PPImRNA. Certainly, the loss of pancreatic PPImRNA can contribute to and sustain the inhibition of insulin biosynthesis, but the initial action of CPH may be post-transcriptional in nature. Studies performed in vitro support this view, and these results will be described later in this section.

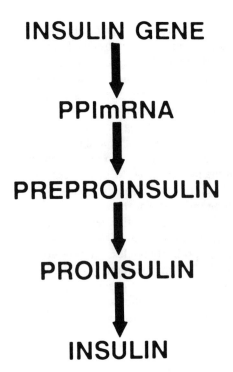

INSULIN GENE

PPImRNA

PREPROINSULIN

PROINSULIN

INSULIN

FIG. 10. Scheme for the synthesis of the insulin gene product pre-proinsulin and its conversion to insulin.

The loss of pancreatic PPImRNA after a dose of CPH is not unique to the rat, as it can be reproduced using the mouse (Table 3). At 12 hours, 73% loss of PPImRNA has occurred, and by 24 hours after CPH administration no significant difference from control is observed. The reduction of PPImRNA over 24 hours in control animals is due to fasting over the experimental period. The effect of CPH on PPImRNA is associated with a loss of insulin in mice (see Fig. 4). These data further substantiate that the effects of CPH-like inhibitors of insulin synthesis are reversible and that species other than the rat are susceptible.

Results obtained from ^{3}H-leucine-incorporation experiments, in which 10 μmol/L CPH was added to isolated pancreatic islets or RINm5F cells, show that the drug can inhibit proinsulin and insulin synthesis without altering cellular levels of PPImRNA (41,42). A 60% inhibition of proinsulin synthesis occurs without a loss of PPImRNA in isolated pancreatic islets treated with CPH. It seems clear from results obtained to date that the ability of CPH and its metabolites to inhibit the synthesis of insulin precursors and lower the cellular content of insulin in primary or clonal cells does not involve a loss of PPImRNA. Rather, an effect on translation appears to be involved in CPH-induced loss of cellular insulin in cell systems and in vivo. It is puzzling why a loss of PPImRNA is observed after CPH treatment in vivo but not in vitro. An indirect mechanism could account for the depletion of PPImRNA in vivo, but there is little information available with which to speculate on its nature.

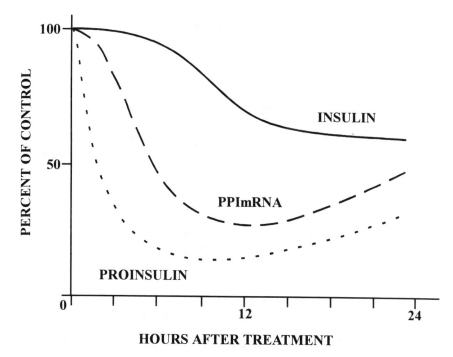

FIG. 11. Depiction of the time course of the decline of pre-proinsulin mRNA (PPImRNA), proinsulin, and insulin in rats after a single 45 mg/kg oral dose of CPH. (Redrawn from data in ref. 42, with permission.)

TABLE 3. *Effects of a Single Oral Dose of CPH (45 mg/kg) on Serum Glucose, Pancreatic PPImRNA, and Insulin Content in Mice.*[a]

Time point (h)	Treatment	Serum glucose (mg/dL)	Pancreatic PPImRNA (% of control at 0 h)[b]	Pancreatic IRI (ng/mg)[c]
0	Water	167.1 ± 12.5	100.0 ± 9.5	203.0 ± 63.0
12	Water	139.4 ± 8.4	88.8 ± 27.6	183.0 ± 44.0
12	CPH	230.9 ± 17.3[d,e]	23.3 ± 1.7[d,e]	251.0 ± 19.0
24	Water	161.8 ± 12.0	55.2 ± 6.0[d]	217.0 ± 36.0
24	CPH	198.9 ± 13.0[d,e]	44.8 ± 6.0[d]	178.0 ± 18.0

[a]Swiss Webster mice (N=4) were sacrificed at 0, 12, and 24 hours after administration of CPH or vehicle (water). Data are presented as the mean ± SEM.

[b]Data are calculated as integrated areas from densitometric scanning of autoradiograms of dot blots and expressed as percentage of the mean control value at the time of treatment (t=0 hour).+

[c]Data are expressed as nanograms (ng) of immunoreactive insulin per milligram (mg) pancreas.

[d]Significantly different from 0-hour control (*P*<0.05).

[e]Significantly different from vehicle control at each time point (*P*<0.05).

Subcellular Dislocation of PPImRNA

The primary gene product in insulin biosynthesis is pre-proinsulin, which is produced by ribosomes bound to membranes constituting the endoplasmic reticulum (57). Pre-proinsulin synthesis is initiated in unbound ribosomes in the cytoplasm, and as the nascent peptide emerges, it becomes associated with a soluble protein, the signal-recognition particle. This stops protein elongation and the complex moves to a receptor on the endoplasmic reticulum. After association with the endoplasmic reticulum, the signal-recognition particle is released and elongation resumes on the membrane-bound ribosome. The growing polypeptide chain that will become pre-proinsulin enters the lumen of the endoplasmic reticulum, and when translation is terminated, the gene product is rapidly converted by a peptidase to the secondary precursor proinsulin. Proinsulin then moves in vesicles from the endoplasmic reticulum to the Golgi area of the cell, where packaging into secretion granules occurs. Once packaging is complete, proinsulin conversion to insulin is initiated by removal of a small peptide fragment (ie, C peptide) to produce the two polypeptide chains of insulin linked by disulfide bridges. This pathway of synthesis and processing is common to many proteins destined for export from cells.

Experiments are now underway in this laboratory to gain evidence for an action of CPH and its analogs on one or more of the post-transcriptional processes involved in insulin biosynthesis. Because ribosomes completing pre-proinsulin synthesis must be bound to the endoplasmic reticulum, we examined the relative fraction of membrane-bound and unbound PPImRNA in RINm5F cells after exposure to CPH and some of its analogs. Cells were exposed for 2 hours to CPH and its active analog 4-DPMP in concentrations known to inhibit insulin synthesis. Treatment of cells with 2-DPMP was also included because this compound does not deplete cellular insulin in RINm5F cells (42). Subcellular fractionation of the cytoplasm of control and treated cells was performed, and the membrane and supernatant fractions were assayed for PPImRNA by dot-blot analysis. The fraction of cytoplasmic PPImRNA associated with the membrane fraction was determined. The results, illustrated in Fig. 12, show that approximately 70% of cytoplasmic PPImRNA in control cells is in the membrane-bound form and that CPH treatment significantly reduced the bound fraction in a concentration dependent manner. The analog 4-DPMP produced an effect on PPImRNA identical to CPH, but the isomer 2-DPMP did not alter the bound fraction (data not shown). These results are consistent with the relative activities of the DPMP isomers to inhibit insulin biosynthesis (40,42) and indicate that CPH-like inhibitors are capable of altering the cytoplasmic localization of PPImRNA. This would occur if ribosome binding to endoplasmic reticulum had been inhibited by the chemicals, resulting in a lowered synthesis of insulin precursors. The dislocation of PPImRNA was reversible, and control values of membrane association were observed by 30 hours after removal of CPH from cultured cells (data not shown).

It appears likely that the observed effects of CPH on the subcellular localization of PPImRNA is associated with the ability of the drug to inhibit insulin

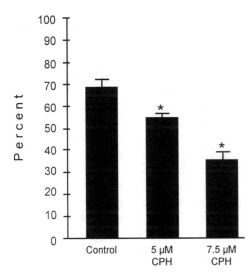

FIG. 12. Percentage of cytoplasmic PPImRNA in the membrane-bound form in control and CPH-treated RINm5F cells.

biosynthesis. The fact that the active CPH analog 4-DPMP produced an effect identical to CPH but the inactive analog 2-DPMP could not produce dislocation of PPImRNA provides some assurance that the apparent reduction in the membrane-bound form of PPImRNA is involved in the inhibitory action of CPH and 4-DPMP on insulin biosynthesis. The time course for reversibility of PPImRNA cytoplasmic dislocation is also consistent with the published time course for recovery of RINm5F cells from the insulin-depleting effects of CPH (40). Further research is needed to gain more direct evidence for an effect of CPH that results in a reduced binding of ribosomes to the endoplasmic reticulum. Possible sites of action would be on initiation, association with signal-recognition article, or binding to the endoplasmic reticulum receptor by the ribosome–signal recognition-article complex. Thus, current results provide a fruitful direction for future research on the ability of chemicals to impact insulin biosynthesis.

SUMMARY AND CONCLUSIONS

The reversible inhibition of insulin synthesis produced by CPH and some of its metabolites and structural analogs represents a remarkable example of target-organ and target-cell toxicity. This is a direct action of these chemicals as it takes place within the insulin-producing cell. The high sensitivity of β-cells in the endocrine pancreas for exhibiting chemical-induced inhibition of hormone synthesis, and the localization of the site of action to the endoplasmic reticulum, are characteristics of the toxicity that make it unusually specific.

The activity of CPH and its analogs to directly inhibit insulin secretion through a calcium-blocking action probably lacks the same degree of specificity that exists for the inhibition of insulin synthesis. This can be said because CPH is capable of inhibiting other calcium-related events, such as growth hormone and ACTH secretion. The inability of animals treated with CPH or its analogs to control blood glucose is primarily due to a lack of adequate insulin secretion brought about, in large measure, by deficiencies in cellular stores of the hormone.

Available knowledge does not provide an explanation for the cellular and subcellular specificity involved in the action of CPH and its analogs. It is unlikely that cell specificity is due to specific or selective localization of the chemicals in the endoplasmic reticulum of β-cells. Lipophilic amines generally cross membranes easily and are bound to intracellular components. Studies of the relative uptake of CPH and its analogs by the different cells composing the endocrine pancreas have not been performed, so that specificity based on factors related to the fate of chemicals in the pancreas cannot be ruled out. However, it seems likely that the specificity will be understood in concert with elucidation of the biochemical mechanism for CPH-induced inhibition of insulin biosynthesis.

The rat, a sensitive species to the toxicity of CPH in the endocrine pancreas, converts the drug to metabolites that have greater potencies than the unchanged compound for inhibiting insulin biosynthesis. The major metabolite present in tissues of the rat is DMCPH-epoxide, an *N*-demethylated, stable epoxide with 20 times the inhibitory potency of CPH. That metabolic product undoubtedly contributes to the action of CPH and is one reason why the rat is very susceptible to its diabetogenic effects. The mouse also exhibits pancreatic insulin depletion after CPH but does not produce large amounts of DMCPH-epoxide, showing that the metabolite is not the sole determinant of sensitivity to the effects of CPH. Humans do not excrete DMCPH-epoxide as a major metabolite in the urine after administration of CPH, and this provides some indication that the diabetogenic effect of the drug is not a serious threat when it is used clinically. However, evidence obtained from human studies indicates that the chemical has the potential to be diabetogenic in man.

Immature rats exhibit higher sensitivity than adult animals to the insulin-depleting action of CPH and its active analog 4-DPMP. The increased susceptibility of the developing and young animal is due in part to age-related differences in the toxicokinetics of CPH, but available data indicate that additional factors may also contribute. While the action of CPH in adult animals is reversible, this is not the case for effects produced in fetal animals undergoing transplacental exposure. The abnormal glucose tolerance and excessive pancreatic content of insulin in the adult offspring of CPH-treated pregnant animals is an important observation. Chemical insult of the developing endocrine pancreas can lead to an apparently permanent dysfunctional state in the adult animal. While the characteristics and mechanism of this abnormality have not been fully explored, it is necessary to do so because chemical "triggers" for certain forms of diabetes have been suspected for a long time.

The biochemical mechanism by which CPH-like chemicals produce a depletion of pancreatic insulin is being uncovered. There seems little doubt that a direct inhibition of insulin synthesis by these chemicals is responsible for the loss of insulin. This effect is not due to a general cytotoxic action in β-cells, because it is reversible. Current evidence indicates that an action of CPH at the level of translation is involved. Direct exposure of insulin-producing cells to CPH or 4-DPMP results in a dislocation of insulin mRNA (PPImRNA) within the cytoplasm of the cell, as less mRNA is found to be associated with cytoplasmic membranes. This effect could result from alteration of ribosome binding to endoplasmic reticulum, and this would result in an inhibition of hormone synthesis. The dramatic morphologic changes that occur in the endoplasmic reticulum of β-cells during treatment of animals with the chemicals is entirely consistent with the biochemical evidence that suggests an action at that organelle.

An apparent secondary consequence of the initial action of CPH-like chemicals in vivo is the decline in PPImRNA. This is not observed in primary or clonal insulin-producing cells exposed to the chemicals. Thus, the decline of insulin-specific mRNA can be considered an indirect effect resulting from animal treatment. An alternative explanation is that a metabolite of CPH has the ability to decrease synthesis or increase degradation of PPImRNA. No such activity has been detected in cells exposed to the known metabolites of the drug. The indirect relationship between chemical-induced inhibition of insulin synthesis and the subsequent decline in PPImRNA remains unknown.

In conclusion, it must be pointed out that studies of mechanisms by which chemicals cause toxicity usually enhance the understanding of the normal physiology and biochemistry of living systems. It is very likely that the reversible chemical inhibitors of insulin synthesis discussed in this chapter will be used as tools with which to build a better understanding of the functioning of the insulin-secreting β-cell. CPH has already been valuable in experiments designed to provide information regarding a differential regulation for the expression of the two different insulin genes in the rat (20). Other possible uses for these chemicals include their employment in studies of the role of fetal insulin in growth and development, regulation of normal cellular levels of PPImRNA, and elucidation of new factors controlling the post-transcriptional events of insulin biosynthesis.

ACKNOWLEDGMENTS

The research described from this laboratory was conducted in collaboration with excellent graduate students including: J.S. Wold, D.E. Rickert, K.L. Hintze, S.A. Chow, K.A. Kennedy and C.P. Miller. All of those scholars continue to be productive scientists. Grant support for their research was obtained from the National Institutes of Health and the Juvenile Diabetes Foundation.

REFERENCES

1. Assin R, Larger E. The role of toxins. In: Leslie RDG, ed. *Causes of diabetes, genetic and environmental factors*. Chichester, UK: John Wiley and Sons; 1993:105–123.
2. Beliles RP. The subchronic toxicity of 5-benzyl-11-[4-(N-methylpiperidylene)]-5,6-dihydromorphanthridine hydrogen maleate. *Toxicol Appl Pharmacol*. 1971;18:451–456.

3. Bergen SS. Appetite stimulating properties of cyproheptadine. *Am J Dis Child*. 1964;108:270–273.
4. Boillot D, Int'Veld P, Sai P, et al. Functional and morphological modifications induced in rat islets by pentamidine and other diamidines in vitro. *Diabetologia*. 1985;28:359–364.
5. Chatterjee AK, Fischer LJ. Age-related susceptibility to the insulin-depleting action of 4-diphenyl-methylpiperidine in young rats. *Life Sci*. 1988;43:151–159.
6. Chow SA, Fischer LJ. Postnatal changes in the insulin-depleting action and disposition of cyproheptadine in rats. *Dev Pharmacol Ther*. 1991;16:150–163.
7. Chow SA, Fischer LJ. Alterations in rat pancreatic B-cell function induced by prenatal exposure to cyproheptadine. *Diabetes*. 1984;33:572–575.
8. Chow SA, Fischer LJ. Susceptibility of fetal rat endocrine pancreas to the diabetogenic action of cyproheptadine. *Toxicol Appl Pharmacol*. 1986;84:264–277.
9. Chow SA, Fischer LJ. Metabolism and disposition of cyproheptadine and desmethylcyproheptadine in pregnant and fetal rats. *Drug Metab Dispos*. 1987;15:740–748.
10. Chow SA, Falany JL, Fischer LJ. Cyproheptadine metabolites inhibit proinsulin and insulin biosynthesis and insulin release in isolated rat pancreatic islets. *Cell Biol Toxicol*. 1989;5:129–143.
11. Chow SA, Rickert DE, Fischer LJ. Evidence that drug metabolites are involved in cyproheptadine-induced loss of pancreatic insulin. *J Pharmacol Exp Ther*. 1988;246:143–149.
12. Clark WR, Rutter WJ. Synthesis and accumulation of insulin in the fetal rat pancreas. *Dev Biol*. 1972;29:468–481.
13. DeLaFuente M, Alia M. The teratogenicity of cyproheptadine in two generations of Wistar rats. *Arch Int Pharmacodyn*. 1982;257:168–176.
14. Donatsch P, Lowe DA, Richardson BP, Taylor P. Mechanism by which cyproheptadine inhibits insulin secretion. *Br J Pharmacol*. 1980;70:355–362.
15. Egge AC, Rogal AD, Varma MM, Blizzard RM. Effect of cyproheptadine on TRH-stimulated prolactin and TSH release in man. *J Clin Endocrinol Metab*. 1977;44:210–213.
16. Engelhardt EL, Zell HC, Saari WS, et al. Structure activity relationships in the cyproheptadine series. *J Med Chem*. 1965;8:829–835.
17. Fischer LJ, Thies RL, Charkowski D, Donham KJ. Formation and urinary excretion of cyproheptadine glucuronide in monkeys, chimpanzees, and humans. *Drug Metab Dispos*. 1980;8:422–424.
18. Fischer LJ, Wold JS, Rickert DE. Structure-activity relationships in drug-induced pancreatic islet cell toxicity. *Toxicol Appl Pharmacol*. 1973;26:288–298.
19. Gazdar AF, Chick WL, Oie HK, et al. Continuous, clonal, insulin- and somatostatin-secreting cell lines established from a transplantable rat islet cell tumor. *Proc Natl Acad Sci U S A*. 1980;77:3519–3523.
20. Giddings SJ, Carnaghi LR, Fischer LJ, Miller CP. Differential regulation of rat insulin I and II mRNA synthesis: effects of fasting and cyproheptadine. *Mol Endocrinol*. 1991;4:549–554.
21. Golander A, Spirer Z. Inhibition of the insulin response to glucose after treatment with cyproheptadine. *Acta Paediatr Scand*. 1982;71:485–487.
22. Gold G, Pou J, Nowlain RM, Grodsky GM. Effects of monensin on conversion of proinsulin to insulin and secretion of newly synthesized insulin in the isolated rat islet. *Diabetes*. 1994;33:1019–1024.
23. Hucker HB, Balletto AJ, Staufer SC, Zacchei AG, Arison BH. Physiological disposition and urinary metabolites of cyproheptadine in dog, rat and cat. *Drug Metab Dispos*. 1974;2:406–415.
24. Halban PA, Wollheim CB, Blondel B, Niesor E, Renold AE. Perturbation of hormone storage and release induced by cyproheptadine in rat pancreatic islets in vitro. *Endocrinology*. 1979;104:1096–1106.
25. Hill RS, Boyd AE. Perfusion of a clonal cell line of simian virus 40-transfected beta cells, insulin secretory dynamics in response to glucose, 3-isobutyrl-1-methylxanthine and potassium. *Diabetes*. 1985;34:115–120.
26. Hintze KL, Aboul-Enein HY, Fischer LJ. Isomeric specificity of diphenylmethylpiperidine in the production of rat pancreatic islet cell toxicity. *Toxicology*. 1977;7:133–140.
27. Hintze KL, Baker Grow A, Fischer LJ. Cyproheptadine-induced alterations in rat insulin synthesis. *Biochem Pharmacol*. 1977;26:2021–2027.
28. Hintze KL, Baker Grow A, Fischer LJ. Role of the pituitary in cyproheptadine-induced pancreatic beta-cell toxicity. *Experientia*. 1977;33:1495–1496.
29. Hintze KL, Wold JS, Fischer LJ. Disposition of cyproheptadine in rats, mice and humans and identification of a stable epoxide metabolite. *Drug Metab Dispos*. 1975;3:1–9.
30. Hruban A, Rubenstein AH, Slesers A. Alterations in pancreatic beta cells induced by cyclizine. *Lab Invest*. 1972;26:270–277.

31. Ishibashi M, Fukushima T, Yamaji T. Cyproheptadine-mediated inhibition of growth hormone and prolactin release from pituitary adenoma cells of acromegaly and gigantism in culture. *Acta Endocrinol.* 1985;109:474–480.
32. Jahr H, Beckert R, Reiher H, Besch W, Zuhlke H. Cyproheptadine inhibits (pro)insulin biosynthesis and secretion of isolated human pancreatic islets. *Horm Metab Res.* 1981;13:359.
33. Joost HG, Beckmann J, Holze S, Lenzen S, Poser W, Hasselblatt A. Inhibition of insulin and glucagon release from the perfused rat pancreas by cyproheptadine (Periactinol, Nuran). *Diabetologia.* 1976;12:201–206.
34. Karam JH, Lewitt PA, Young CW, et al. Insulopenic diabetes after rodenticide (Vacor) ingestion: a unique model of acquired diabetes in man. *Diabetes.* 1980;29:971–978.
35. Kennedy KA, Halmi KA, Fischer LJ. Urinary excretion of a quaternary ammonium glucuronide metabolite of cyproheptadine in humans undergoing chronic drug therapy. *Life Sci.* 1977;21:1813–1820.
36. Lamberts SWJ, Verleun T, Bons EG, Uitterlinden P, Oosterom R. Effect of cyproheptadine, desmethyl-cyproheptadine, γ-amino-butyric acid and sodium valproate on adrenocorticotrophin secretion by cultured pituitary tumor cells from three patients with Nelson's syndrome. *J Endocrinol.* 1983;96:401–406.
37. Longnecker DS, Wold JS, Fischer LJ. Ultrastructural study of alterations in beta cells of pancreatic islets from cyproheptadine-treated rats. *Diabetes.* 1972;21:71–79.
38. Malaisse WJ. The endocrine pancreas as a target organ for toxicity. In: Cohen GM, ed. *Target Organ Toxicity.* Boca Raton, fla: CRC Press; 1986:143–158.
39. Malaisse-Lagae F, Amherdt M, Ravazzola M, et al. Role of microtubules in the synthesis, conversion and release of (pro)insulin: a biochemical and radioautographic study in rat islets. *J Clin Invest.* 1979;63:1284–1296.
40. Miller CP, Fischer LJ. Cyproheptadine-induced alterations in clonal insulin-producing cell lines. *Biochem Pharmacol.* 1990;39:1983–1990.
41. Miller CP, Giddings SJ, Chatterjee AK, Fischer LJ. Rapid alteration of pancreatic proinsulin and pre-proinsulin messenger ribonucleic acid in rats treated with cyproheptadine. *Endocrinology.* 1991;128:3040–3046.
42. Miller CP, Reape TJ, Fischer LJ. Inhibition of insulin production by cyproheptadine in RINm5F rat insulinoma cells. *J Biochem Toxicol.* 1993;8:127–134.
43. Molello JA, Barnard SD, Thompson DJ. Pancreatic beta cell vacuolation in rats after oral administration of hexamethylmelamine. *Toxicol Appl Pharmacol.* 1984;72:255–261.
44. Perrone C, Bricaire F, Leport C, et al. Hypoglycemia and diabetes mellitus following parenteral pentamidine mesylate treatment in AIDS patients. *Diabet Med.* 1990;7:585–589.
45. Porter CC, Arison BH, Gruber VF, Titus DC, Vandenheuvel WJA. Human metabolism of cyproheptadine. *Drug Metab Dispos.* 1975;3:189–197.
46. Pray GA, Halban A, Wollheim CB, Blondel B, Strauss AJ, Renold AE. Regulation of immunoreactive-insulin release from a rat cell line (RINm5F). *Biochem J.* 1983;210:345–352.
47. Rall T, Schleifer LS. Drugs effective in the therapy of epilepsies. In: Gilman AG, Goodman LS, Rall TW, Murad F, eds. *The Pharmacological Basis of Therapeutics.* 7th edition. New York, NY: Macmillan, 1985;446–472.
48. Richardson BP. Failure of cyproheptadine to induce pancreatic beta cell lesions in hypophysectomized rats. *Diabetologia.* 1974;10:479–483.
49. Richardson BP, Turcot-Lemay L, McDaniel ML, Lacy PE. Pancreatic β-cell changes induced by cyproheptadine in vitro. *Lab Invest.* 1975;33:509–513.
50. Rickert DE, Fischer LJ. Cyproheptadine and beta cell function in the rat: insulin secretion from pancreas segments in vitro. *Proc Soc Exp Biol Med.* 1975;150:1–6.
51. Rickert DE, Burke J, Fischer LJ. Cyproheptadine-induced depletion of insulin in the rat. *J Pharmacol Exp Ther.* 1975;193:585–593.
52. Rickert DE, Fischer LJ, Burke JP, et al. Cyproheptadine-induced insulin depletion in rat pancreatic beta cells: demonstration by light and electron microscopic immunocytochemistry. *Horm Metab Res.* 1976;8:430–434.
53. Santerre RF, Cook RA, Crisel RMD, et al. Insulin synthesis in a clonal cell line of simian virus 40-transformed hamster pancreatic beta cells. *Proc Natl Acad Sci U S A.* 1981;78:4339–4343.
54. Sodoyez-Goffaux F, Sodoyez JC, DeVos CJ, Foa PP. Insulin secretion and metabolism during the perinatal period in the rat: evidence for a placental role in fetal hyperinsulinemia. *J Clin Invest.* 1979;63:1095–1102.

55. Stiel JN, Liddle GW, Lacy WW. Studies of the mechanism of cyproheptadine-induced weight gain in human subjects. *Metabolism*. 1970;19:192–200.
56. Weinstein D, Ornoy A, Ben-Zur Z, Pfeifer Y, Sulman FG. Teratogenicity of cyproheptadine in pregnant rats. *Arch Int Pharmacodyn*. 1975;215:345–349.
57. Welsch M, Scherberg N, Gilmore R, Steiner DF. Translational control of insulin biosynthesis. *Biochem J*. 1986;235:459–467.
58. Wold JS, Fischer LJ. The tissue distribution of cyproheptadine and its metabolites in rats and mice. *J Pharmacol Exp Ther*. 1972;183:188–196.
59. Wold JS, Longnecker DS, Fischer LJ. Species dependent pancreatic islet toxicity produced by cyproheptadine: alterations in beta cell structure and function. *Toxicol Appl Pharmacol*. 1971;19:188–201.
60. Yamamoto H, Uchigata Y, Okamoto H. Streptozotocin and alloxan induce DNA strand breaks and poly(ADP-ribose) synthetase in pancreatic islets. *Nature*. 1981;294:284–286.

Endocrine Toxicology, 2nd ed.,
Edited by J. A. Thomas and H. D. Colby
Copyright © 1997 Taylor & Francis

12

Epidemiologic Evidence for Toxic Effects of Occupational and Environmental Chemicals on the Testes

Lowell E. Sever

Battelle Seattle Research Center, Seattle, Washington 98105

INTRODUCTION

Interest is increasing regarding the potential reproductive effects of exposure to occupational and environmental chemicals. From concerns about teratogenic effects of such chemicals, attention has expanded to examine reproductive toxicity in males and females. Awareness of the effects of environmental and occupational chemical exposures on male reproductive function has increased. This is a result of animal studies and of occupational exposures in which toxic substances made workers sterile and/or impotent. Issues of reproductive toxicology promise to be major ones in environmental and occupational health in the decade to come.

This chapter focuses on evidence for the effects of occupational chemicals on male reproduction, primarily in light of human data from epidemiologic studies. Animal studies are illustrative, but the theme is the human experience.

Reproductive function is examined as an indicator of toxic effects. When it is possible, we consider direct evidence for toxic damage to the testes. For some substances, the only data available consist of information on impaired reproductive function. For others, we discuss findings with regard to sperm analysis. It is not implied that the mode of action of these chemicals is necessarily by a direct effect on the testes. Rather, we address the general problems of male reproductive toxicology, with attention to the specific mechanisms when they are recognized.

Mattison (60) suggests that reproductive toxicants may act directly either because of similarity to an exogenous compound such as a nutrient or hormone or because of chemical reactivity, as in the case of an alkylating agent, denaturant, or chelator. Other reproductive toxicants may act indirectly, requiring metabolic processing before having a toxic effect.

Testicular toxicants are difficult to evaluate because of other factors of potential importance to male reproductive function. These include concomitant exposure to drugs and chemicals and the effects of general health on male reproductive function. Male infertility can be induced by chemicals that directly affect spermatogenic cells or indirectly via the hormonal and/or central and peripheral nervous systems.

To understand the effects of exogenous substances on male reproductive function, it is important to consider the structure and function of the reproductive system. In the original version of this chapter (90), a brief review of relevant structure, function, and hormonal control was provided; the anatomy of the testis and its histologic structure were described, and the discussion focused on the testis from the point of view of exocrine and endocrine functions and its relationship to other endocrinologic organs. These points are not discussed further here. Methods for assessing human testicular function, including reproductive histories, sperm analysis, assessment of hormonal status, and histologic studies described in the earlier work (90) are summarized here. The concentration in this chapter consists of a review of specific chemicals shown to affect reproduction in the human male, condensing material discussed in Sever and Hessol (90) and adding information developed during the past 10 years.

ASSESSING EFFECTS OF CHEMICALS ON MALE REPRODUCTION

There are several ways that the effects of an agent on male reproduction can be manifest. These include symptoms such as impotence or reduced libido, reduced fertility, alterations in sperm, changes in hormonal production (or action), and adverse reproductive outcomes such as spontaneous abortions or birth defects. In many instances, the pathways leading from chemical exposure to these manifestations are unknown.

There are several methods by which the effects of chemicals on the testes can be assessed. Some involve examination of reproductive function and others consider direct evidence for cellular damage. Although it would be of greatest interest to be able to collect direct toxicologic evidence (eg, hormonal assays or biopsies), the application of such methods has been limited in human studies involving occupational and environmental exposures. Thus, although their clinical usefulness has been demonstrated, there are limitations to the availability of such methods in population-based studies. In this chapter, we summarize four general ways of assessing male reproductive toxicity: (1) evaluation of reproductive history, (2) evaluation of sperm, (3) determination of blood hormone levels, and (4) assessment of testicular histology.

Reproductive History

The first stage of any investigation of reproductive toxicity in humans is likely to include the collection of information regarding reproductive history. While the occupational medical history should include questions on reproductive outcome for male workers, as well as for females, such information has not routinely been collected.

By purposeful collection and analysis of reproductive history information through questionnaires, important data can be obtained on infertility and adverse pregnancy outcomes. The use of well designed questionnaires allows the ascertainment of multiple reproductive outcomes, such as infertility, time to pregnancy, birth defects, and spontaneous abortions, with the use a single instrument. At the same time, questionnaires allow the collection of exposure data and information on potential confounders. Questionnaires and analytical methods have been developed that allow comparison of the fertility of exposed workers with population norms (56,113). On the negative side, data obtained through the use of such questionnaires may be subject to poor memory, reporting bias, or the respondent's unwillingness to provide accurate information.

Sperm Analysis

Sperm analysis is one of the most commonly employed methods for studying testicular function in man. One reason sperm analysis is used for evaluating the effects of testicular toxicants is that spermatogenic cells at any stage of differentiation can be directly or indirectly damaged by chemicals that interfere with various sites in the endocrine or exocrine systems (54). The result of damage to spermatogenic cell differentiation is interference with the production of normal spermatozoa. This can result in azoospermia, oligospermia, or the production of morphologically abnormal sperm or genetic mutations that may be associated with fetal wastage, congenital malformations, and/or genetic disorders.

Sperm evaluation usually consists of sperm count, motility, morphology, and semen volume. Some investigators also use sperm penetration assays as a measure of seminal fertility, and the double Y-body test is coming into increasing use (115). There are problems, however, with sperm analysis, beginning with the procurement of the specimen through placing the results within a normal range. There are also variations in sperm output in the same individual, depending on when sampling occurs. Sperm output may drop owing to systemic or localized infections, stress, allergic reactions, and other causes. Nevertheless, sperm analysis can be very effective for detecting testicular dysfunction, especially in the presence of azoospermia or oligospermia.

A number of relatively new techniques have been developed for sperm evaluations. These include standardized computer-based scoring systems and videotaping of sperm trajectories and motility patterns (44).

Hormonal Evaluations

Measuring levels of circulating hormones is a useful procedure in examining the effects of suspected reproductive toxicants. Commonly measured are blood levels of the gonadotropins, luteinizing hormone (LH) and follicle-stimulating hormone (FSH), and the androgenic hormone testosterone. Elevated gonadotropin levels are evidence of testicular disease (1). Leydig cell dysfunction often results in elevated LH production; elevated plasma FSH levels are frequently found in men with damage to the seminiferous epithelium. In individuals with severe oligospermia or azoospermia, elevated FSH levels are proof of severe tubular damage and a reduction in all the germinal elements, including spermatogonia (1). It should be noted, however, that serious disturbances in spermatogenesis have been observed in men with "normal" FSH levels (91).

The normal range for testosterone levels is extremely broad and the presence of blood levels within this range is often interpreted as indicating normal Leydig cell function. This may not be the case, however, as functional tests, such as stimulation by human chorionic gonadotropin (hCG), often demonstrate Leydig cell compensation whereby normal amounts of testosterone are produced despite intrinsic cell damage (91).

Hormonal analyses are useful in evaluating the toxic effects of chemicals on the testes, but significant damage can exist in the presence of "normal" hormonal values. Hormonal analyses are an important component of the armamentarium for studies of male reproductive toxicity but must be interpreted along with other evidence regarding reproductive function. The results of hormonal analyses in studies of specific chemicals are considered below.

Testicular Histology

Histologic evaluation of testicular tissue obtained by biopsy has the potential to determine cytotoxic effects of chemicals on the testes. Testicular biopsy can be used to determine if the structure of the testis is histologically normal. In addition, histochemical procedures can be used to demonstrate chemical changes at the cellular level.

Few studies of occupational or environmental exposures have utilized such techniques, although they are frequently used in studies of infertility when azoospermia or severe oligospermia is present (26). Histologic examination of the testis and quantitative analysis of spermatogenesis have potentially important roles in studies of the effects of exposure to environmental and occupational toxic agents on spermatogenesis (91). An extensive discussion of methods for assessment of male reproductive toxicology is included in a recent monograph on biological markers from the National Research Council (65).

OCCUPATIONAL AND ENVIRONMENTAL CHEMICALS AFFECTING REPRODUCTION IN THE HUMAN MALE

Occupational and environmental chemicals shown to have an effect on male reproductive function are limited in number. There are even fewer chemicals whereby specific changes in testicular function or spermiogenesis have been observed in the male reproductive system. The following discussion considers the specific chemical agents that we believe act as male reproductive toxicants.

Dibromochloropropane

The discovery that dibromochloropropane (DBCP) is toxic to the male reproductive system has stimulated much of the subsequent research in this area. Commercially produced beginning in 1956, DBCP is a highly persistent, lipophilic, brominated organochlorine that has been used as a fumigant against nematodes for a wide variety of plants. Applied as a liquid by several different methods, DBCP volatilizes and has a fumigating action once in the soil (3). In California, DBCP was used mainly on grapes, peaches, citrus fruits, and tomatoes; in the Carolinas it was used on peaches and soybeans; in Central America and Israel, on bananas; and in Hawaii, on pineapples (104). In 1977, DBCP was clearly demonstrated to be associated with sterility and low sperm counts in exposed workers. Its use in the United States was subsequently suspended, with the exception of use on pineapple fields in Hawaii (3). All use of DBCP in the United States was banned by the U.S. Environmental Protection Agency in 1985 (109). The risks associated with DBCP exposure and the relevant regulatory activities have been reviewed in several publications (3,4,39,55,85,94,104,107).

Numerous studies have been conducted on the effects of DBCP on male reproductive function. To summarize the evidence regarding the toxicity of DBCP to the male reproductive system, it is necessary to examine the reproductive history information from various studies, review the evidence from sperm analyses of exposed workers, and subsequently consider data from hormonal evaluations and studies of testicular histology.

Reproductive History

The recognition of the possible effects of DBCP on male reproductive function came not from scientists but from workers. The work force of the Occidental Chemical Company plant in Lathrop, California, in the area where DBCP was processed, was small. Although the workers were young and wanted children, they noticed that there was a paucity of children conceived by the men after they had started to work in the DBCP-handling area of the factory (104,107,116). It was the perception of impaired fertility by the workers that led to semen analyses and to the identification of a high rate of azoospermia and severe oligospermia.

In the original publication on the Occidental Chemical Company workers, Whorton et al. (105) reported on 36 male workers who were exposed to DBCP. They noted the reported infertility, but the only additional reproductive history information included was that seven of the 36 men had never fathered children. It appears that since infertility was the reason the study was initiated and semen analyses were carried out, reproductive history information was not published at that time. The authors did report, however, that none of the men had loss of libido or difficulty with erection or ejaculation.

Potashnik et al. (70) studied six DBCP production workers in Israel. It is not clear how these cases were identified; of the six, three reported decreased libido, two reported infertility, and one reported impotence. Thus, in contrast to the original series reported by Whorton et al. (105), these workers had problems of sexual dysfunction as well as infertility. The number of pregnancies for the wife of each worker was reported, but no information was provided regarding the timing of the pregnancies in relation to DBCP exposure.

Glass et al. (28) studied a group of pesticide applicators that included individuals with varying levels of exposure to DBCP. Nine men out of 96 who had semen analyses reported clinical infertility, which was defined as 1 year of unprotected coitus without conception. There was no relationship between clinical infertility and DBCP exposure.

Kahn and Whorton (42) challenged the assertion by Glass et al. (28) that infertility was not a problem among the applicators. They questioned the usefulness of "clinical infertility," based on a questionnaire, in assessing reproductive effects. In response, Glass (27) defended the use of clinical infertility in studies of this type, particularly when combined with other indicators of reproductive toxicity.

Perhaps the most important information on the effects of DBCP on applicators comes from a report on sterility among banana plantation workers in Costa Rica (94). Approximately 1500 male workers from the Atlantic banana-growing region of Costa Rica had been diagnosed as infertile as a result of DBCP exposure. It is estimated that 20–25% of the banana workers in this area were affected by mid-1990 (94). Exposure could not be quantified among these pesticide applicators but the application methods employed would have led to prolonged high level exposures. None of the workers wore protective clothing during applications, and they did not use safety precautions such as avoiding spills and washing after work. Because of the application techniques employed, workers continually inhaled DBCP and contacted DBCP through their hands, arms, legs, and feet. In addition, DBCP was applied throughout the year except for a 2–3 month period. Therefore, applicators had the potential for high levels of exposure over prolonged periods of time.

There is limited information on reproductive outcomes among workers exposed to DBCP. Kharrazi et al. (45) studied a group of 62 married banana workers from Israel who were exposed to DBCP. Data were collected from the workers on exposure to DBCP and on the reproductive histories of their wives. Data on pregnancy outcomes were also obtained from hospital records. The pregnancy outcomes among the wives of the 62 workers were compared with a subset of 16 workers whose wives conceived both before and after exposure to DBCP. There were no significant differences between the number of pregnancies, number of live births, or mean age of the mother in the before and after DBCP exposure groups. There was, however, a significant difference in the rate of spontaneous abortions between the before (6.6%) and after (19.8%) DBCP exposure groups.

This difference was even more pronounced in the subset of wives who conceived both before (5.9%) and after (27.5%) exposure.

In a follow-up study 8 years after their initial assessment of the effects of DBCP exposure, Potashnik, Yanai-Inbar, and co-workers (73) examined the outcomes of pregnancies fathered by members of their cohort. The spontaneous abortion rate among exposed pregnancies was virtually identical to that observed for pre-exposed and unexposed conceptions (13.6% versus 13.4%). The mode of delivery and birthweights of the children born during exposure and recovery periods were normal, and there was no increased risk of congenital malformations (72). The finding of no increased risk of spontaneous abortion contrasts with the earlier study by Kharrazi et al. (45).

Potashnik and Phillip (72) studied birth defects and health status among children conceived during or after paternal exposure to DBCP. They did not observe any increase in birth defects among 34 children evaluated, whose general health status was unremarkable.

Potashnik and colleagues carried out studies of sex ratio among offspring of DBCP-exposed workers (29,71,73). The results can be summarized as follows: In 51 births among the unexposed workers and the exposed workers prior to exposure, the prevalence of males was 52.9%. Among offspring conceived by exposed men during exposure, the rate of males was 35.2%, while the rate among azoospermic and ogliospermic men during recovery of spermatogenesis was 21% (73). These results represent a statistically significant decrease in the number of male births. The decrease in sex ratio prior to the onset of severe testicular dysfunction and infertility is interpreted as a possibly early effect on reproductive performance (71). This suggests that DBCP may be particularly toxic to Y chromosome–bearing sperm cells (109) and that there is a late restoration of fertility potential for such cells (73).

To our knowledge, there has been no evaluation of reproductive outcome in the studies of production workers in the United States.

Finally, with regard to reproductive history data, we consider the approach used by Levine et al. (56), in which the number of births to exposed workers is compared with the number of births expected as derived from national birth probabilities. The method is based on the concept of a standardized fertility ratio (observed:expected births), which can be compared for exposed and unexposed periods of workers' employment.

Levine et al. (57) validated their methodology by analyzing data on the DBCP-exposed workers originally studied by Whorton et al. (105). The standardized fertility ratio (SFR) from data available in 1977 for the at-risk exposed workers was 0.75, significantly lower than the ratios for the not-at-risk period (SFR = 1.88), or the portion related to employment in other areas of the factory (SFR = 2.16). Levine et al. (57) stressed that with use of a simple reproductive history questionnaire and their method, it would have been possible to detect occupationally induced infertility in these workers well in advance of the actual time of discovery.

Regarding the identification of reproductive toxicity of DBCP by reproductive history, a quotation from Marvin Legator (55) is particularly appropriate:

> Not only would a simple sperm analysis have indicated a problem, but the most elementary questionnaire, taken in conjunction with a physical examination by an industrial physician, should have been enough to alert management to the existing problem. It is also hard to understand how in this time of sophisticated computer technology, epidemiologic studies, and a general concern of management for the health of their workers, that the DBCP problem was brought to light by employees discussing their inability to raise a family.

Sperm Analysis

It was through the analysis of semen samples from the infertile Occidental Chemical Company workers that the reproductive toxicity of DBCP was established (105). In the Lathrop, California, facility, 39 workers in the agricultural chemical division, where DBCP was formulated, were identified (105). The workers included three females and 36 males, 25 of whom were nonvasectomized. Semen specimens were collected from the nonvasectomized males.

Of the 25 nonvasectomized men, 14 had azoospermia or oligospermia. Eleven men (group A) had sperm counts ≤1 million/mL; 11 men (group B) had normal counts >40 million/mL; and three men had counts of 10–30 million/mL. A striking relationship was found between sperm count and duration of exposure. The men in group A had a mean sperm count of 0.2 million/mL and a mean exposure time of 8 years; for group B, the mean sperm count was 93 million/mL, and mean exposure time, 0.08 years. In other words, workers with sperm counts ≤1 million/mL had been exposed at least 3 years, whereas no one with a count >40 million/mL had been exposed for more than 3 months (105). Thus, there is a clear relationship between duration of exposure and oligospermia and azoospermia.

A second study of the Occidental Chemical Company facility was conducted, in which an attempt was made to study testicular function in all male employees (106). The total male population at risk was 310, of whom 196 agreed to be examined, including the original 36 workers described above. A total of 142 men provided semen samples for analysis. It was not possible to establish actual levels of exposure to DBCP. Exposure could occur at several locations in the plant, and the movement of workers within the plant created problems in assessing the duration of exposure for individual workers. Best estimates of total months of potential exposure to DBCP were made for each worker.

Of the 142 men who provided semen samples, 107 were classified as "ever" exposed, and 35 were classified as "never" exposed. For the ever-exposed group, the median sperm count was 46 million/mL; for the never-exposed group, the median count was 79 million/mL. Of the exposed workers, 13.1% were azoospermic, 16.8% were severely oligospermic, and 15.8% were mildly ogliospermic. Among the nonexposed workers, 2.9% were azoospermic, none was severely oligospermic, and 5.7% were mildly oligospermic. The authors also looked at the ratio of oligospermia to normospermia in 126 men for whom information on months of potential DBCP exposure was available. There was an increasing ratio of men with sperm counts < 20 million/mL with increasing time of exposure (107). Thus, there were clear-cut differences in both the median sperm counts and the distributions of counts between the exposed and unexposed men.

As a result of these findings at the Lathrop, California, plant, studies were also conducted of workers at other DBCP-manufacturing facilities. Milby and Whorton (63) presented data from sperm analyses of a group of 85 DBCP workers, which they compare with analyses from a control group of 84 unexposed workers. No information on the population from which these workers came was provided, except that they came from a single plant "engaged in the manufacture, processing or formulation" of DBCP. Men were classified into two exposure groups on the basis of job categories; there were major differences in participation rates between the exposed and unexposed groups. For the exposed group, the median sperm count was 46 million/mL, the rate of azoospermia 1.4%, and the rate of oligospermia 15.5%. For the unexposed group, the median sperm count was 88 million/mL, the rate of azoospermia 2.9%, and the rate of oligospermia 5.9%. These differences in distribution were reported to be statistically significant.

Egnatz et al. (19) conducted evaluations of Dow Chemical workers previously exposed to DBCP and of nonexposed workers. These were workers from the Michigan division of Dow, where DBCP had been manufactured from 1957 through 1975. The exposure group consisted of 232 chemical workers who were classified into four production and two nonproduction subdivisions. These groups were further categorized by time since last exposure: less than 5 years or 5 years or more. Frequency distributions indicated a tendency toward a higher percentage of low sperm counts in the exposed employees relative to the nonexposed group. In the subgroup of production workers with recent direct exposure, sperm counts were inversely correlated with exposure duration.

Whorton (104) presented data from a Magnolia, Arkansas, Dow Chemical plant where DBCP was produced. Of 61 exposed men examined, 32.8% were reported to be azoospermic. Only 4% of controls had azoospermia. An additional 44.3% of the exposed group had sperm counts < 50 million/mL. Babich et al. (3) stated that Dow Chemical reported a 24.2% rate of azoospermia among the DBCP-exposed workers at the Magnolia plant and a 30.2% rate for oligospermia. They noted that the duration of exposure at that plant was only 20 months. It is not clear why there is a discrepancy between the data presented by Whorton (104) and those presented by Babich et al. (3).

Kapp and associates studied Y-bodies in sperm among DBCP workers in the Magnolia, Arkansas, plant (43). The use of the double Y-body test detects Y-chromosome nondisjunction through fluorescent staining. Kapp et al. (43) reported a mean of 3.8% double Y-bodies among DBCP-exposed workers compared with a mean of 1.2% for unexposed individuals. There was a statistically significant difference between the exposed and unexposed groups in the distribution of double Y-bodies.

Another United States producer of DBCP was the Shell Chemical Company, with two production facilities located in Denver, Colorado, and Mobile, Alabama. The Denver plant produced DBCP from 1956 to 1976, whereas the Mobile plant was in production only from 1976 to July 1977 (59). At Denver, 64 DBCP-exposed and 20 unexposed workers were studied. At Mobile, 71 DBCP-exposed workers and 37 unexposed workers were studied.

Among the Denver workers, 21.9% of the exposed group had sperm counts of less than 20 million/mL, compared with 10% of the controls. In Denver, 7% of the exposed workers had azoospermia, compared with none of the controls. The differences in sperm count between the exposed and unexposed Denver workers were not, however, statistically significant. When the data on sperm count were examined by adjusted hours of DBCP exposure, Denver employees with greater than 1,000 hours of exposure had a significantly lower sperm count.

The results from the Mobile, Alabama, plant are quite different from those of Denver. Of the exposed workers in Mobile, 16.9% had sperm counts < 20 million/mL, compared with 8.8% of the controls. The frequency of azoospermia was lower in Mobile (2%) than in Denver, and again there were no azoospermics among the controls. Unlike Denver, there were highly statistically significant reductions in sperm count among the exposed workers. The median sperm count in the exposed group was 45.6 million/mL compared with a median of 84 million/mL in the unexposed. In terms of levels of exposure, employees exposed to less than 40 adjusted hours of DBCP did not have significantly reduced sperm counts, whereas those with more than 100 hours did have reduced counts.

The authors note that the results showing DBCP-exposed workers at the Mobile plant to have a significantly lower sperm count than the exposed Denver workers were somewhat surprising, given the fact that the average Denver worker was exposed for more hours than the average Mobile worker (59). They suggested that this may be due to the possibility that some of the Denver workers, who had not been exposed to DBCP since 1976, had regained some of their lost testicular function. Conversely, the more recently exposed Mobile workers still showed the acute effects of DBCP exposure at the time of the study, and thus the reduced sperm counts were observed. The data, interpreted in this fashion, support the suggestion that the reproductive toxicity due to DBCP may be reversible to some degree (a point we discuss below).

Sperm analyses were also carried out on DBCP production workers in Israel (69,72). In the original study of six workers, all had azoospermia that followed periods of DBCP exposure of 3–10 years (70). In a subsequent larger study, Potashnik et al. (74) examined 23 workers exposed to DBCP during production. The workers were classified into three groups on the basis of sperm counts. Group A consisted of 12 workers with azoospermia. All of these workers had been directly involved in DBCP production and had exposure times ranging from 100 hours to more than 6,700 hours. In five members of this group, the most recent exposure had been 1–5 years earlier. Group B consisted of six workers with oligospermia, with sperm counts in the range of 0.5–10 million/mL. The exposure times for this group ranged from 34 hours to 95 hours, and three members of the group had had their last exposure 1–2 years previously. Group C consisted of five employees with normal sperm counts (20.5–65 million/mL) who were involved in packing DBCP and whose exposures were recent but shorter. Thus, these findings reveal a close correlation between exposure time and sperm counts. Severe impairment of spermatogenesis was present in 78% of the exposed workers studied.

In addition to the studies that examined DBCP-production workers, there are studies that examined applicators or agricultural workers. These studies are important in that they demonstrate DBCP's effects on spermatogenesis at levels of exposure potentially lower than those observed in the production process.

Glass et al. (28) studied sperm counts of pesticide applicators from 20 California firms that had been heavy users of DBCP from 1976 to 1977. Accurate quantification of exposure was not possible, and the workers were grouped by days of DBCP use in the current year. There were 22 men with no exposure, 19 men with 1 day to 2 weeks of exposure, 31 men with exposure between 2 weeks and 2 months, and 24 with exposure of more than 2 months. The number of past years of exposure was also determined.

Glass et al. (28) reported a significant trend of sperm count decline with increasing exposure. By individual exposure groups, only those with greater than 2 months' exposure had significantly lower sperm counts. In this group, 14 men had sperm counts ≤40 million/mL, and four of these men had azoospermia. There was a nonsignificant trend for decreased sperm count with past exposure that was confounded by recent exposure. The authors noted that they expected men with several years' exposure to be more severely affected than men with only recent contact. Since that was not observed, they suggested that the effects of DBCP may be reversible in men with mild sperm count depression.

Kahn and Whorton (42) questioned the analysis of the sperm count data presented by Glass et al. (28). Kahn and Whorton (42) compared the distribution of sperm counts for the applicators with a control population assembled from chemical workers not exposed to testicular toxicants. They reported significant differences between the applicators as a group, those exposed for 2 weeks to 2 months, and those exposed for more than 2 months, and the controls, when the distributions of sperm counts are analyzed. Thus, Kahn and Whorton (42) believe that exposure has an effect on sperm count at levels lower than the effect levels suggested by Glass et al. (28).

In response to Kahn and Whorton (42), Glass (27) challenged the appropriateness of an external control population when internal controls were studied. He notes several reasons why the controls (unexposed group) they studied were a better reference population than the control population of Kahn and Whorton (42).

Sandifer et al. (80) studied agricultural workers, including formulators, applicators, farmers, and farm workers, who were potentially exposed to DBCP. Six of eight formulators and 13 of 43 users were oligospermic, with sperm counts <20 million/mL. The authors assessed exposure by dividing the total number of pounds of DBCP used by the number of days in which it was used.

A significant negative correlation was demonstrated between sperm count and the index of exposure.

A third study of agricultural workers exposed to DBCP is a one by the National Institute for Occupational Safety and Health (NIOSH) among pineapple-plantation workers in Hawaii (50). This study included industrial-hygiene monitoring and prospective medical evaluation. Three groups of workers had different levels of DBCP exposure: 35 field workers who applied DBCP, 27 maintenance workers who repaired fumigation tractors, and 29 unexposed plantation workers. Three semen specimens were collected from each participant: one before the fumigation season, one midway through, and one approximately 3 weeks after the season. Exposure to DBCP in the low concentrations present in this situation was found to produce significant effects on sperm count.

In summary, extensive data from several studies show a marked effect of DBCP on sperm production, with important relationships between sperm counts and duration of exposure. It is interesting to note that there does not appear to be evidence for increased rates of abnormalities of sperm morphology associated with DBCP exposure. One study showed an increase in double Y-bodies among exposed workers (43).

Hormonal Evaluations

In the original study of the Occidental Chemical Company plant, Whorton et al. (105) found that the exposed men who had oligospermia or azoospermia had elevated blood levels of follicle-stimulating hormone (FSH) and luteinizing hormone (LH) compared with men who had normal sperm counts. The high FSH levels are consistent with impaired spermatogenesis in these individuals. The serum testosterone levels were similar for the two groups, and the cause of the elevated LH is not known.

In the more complete study of the Occidental workers (106), additional workers were studied for changes in hormonal levels. Whorton et al. (106) found that exposure was directly related to FSH and LH blood levels, which were inversely related to the log of sperm count. There were no associations with testosterone levels. From a predictive point of view, they found that FSH alone was as good a predictor of effect as a combination of the three hormones, provided that a large percentage of the workers had azoospermia. However, if the azoospermic males were excluded, then FSH was of little value in detecting oligospermia. The authors concluded that the hormonal data showed no evidence of an alteration of the pituitary–testes axis.

In the follow-up assessment of the Occidental workers, Whorton and Milby (110) determined changes in FSH levels between 1977 and 1978. There was a significant increase in the mean FSH level for 11 azoospermic men during the follow-up period. Of eight men with vasectomies, two had normal FSH levels and six had elevated levels, with four of the six men having had potential DBCP exposure of greater than 4 years. The authors interpreted the observed increases in FSH following termination of exposure as being consistent with increasing testicular dysfunction, at least of the FSH pituitary–testicular axis.

Hormonal levels were also studied in workers at the Dow Chemical Company, Midland, Michigan, by Egnatz et al. (19). High FSH and LH levels were found among potentially exposed workers relative to the comparison group. FSH levels in the production group and LH levels in both production and nonproduction groups were significantly elevated. In the production subgroup with recent direct exposure, duration of exposure was highly positively correlated with FSH. In addition, there was a highly significant negative correlation between sperm count and FSH levels. In this subgroup, mean values for both sperm count and FSH levels were within normal limits.

In their studies of Shell Chemical Company employees in Denver and Mobile, Lipshultz et al. (59) measured serum FSH, LH, and testosterone levels. They reported only on FSH levels, believing that it more closely reflected abnormalities in spermatogenesis. They found that the mean serum concentration of FSH was significantly higher at both the Denver and Mobile facilities for the exposed versus the unexposed cohorts. The significance decreased by ten levels of magnitude when the group with shorter but more recent exposure (Mobile) was compared with the workers from the plant with the longer history of chemical production (Denver).

Additional information on hormonal evaluations of the Shell workers comes from the study by Lantz et al. (52). They examined 14 oligospermic men from the Mobile plant. This was the plant with the shorter, more recent exposures. Thirteen of the 14 men had normal basal serum LH levels and a normal LH response following administration of LH-releasing hormone (LH-RH). Mean LH levels were significantly elevated in a group of exposed workers who also had extratesticular abnormalities (group 1), but they were not elevated in the group without abnormalities (group 2). For both groups, the mean testosterone concentrations were significantly lower than in control subjects. With regard to FSH, the mean basal level in group 1 was significantly higher than in controls, and the FSH response following LH-RH was greater. The authors interpret their results as suggesting that mild abnormalities of the Leydig cells may be related to DBCP exposure.

Potashnik et al. (70) evaluated hormonal levels in their original six subjects. They reported significantly elevated FSH levels and normal LH and testosterone concentrations in those workers who had azoospermia. In the expanded study of the Israeli workers, Potashnik et al. (74) found that plasma FSH levels were significantly higher than the upper limit of normal in ten members of the azoospermic group. Two men in this group, with relatively short exposure times, had normal FSH levels. Plasma FSH levels in the group of oligospermic workers were normal. Plasma LH and testosterone levels were normal in both groups, with the exception of one azoospermic worker who had a low testosterone level and a high level of LH. Since normal FSH levels were found in the oligospermic workers, the authors suggested that plasma FSH levels are of limited value as a sensitive indicator for predicting the gonadotoxic effect of DBCP.

Sandifer et al. (80) measured FSH, LH, and testosterone levels in DBCP-exposed agricultural workers. They found significant differences between exposure groups in FSH and LH levels but not in testosterone levels. Significant negative correlations were observed between FSH and LH levels and sperm counts. FSH levels showed a definite trend toward abnormality. The authors suggested that high levels of FSH could serve as a reliable indicator of testicular function; elevated FSH levels almost always indicate low sperm counts. The presence of normal hormonal levels, however, does not rule out the possibility of impaired spermatogenesis.

Glass et al. (28) studied FSH and LH in their group of DBCP applicators but reported only on hormonal levels in relation to days of exposure in the current year. A statistically significant trend for increasing FSH levels with increasing exposure was observed. The association with LH levels was similar but not significant.

In summary, the data from the studies reviewed suggest an important relationship between DBCP exposure, FSH levels, and sperm counts. In addition, there is some evidence for an effect of DBCP exposure on LH levels. It appears that high FSH levels may be a useful indicator of altered spermatogenesis and damage to the seminiferous tubules. Since such damage can occur in the absence of altered FSH levels, normal levels of FSH cannot be interpreted as indicating a lack of an effect of DBCP exposure.

Testicular Histology

Testicular histology was evaluated in workers from three of the exposed groups, including individuals from the Occidental Chemical Company plant, the Mobile facility of Shell Chemical Company, and the Israeli manufacturing facility.

Whorton et al. (106) reported on the results of bilateral, open testicular biopsies in 10 workers. In the most severe cases, there was generalized absence of all spermatogenic activity, and the seminiferous tubules were devoid of spermatogonia. In the less severely affected, there was a decrease in the amount of cellularity within the seminiferous tubules.

Biava et al. (5) presented more detailed information regarding the 10 testicular biopsies. The individuals were classified into three groups on the basis of sperm counts. Three individuals had normal sperm counts and normal testicular histology. Two of these three individuals had only short exposures to DBCP. The second group consisted of two individuals who were azoospermic and had the longest history of DBCP exposure. In both of these men, the seminiferous tubules were devoid of germ cells. The Sertoli cells were normal, and there was no evidence of cellular necrosis. The intercellular junctions were unchanged. The third group consisted of five workers with reduced sperm counts and exposures to DBCP intermediate to those of the other two groups. Specimens from these men demonstrated moderately to markedly decreased sperm formation, and spermatogenic cells were observed in only a minority of the tubules. Aside from the changes in spermatogenic activity, no consistent histologic features were observed in the biopsies from the three groups.

Biava et al. (5) suggested that suppression of spermatogenesis might be related to a failure of the normal process of spermatogonia renewal at the stem-cell level. Under those conditions, spermatogenesis would be impeded at its earliest stage. As the stem-cell pool became depleted, the number of differentiating and mature sperm cells would be correspondingly reduced. If failure of the stem-cell renewal process was caused by DBCP, it would indicate that stem cells were selectively sensitive to DBCP or its metabolites.

Lantz et al. (52) performed testicular biopsies on 14 workers from the Mobile facility of Shell Chemical who suffered from oligospermia. Group 1 included four men with reduced late spermatids and spermatozoa; the other three exhibited markedly impaired spermatogenesis. There was focal hyalinization of the tubular walls in most of the biopsies. In group 2, all biopsies showed some tubules with fairly complete cell associations and the production of some spermatozoa, with the exception of one man with an elevated FSH in whom spermatogenesis was severely compromised. In their study, the predominant finding was some reduction in all cell types. This supports the suggestion of Biava et al. (5) that DBCP affects the renewal of spermatogonia.

The final group studied by testicular biopsy was the Israeli production workers (70,74). Twelve individuals with azoospermia underwent testicular biopsy. All histologic sections revealed complete atrophy of the seminiferous epithelium, and Sertoli cells only lined the majority of the tubules. No evidence of active spermatogenesis was found. The Leydig cells were normal in appearance. A similar histologic picture was observed in biopsies from two men with oligospermia, although there was some evidence of active spermatogenesis.

One of the subjects who had a testicular biopsy reported in the study of Potashnik et al. (70) underwent a second biopsy eight years later. The initial biopsy showed severe damage to the seminiferous tubules with sporadic preservation of spermatogenesis and large groups of Leydig cells in the interstitial tissue. The second biopsy revealed all stages of spermatogenesis, with spermatozoa in more than one third of the tubules.

In summary, histologic evaluation of testicular tissue obtained by biopsy from men exposed to DBCP showed a selective decrease or loss of spermatogenic cells without any other consistent testicular defect. In severely affected workers, spermatogenic cells were absent from the seminiferous tubules, with only Sertoli cells remaining. In the less severely affected workers there was a decrease in spermatogenesis. These histologic studies suggest a direct DBCP effect on the seminiferous tubules and on the spermatogonia.

Recovery of Testicular Function

Following recognition of DBCP's effects on sperm counts, there has been considerable interest in the possibility of recovery of testicular function following termination of exposure. This has been considered in some of the studies discussed above and has been the central topic of several additional studies.

Whorton and Milby (110) examined recovery of testicular function in 21 of the men from the Occidental Chemical Company who had DBCP-related sperm count depression (105,106). One year after termination of exposure, none of the 12 men with azoospermia showed improvement in sperm count; they remained azoospermic. Of the nine restudied individuals who had oligospermia in 1977, three of four men with prior counts <10 million/mL showed improvement, with two being normospermic (count >20 million/mL). Five men had had counts in the 10–19 million/mL range in 1977, and four of these men were normospermic in 1978. With regard to the effect of duration of exposure, 11 of 12 men with 4 or more years of exposure were azoospermic in 1977 and remained so 1 year later; the remaining man was oligospermic and remained so. Seven of nine men exposed for less than 4 years showed some recovery.

Lantz et al. (52) studied the recovery of testicular function among a group of the Shell Chemical workers who had been studied earlier by Lipshultz et al. (59). Sperm counts were compared for three periods following exposure: 1–6 months, 6–12 months, and 18–21 months. Following cessation of DBCP production, a statistically significant increase in sperm count was demonstrated when the counts at 18–21 months were compared with the counts at 1–6 months. One subject who was azoospermic remained so. Five men had more than a 2-fold increase in sperm counts. The authors suggested that the improved semen quality following the last DBCP contact indicates the regenerative capacity of the testes if impairment in semen quality following DBCP insult is recognized early enough.

Whorton (108) presented additional information on recovery of testicular function as reflected in sperm analyses. Cited are two unpublished studies that report recovery to normospermic ranges for some previously azoospermic men. Both studies found relatively quick improvements in oligospermic men following cessation of exposure. Whorton (108) also noted that two evaluations of pineapple workers 6 months after cessation of DBCP use showed no differences between exposed and unexposed workers.

Since the publication of our original review in 1985, several investigators have studied the long-term impact of DBCP on sperm counts and FSH levels. For example, Eaton et al. (17) carried out an assessment of members of the original cohort studied by Whorton et al. (105). Two of eight men who were azoospermic in the initial assessment produced sperm 5–8 years after termination of exposure. Among the men with depressed sperm counts, there was no increase in sperm production. Thus, for most of the affected men, there appeared to be no major changes in testicular function based on sperm counts. Similar results were reported for FSH; elevated serum FSH levels did not drop in oligospermic or azoospermic men (17).

Following the publication of these results, Lanham (51) presented preliminary data on follow-up of DBCP-exposed Dow Chemical workers. Lanham found that out of 26 azoospermic workers who were followed-up for 9 years, 19 had a return of sperm production and 15 of these had counts >20 million/mL. Out of a group of 17 workers who had been oligospermic (counts <20 million/mL) in their initial assessment, 14 who were followed-up all had counts >20 million. Among the workers who recovered sperm production, FSH levels returned to normal, except for three initially azoospermic workers who became ogliospermic. The workers who were still azoospermic at 9 years continued to have elevated FSH levels.

Schenker et al. (82) attributed the reported differences in recovery of testicular function in the two studies to differences between the cohorts in duration of DBCP exposure. The Dow Chemical workers had up to 18 months of exposure, while those studied by Eaton et al. (17) had exposures of up to 15 years.

Subsequently, Olsen et al. (69) presented detailed information on recovery of spermatogenesis among the Dow Chemical workers. Among the 19 azoospermic men who recovered sperm production, 13 achieved normospermic levels, although their counts were significantly lower (mean, 44.4 million/mL) than those among 17 formerly ogliospermic men who recovered to normospermic levels (mean, 88.8 million/mL). Interestingly, duration of exposure and categorization of exposure (high, moderate, or low) were not predictive of recovery, but job category was. Among those with spermatogenesis recovery, there was increased testicular size (testicular atrophy had been associated with azoospermia) and decreased FSH and LH levels. FSH levels were initially higher among the azoospermic men.

Whorton and Foliart (109) summarized the results of long-term follow-up of DBCP-affected men. Recovery of sperm production was found within 12–16 months from last exposure in most men diagnosed as ogliospermic. For azoospermic men, particularly those with elevated FSH levels, there is limited evidence for recovery of spermatogenesis.

Testicular Effects of DBCP in Animals

There has been considerable discussion regarding the fact that there was convincing animal evidence of the toxicity of DBCP to the testes well before the first workers presented with infertility (3,39,55,116). Although beyond the scope of this discussion, it should also be noted that carcinogenicity and mutagenicity of DBCP in animals have also been established (3,55).

Animal studies can play an important role in the identification of reproductive toxicants, but only if careful attention and evaluation are directed toward their results.

Summary

DBCP is a potent reproductive toxin to the human male, presumably by a direct effect on the spermatogonia and on the seminiferous tubules, resulting in the reduction of spermatogenesis. Presenting clinically as infertility, sperm analysis reveals a consistent pattern of azoospermia or oligospermia with a dose–response relationship. Following cessation of exposure, there is some tendency for a resumption of normal spermatogenesis, particularly in those individuals with oligospermia. The hormonal patterns in those with DBCP exposure and reduced sperm production are characterized by elevated levels of FSH, representative of tubular damage and of reduction in spermatogonia. The testicular biopsies performed show a deficit of spermatogenic cells, as would be expected given the results of sperm analyses and hormonal evaluations.

DBCP has been considered a prototypic agent against which other male reproductive toxicants can be compared. In addition, studies of DBCP have utilized multiple approaches for assessing the effects of chemicals on male reproduction. Just as thalidomide has become a model agent of drug teratogenesis, DBCP has become a model for male reproductive toxicity.

Ethylene Dibromide

Ethylene dibromide (EDB) has been used in the United States as a scavenger in leaded gasoline and as an active ingredient in a number of pesticides used as fumigants. The use of EDB was restricted in the 1980s because of a variety of concerns regarding its toxicity, including reproductive toxicity in males. A limited number of studies of male reproductive toxicity have been conducted, and EDB should be considered a reproductive toxicant for humans. We did not include EDB among the recognized toxicants to the testes in our original review but believe it needs to be recognized as such. Here we consider the results from three studies: (1) a fertility study in workers exposed to EDB in the production of pesticides (113), (2) a longitudinal study of short-term exposure among forestry pesticide applicators (84,83), and (3) a cross-sectional study of chronic exposure among papaya workers (76,83).

Wong and co-workers (113) evaluated reproductive performance in a cohort of workers from four EDB-manufacturing plants. Information on demographic variables and numbers of live births to the workers' wives was collected for 297 couples, using a standardized questionnaire. The number of expected births for workers at each plant was calculated using the numbers of person-years at risk of pregnancy and national tables of birth probabilities specific for age, parity, year, and race. The observed number of births was compared with the expected number. For one of the four plants, the observed number of births was significantly less than the expected number. When the four plants were combined, there were no significant differences between the observed births for the exposed workers and the expected number of births. The authors concluded that the data from one of the plants suggested that EDB had a negative impact on fertility and that the study had sufficient statistical power to detect a 20% decrease in fertility at the four plants, if such a reduction had been present.

In a longitudinal study of 10 EDB-exposed forestry workers (84), semen parameters prior to short-term high exposure were compared with those following exposure and with those of nonexposed workers. Sperm velocity decreased in all ten exposed workers, and semen volume was decreased in nine. These changes were statistically significant.

The final EDB study is a study of semen quality in papaya workers in Hawaii (76,83,84). The exposed group consisted of 46 men employed in papaya fumigation. The comparison group consisted of 43 men who worked in a sugar refinery and who had no EDB exposure. Multiple semen parameters were studied and regression models controlled for potential confounders. While there were no statistically significant differences in mean sperm concentration, a significantly higher proportion of exposed men had oligospermia (sperm count <20 million/mL). The effect of exposure on sperm count per ejaculate was highly statistically significant. There were also statistically significant differences in the percentages of viable sperm and motile sperm, with lower percentages in the exposed group. Finally, the exposed group had significantly higher rates of some types of morphologically abnormal sperm. There was limited evidence for an effect of duration of exposure on viability and motility. But there were no differences between workers who had potentially higher peak exposures than other workers in the exposed group.

These findings suggest a deleterious effect of EDB exposure on semen quality. They are also consistent with an effect of current EDB exposure rather than cumulative exposure. This is suggested to be due to the constant turnover of sperm production. Comparing the longitudinal study of forestry workers and the cross-sectional study of papaya workers indicates that longer-term EDB exposure resulted in effects on sperm motility and viability, suggesting that the short exposure may slow sperm velocity but longer exposures cause immotility and cell death (84).

Chlordecone

Chlordecone (Kepone) is a highly stable chlorinated hydrocarbon pesticide introduced in 1958 as an insecticide and fungicide (20). Its manufacture and use were terminated in the United States in 1977 because of its acute toxicity. A chronological history of chlordecone is developed in a review paper by Huff and Gerstner (34).

Three groups of workers had potential for occupational exposure to chlordecone: manufacturers, formulators, and applicators. Studies have focused on manufacturing facilities because of the high exposure levels. Studies of exposed manufacturing workers are reviewed by Epstein (20) and there is a clear pattern of clinical illness (eg, "Kepone shakes") associated with high levels of exposure.

Three clinical-epidemiologic studies include data on reproductive toxicity. All three of these studies were carried out on workers who had been employed at the Life Science Products Company in Hopewell, Virginia. Cannon et al. (8) studied a broad variety of clinical signs and symptoms, laboratory tests, and blood chlordecone levels among current and former workers and comparison groups. Totals of 33 current chlordecone workers and 100 former workers were studied and compared with family members, former employees of the Allied Chemical Corporation (the other United States firm that had manufactured chlordecone), and residents of Hopewell chosen randomly from among houses in stratified distances from the plant. Of interest here is the fact that the investigators reported that among the individuals with symptoms of the "Kepone shakes," sperm counts showed oligospermia, with a predominance of abnormal and nonmotile forms. No additional information relative to testicular toxicity was provided.

Taylor et al. (92) discussed clinical observations of chlordecone intoxication in humans, again based on study of the Hopewell workers. Their focus was on 23 workers with serum chlordecone levels of 2000 ng/mL or greater and chronic chlordecone intoxication. They reported that "in 13 patients, sperm specimens showed a substantial reduction in motility: in most of these the sperm count was less than expected" (92). These results were not further quantified. They also state that testicular biopsy in three patients revealed considerable reduction in spermatids, secondary spermatocytes, and spermatozoa. In their discussion, the authors make reference to "infertility reported by the workers," but no data are provided.

The third study with data relevant to reproductive toxicology is that of Cohn et al. (14) on the treatment of chlordecone poisoning. They studied a group of 32 former employees at the Hopewell plant who had symptoms of chlordecone poisoning and blood chlordecone levels >600 ng/mL. The authors examined sperm counts in relation to blood chlordecone levels and reported that in 19 of 20 subjects with levels >1000 ng/mL, the motile sperm count was <25 million/mL. In 21 subjects with blood chlordecone levels <1000 ng/mL, there were seven with sperm counts described as "abnormal," although abnormal was not defined. The difference in the proportions of abnormal sperm counts in the two exposure groups was statistically significant. In 12 of 13 subjects whose blood chlordecone levels decreased, the count of motile sperm increased. No detailed information on sperm counts or changes were provided by the authors. Barlow and Sullivan (4) interpreted the findings of Cohn et al. (14) to indicate that in the majority of cases recovery from oligospermia is to be expected following chlordecone poisoning. Relevant to this point is that, according to Epstein (20), testicular atrophy was not noted on clinical examination of the chlordecone-poisoned workers.

Finally, with regard to human studies, Guzellan (cited in ref. 34) reported that semen analyses of 14 workers exposed to chlordecone showed abnormal sperm morphology, decreased sperm motility, and oligospermia, allowing the conclusion that these patients were sterile. No additional information is available, and it is not clear what subjects are represented in this report.

In summary, the studies of male workers with high levels of exposure to chlordecone show that these individuals frequently have abnormalities in sperm count, morphology, and motility. In addition, there is evidence from one study (92) for histologic alterations of spermatogenesis. Of interest and importance, to our knowledge there are no published data on pregnancy outcome among the workers studied and no mention is made of reproductive history information in the questionnaires described by Cannon et al. (8). The human data suggest a direct effect of chlordecone on the testes. The reported alterations in spermatogenesis and the histologic evidence of altered germinal epithelium are compatible with such a toxic effect. We did not identify any more recent studies of reproductive effects of chlordecone than those discussed above from our original chapter.

Lead

The effects of lead on the reproductive system of the human male have not been studied as extensively as DBCP, although evidence of the deleterious effects of lead on human reproduction dates back to the ancient Roman and Greek civilizations (25). Most of the scientific literature considering the effects of lead on the reproductive system has dealt with the female, as heavy metals are known teratogens and abortifacients (30). There is historical evidence, however, that lead may decrease the fertility of exposed male workers and may effect the reproductive performance of their wives (78). Studies have shown both a reduction in the number of offspring in families of workers occupationally exposed to lead (9) and an increase in the miscarriage rate among women whose husbands were exposed (48).

Lancranjan et al. (48) studied 150 male workers at a lead storage battery plant. Workers were divided into four exposure groups: (1) 23 men with lead poisoning (mean blood lead, 74.5 µg/dL); (2) 42 men with moderately increased lead absorption (mean blood lead, 52.8 µg/dL); (3) 35 men with slightly increased lead absorption (mean blood lead, 41 µg/dL); and (4) a group of 50 men with "physiologic absorption" of lead. Semen analyses and endocrinologic analyses of 17-ketosteroids and total urinary gonadotropins were carried out on volunteers.

Semen analyses showed increased incidence of teratospermia, asthenospermia, and hypospermia among the workers in the three exposure groups. The incidence of teratospermia showed a dose–response relationship. Increased frequencies of asthenospermia, hypospermia, and teratospermia were associated with decreased fertility in the moderate and high lead-exposure groups. Of the lead-poisoned workers, 75% were hypofertile and 50% were infertile, on the basis of accepted criteria.

Studies failed to show any influence of lead absorption on androgen secretion. Similarly, tests for urinary gonadotropins did not reveal any differences between groups. The investigators interpreted these results as excluding an effect of lead on the hypothalamic–pituitary axis.

Lancranjan et al. (48) concluded that (1) increased lead absorption is associated with alterations in spermatogenesis leading to decreased fertility; (2) Leydig cell androgen production is not affected by exposure to lead; and (3) the observed effects of lead on spermatogenesis are produced by direct toxic effects on the testes and not through the hypothalamic–pituitary axis.

The findings of Lancranjan et al. (48) can be compared with those of Braunstein et al. (6) from a clinical study of a group of chronically lead-poisoned men. Six men were studied who had clinical lead-poisoning after 2–11 years of exposure to lead in a secondary lead smelter. All six reported decreased libido and frequency of intercourse. An additional four men with chronic lead exposure in the same smelter but without clinical lead poisoning were also studied. Three of these four reported some decrease in libido and frequency of intercourse. A control group consisted of nine volunteers of similar socioeconomic background.

For all individuals, measurements were made of blood and urine lead levels and of serum levels of testosterone, FSH, LH, estradiol, prolactin, and testosterone-binding globulin–binding activity. Semen samples were obtained on two separate days following a variable period of abstinence. The two most severely lead-poisoned men had testicular biopsies (6).

The blood lead levels of the lead-poisoned and lead-exposed men were significantly higher than those of the control group. The sperm counts in the lead-poisoned and lead-exposed groups ranged from normal to severely oligospermic. There were no significant differences among groups in the occurrence of morphologically abnormal sperm. Basal serum testosterone levels were significantly reduced in the lead-poisoned and lead-exposed groups. They had normal basal levels of FSH, LH, estradiol, and prolactin. Microscopic examination of the testicular tissue from the two lead-poisoned workers showed histologic changes indicative of peritubular fibrosis and oligospermia (6).

The authors (6) concluded that lead may affect the male reproductive system through both the hypothalamic–pituitary axis, resulting in abnormal LH secretary dynamics and, at the testis itself, in peritubular fibrosis and oligospermia. Since the lead-poisoned workers had been on chelation therapy with calcium ethylenediaminetetraacetic acid (EDTA), it is possible that some of the reproductive abnormalities noted were related to that treatment.

There are important differences between the findings of Lancrajan et al. (48) and Braunstein et al. (6). Although both studies reported depressed sperm counts, they differed in the presence of morphologically abnormal sperm. In addition, they differed in terms of whether there is an effect on androgen production and whether the hypothalamic–pituitary axis is affected. They tended to agree, however, regarding a direct effect of lead on the seminiferous tubules and on spermatogenesis.

Since the publication of our original review, several studies have considered the effects of male lead exposure on fertility and reproductive outcome, semen parameters, and endocrinologic status. We summarize these recent studies here. In addition, several reviews have considered the reproductive toxicity of lead in males (95,111,112).

With regard to fertility, Coste et al. (15) studied live births among a cohort of battery factory workers in France. Blood lead levels and work location were used to establish four exposure groups, one without lead-exposed jobs and three with jobs that involved lead exposure, with strata based on blood lead levels. The outcome of interest was infertility, defined by the nonoccurrence of live birth during one observed year. This study found no association between lead exposure and infertility after controlling for potential confounding. In this population, exposed subjects with blood lead levels >60 µg/dL had more live births, but the mean blood lead level among all exposed workers was relatively moderate (46.3 ± 15.2 µg/dL) and only 17% of the exposed person-years were in the higher category of lead absorption.

Gennart et al. (24) also studied fertility in lead battery factory workers. Their exposed cohort in Belgium was compared with a group of unexposed workers. The mean blood lead levels in their exposed workers was 46.3 ± 11.2 µg/dL, almost exactly the same as the mean in the French study by Coste et al. (15). Exposure was characterized by two dichotomous variables identifying the years of fertility of the exposed worker's wife before and after exposure.

Gennart et al. (24) found that the ratio of the observed birth rate to the age-standardized expected birth rate was significantly reduced in the lead workers during exposure, compared with the unexposed. Logistic regression analysis showed no significant differences between the groups prior to exposure. A statistically significant negative association between exposure and the probability of a live birth was found among the lead workers. Exposure intensity and duration were not found to be significantly associated with fertility, but there was a tendency toward a lower odds ratio with increasing duration of exposure.

The results of this study are compatible with suggestions that testicular toxicity can occur in lead-exposed workers without overt symptoms of lead poisoning. The findings stand in contrast with those of the study by Coste et al. (15), and Gennart et al. (24) suggest this may be due to differences in the populations studied or to low-level exposures in the nonexposed workers in the former study. Although blood lead levels were determined for the lead workers, they were not determined for the unexposed group. It is also noted that current blood lead levels may not be indicative of previous levels of exposure.

In additional to these recent studies of fertility in lead-exposed workers, there have been two studies that have examined reproductive outcomes: a study of spontaneous abortions (58) and a study of congenital malformations (79).

Lindbohm et al. (58) carried out a case-control study of spontaneous abortions in wives of men monitored for lead exposure. Lead exposure was determined from biological monitoring records for men in a number of industries in Finland. Spontaneous abortions (cases) and live births (controls) were identified from population registries. In an analysis based on estimated blood lead levels, there was no statistically significant risk of spontaneous abortion in the two highest exposure categories. When subjects were divided into two groups based on the time span between measurement and spermatogenesis, a significant risk of spontaneous abortion was observed in those women whose husbands had blood lead levels ≥ 1.5 µmol/L. The findings of this study suggest that there may be an association between paternal lead exposure and the risk of spontaneous abortion in their wives.

Sallmén et al. (79) carried out a case-control study on congenital malformations in a cohort of men in Finland who were monitored biologically for lead exposure. All types of malformations were studied, and among fathers of cases 37% (10 of 27) had blood lead levels >1.0 µmol/L, compared with 19% (11 of 57) of controls. While the resulting odds ratio was elevated, it did not reach statistical significance. The study was interpreted as providing limited support for the hypothesis that paternal lead exposure is associated with risk of congenital malformation (88). Important for our discussion here is the fact that if such an association should exist, it could represent male-mediated developmental toxicity in which the mechanism is transmission of an agent in the semen as opposed to alterations of the sperm themselves in the testes. This should also be kept in mind in considering potential associations between exposures of men to lead and reduced fertility, as assessed by time to pregnancy, number of live births, or risk of spontaneous abortions.

We are aware of two studies, published since our earlier review, that have examined sperm characteristics in lead-exposed men (2,53). Both of these studies support the findings of the effects of lead on semen parameters discussed earlier.

Assennato et al. (2) compared sperm counts in a small group of Italian battery workers, who were exposed to high airborne lead levels, with those of a group of cement workers. The cumulative frequency distribution of sperm counts among battery workers was significantly shifted downward. This was reflected in a 38% lower median sperm count in the lead workers and a 3-fold increase in the prevalence of oligospermia, defined as a sperm count of ≤ 20 million/mL. There were no significant differences between the groups in LH, FSH, or testosterone levels or in other endocrinologic variables. The authors interpret their findings of effects on semen characteristics in the absence of endocrinologic effects as suggesting a direct toxic effect of lead absorption on the testes.

Lerda (53) studied semen characteristics in a group of 38 workers in an Argentine battery factory. Workers were ranked into three groups, based on their blood lead levels. Sperm counts were significantly lower in all three of the exposed groups than in controls, and the frequencies of asthenospermia and teratospermia were significantly increased. Interestingly, there did not appear to be any associations between dose, as reflected in mean blood lead levels, and the effects on sperm.

As noted above, Assennato et al. (2) examined endocrine function in lead-exposed workers and did not show any significant effects, even though they did observe changes in sperm parameters. Other recent studies also examined endocrine function in lead-exposed workers but did not carry out semen analyses (23,61,67,77).

Rodamilans et al. (77) studied the effects of lead exposure on endocrine function in a group of 23 workers in the Spanish lead-smelting industry. The workers were stratified into three groups on the basis of years of lead exposure: (1) less than 1 year, (2) 1–5 years, and (3) more than 5 years. The controls consisted of a group of volunteers with no history of lead exposure and blood levels similar to those of the general population. The blood lead and zinc protoporphyrin levels of the exposed workers were significantly higher than those of the controls but were not significantly different among the exposure groups. The mean serum lead values in the three groups were in range of 66–76 µg/dL.

When endocrine levels were examined by exposure strata, there were significant differences between the strata with respect to their values compared with the controls. In the highest-exposure group, the serum testosterone level was significantly lower than in the controls, as was the free testosterone index. The serum LH level was significantly higher in the highest-exposure group, while the serum FSH levels were not significantly different. In the middle-exposure group, the free testosterone index was significantly lower, but there was no significant difference in the testosterone levels; LH was significantly higher and there was no difference in FSH. In the lowest-exposure group, there were no significant differences in the testosterone parameters, but the LH values were significantly higher.

The authors (77) interpret their findings as suggesting that the free testosterone index seems to be the best marker of endocrine testicular dysfunction in this population of lead workers. In all of the lead-exposed workers, there was an increase in LH levels. Since there was a significant reduction in serum testosterone only in the group with the longest duration of exposure, the authors suggest that long-term exposure leads to a reduction in testosterone synthesis that cannot be overcome by the hypothalamic–pituitary feedback mechanism. Their findings are interpreted as indicating that hypothalamic–pituitary–testicular axis dysfunction in workers with chronic lead exposure is due early on to direct testicular toxicity affecting testosterone synthesis. With additional periods of exposure, there is an additional toxic mechanism at the hypothalamic or pituitary level.

McGregor and Mason (61) assessed testicular endocrine function in 90 men who were current lead workers and compared them with a referent group with no known lead exposure. They found the mean LH levels to be significantly lower in the exposed group and the mean FSH levels were significantly higher than expected values. The increased FSH was significantly related to blood lead levels; the association was no longer significant when individuals with blood lead levels >47 µg/dL were removed. Multiple regression models suggested that blood lead influences FSH and that the number of years of exposure influenced LH. The subclinical increases in FSH levels observed support the hypothesis of lead-induced damage to the seminiferous tubules at moderate blood lead levels (>47 µg/dL). At these levels, there do not appear to be significant effects on testosterone levels or the free testosterone index.

Another study of endocrinologic effects of lead exposure is that conducted by Ng et al. (67) among lead workers and a comparison group in Singapore. Endocrine values were studied in 122 lead workers, who had a mean blood level of 35.1 µg/dL, and 49 controls. Compared with the nonexposed men, the lead workers had nonsignificantly lower testosterone levels and significantly raised concentrations of LH and FSH. Interestingly, reduced testosterone levels and normal LH concentrations (secondary hypogonadism) were observed in more of the exposed workers ($P=0.05$), and raised LH levels and normal testosterone concentrations (compensated hypogonadism) were significantly more common in the exposed group. FSH and LH concentrations were significantly increased when testosterone levels were normal in the group with less than 10 years of exposure, whereas the group with more than 10 years' exposure had significantly lower LH and FSH levels, comparable with those in the nonexposed. Testosterone, on the other hand, was significantly lower in the 10-year-plus exposure group, when compared with the nonexposed controls. The concentrations of LH and FSH appeared to show an increase with increasing blood lead levels, from 10 µg/dL reaching a peak with a plateau of about 40 µg/dL.

Ng et al. (67) note that raised LH and FSH levels are sensitive indicators of Leydig cell and Sertoli cell failure. Lead may influence testicular function by reducing the production of testosterone or by decreasing the sensitivity of the testes to gonadotropic effects of hormones, which leads in turn to compensatory increases in LH and FSH levels. As the authors point out, men exposed to lead for 10 or more years had low testosterone levels along with normal LH and FSH levels, suggesting a direct action of lead on the testes that leads to reduced testosterone levels. Ng et al. (67) conclude that moderate occupational exposure to lead is associated with small but measurable changes in endocrine function that reflect both primary and secondary effects on the testes and on the hypothalamic–pituitary–testicular axis.

The final study we want to discuss regarding endocrine function in lead-exposed workers in that of Gennart et al. (23), who studied a group of 98 battery factory workers in Belgium. They studied lead-exposed workers with a mean blood level of 51 µg/dL and compared them with 85 controls who did not have occupational lead exposures. The measures of endocrine function, including LH and FSH, did not correlate with lead exposure (blood lead level or duration of exposure) or show significantly different mean values between the exposed group and the controls. Importantly, this study did not evaluate testosterone levels, which have been shown in several of the studies discussed above (67,77) to be affected by lead exposure at relatively low blood levels and in the early stages following exposure. The authors (23) summarize their findings by noting that the lack of correlation between blood lead levels and serum levels of LH or FSH should be interpreted with caution. They suggest that the hypothalamic–pituitary axis may not be affected by moderate lead exposure. They note, however, that it is possible that the normal levels of LH and FSH observed result from an inhibition of the hypothalamic–pituitary axis to the effects of lead on the germinal cells themselves. Unfortunately, this study and the study of Ng et al. (67) did not include any assessment of semen to determine the relationship, or lack of same, between lead exposure, endocrine function, and sperm parameters.

Henderson et al. (33) present data from an unpublished study of 31 men exposed to inorganic lead in a Swedish battery factory. Workers were grouped on the basis of blood lead and zinc protoporphyrin levels. While no differences in sperm count or motility were observed, the investigators did report indications of effects on parameters related to the sperm maturation process, as well as on the prostate and seminal vesicles.

There have also been two reports of reproductive toxicity in groups of workers exposed to tetraethyl lead in gasoline (66,99). In both studies, there were complaints of reduced libido and impotence in men with reduced semen volume, sperm count, motility, and abnormal morphology. In the majority of those studied, urinary androgens were normal. On removal from exposure, potency soon returned, but the sperm counts remained low; there was inadequate follow-up to assess sperm recovery (4).

In summary, there is clear evidence for effects of lead on the male reproductive system, and the data suggest a direct effect on the seminiferous tubules and on spermatogenesis. Effects on gonadotropin or androgen production are less clear, but some studies suggest effects of moderate exposure. The recent epidemiologic studies, which have examined workers with recorded lead levels, have contributed importantly to understanding the reproductive toxicity of lead in the human male.

Carbon Disulfide

Carbon disulfide (CS_2) is primarily used in the production of viscose rayon, and exposure to CS_2 occurs not only in the preparation process but also during the spinning and washing of the viscose. The effects of chronic exposure to CS_2 on androgenic hormone secretion were first suggested by Italian studies, the results of which inspired epidemiologic studies conducted by Lancranjan and associates in 1969 (49) and by Lancranjan in 1972 (47).

In these two epidemiologic studies, semen analysis revealed reductions in sperm counts and altered sperm morphology in workers with occupational exposure to CS_2. In the first study (49), gonadal function was examined in a group of 33 young workers poisoned by CS_2, 31 of them suffering from a sensorimotor toxic polyneuritis. Clinical and endocrinologic examinations included urinary total gonadotropins (23 cases), total neutral 17-ketosteroids (32 cases), and examination of the seminal fluid (31 cases). The laboratory findings were compared with those obtained in controls of the same age. Sperm analysis revealed significantly increased asthenospermia, teratospermia, and hypospermia in the poisoned subjects. The elimination of total neutral 17-ketosteroids was significantly lower in patients than in controls. Urinary total gonadotropin excretion was below normal values in 20 out of the 23 patients studied. The authors suggest possible effects of CS_2 on the hypothalamus and on the testes directly.

In Lancranjan's 1972 study (47), 140 CS_2-exposed workers and 50 controls of the same age without exposure to organic solvents were examined. Workers with conditions potentially related to spermatogenic alterations were excluded. Semen analysis showed significantly increased hypofertility consisting of asthenospermia, hypospermia, and teratospermia in CS_2 workers compared with controls. The author concluded that the high frequency of alterations in spermatogenesis (78%) in patients with chronic CS_2 poisoning without any other cause of hypofertility shows the toxic effects of CS_2 on the testes. A correlation between altered spermatogenesis and the length of exposure was not proved. The author also followed up 18 patients with spermatogenic problems, and 3–30 months after removal from the toxic environment, 12 men (66%) had improved, three (17%) remained the same, and three (17%) showed progressive disorders in spermatogenesis. More specific information is not provided about the length of follow-up for the three patients who showed a deterioration in spermatogenesis.

An additional Italian study (10) of workers at a rayon production plant was undertaken to examine a possible causal relationship between occupational exposure to CS_2 and certain disorders or metabolic disturbances. A total of 308 workers was divided into seven CS_2-exposure groups, based on past and present exposure to CS_2. Thyroid function, sex hormones, and sexual behavior were evaluated. The authors concluded that (1) thyroxine levels were reduced in CS_2-exposed workers; (2) LH and FSH were significantly reduced in exposed subjects, whereas testosterone was not; and (3) sexual activity was significantly reduced in the exposed workers without any correlation with hormonal deficit. After discontinuing heavy exposure to CS_2, alterations of hormonal balance did not seem to persist; however, sexual activity remained reduced. The authors suggest that the primary action of CS_2 is on pituitary activity.

NIOSH undertook a comprehensive industrial hygiene and medical survey to evaluate a group of workers who had at least 1 year of CS_2 exposure and to compare them with unexposed controls from the same plant. Semen analysis was included to ascertain if the previous reports of impaired semen quality would be confirmed at the current exposure levels (62). For 86 CS_2-exposed workers and 89 control workers, there were no statistically significant differences in sperm count, morphology, or semen volume. Lack of significant differences remained when the control group was compared with the exposed group as a whole and with each individual exposure subgroup. The author concluded that the lack of significant differences between the control and the CS_2-exposed group was a reflection that CS_2 at its current exposure levels did not cause changes in the semen parameters. However, the low rate of participation (50%) in the semen evaluation opens the possibility that, had more workers participated, the results might have been different. Another concern is that there may have been differences introduced as a result of varying length of employment between the exposure groups; the control and other (non-CS_2) exposure groups had a much longer mean employment than the CS_2-exposed groups. Nonetheless, all workers had to have been employed for at least 12 months to participate in the study, and theoretically this should have been long enough to cause effects.

In a review paper, Schrag and Dixon (85) note that although the study by Meyer (62) was negative, data from other studies seem to support the inclusion of CS_2 among recognized male reproductive hazards. While we agree with this assessment, more recent data again raise questions about the strength of this association.

The issue of the effects of CS_2 on male reproductive function was addressed recently by a study of viscose-rayon workers in Belgium (96). A group of 116 exposed workers was compared with a group of 79 other workers (nonexposed men). A self-administered questionnaire was used to collect information on sexual behavior and reproduction. Semen samples were collected from 43 of the exposed and 35 of the nonexposed men. While there were no significant differences in impaired libido between the exposed the unexposed workers, subjects with high present exposure or with high cumulative exposure presented significantly more often with this complaint. The exposed men did report significantly more impotence. Significant associations were found between CS_2 exposure and decreased libido in adjusted multiple logistic regression analyses. No effects were noted on fertility or semen parameters. The only significant finding with regard to semen was an increase in the frequency of round cells in the nonexposed subjects. The authors note that their sample size is small and thus the statistical power to observe an effect is low, but their findings are consistent with those of Meyer (62).

Endocrinologic effects of CS_2 exposure were also studied in the Belgian viscose-rayon workers (97). There were no statistically significant differences between the exposed and unexposed workers in thyroxin, LH, FSH or testosterone levels. The median prolactin levels were found to be significantly lower in the exposed workers, but this disappeared following adjustment for potential confounders. The authors suggest that their findings could differ from the studies reporting positive endocrinologic findings because of differences in exposure levels, selection bias, or the presence of potential confounders.

In summary, the data on CS_2 exposure at high levels support the suggestion that this substance is toxic to the male reproductive system. Sperm analyses and hormonal evaluations indicate that effects on both the testis and the pituitary/hypothalamus may be involved. The studies showing no effect on sperm parameters or hormonal levels at low exposure levels indicate the possible importance of a threshold for reproductive toxicity associated with exposure to this substance.

Vinyl Chloride

Vinyl chloride monomer, also known as chloroethylene, is widely used in the plastics industry, in organic synthesis, and in the production of vinyl resins (4). One of the major uses is in the production of polyvinyl chloride. Exposure of workers to vinyl chloride has been associated with a distinctive tumor type, angiosarcoma of the liver, as well as with cancers of the brain, lung, and hematolymphopoietic system (35). It has also been shown to be a transplacental carcinogen in rats.

In 1976, Walker (101) presented evidence showing loss of libido in men exposed to high levels of vinyl chloride monomer. The study involved 37 men aged 26–59 years and employed for periods ranging from 9 months to 5.5 years in a plant where polyvinyl chloride was manufactured from vinyl chloride; of these men, 13 suffered from loss of libido. Earlier, Walker (100) described the men as suffering from impotence, but no further information was given. Because of other symptoms, it was not clear if the reported loss of libido or potency was a specific effect of vinyl chloride toxicity or related more to general effects of exposure (4).

The greatest interest in vinyl chloride as a reproductive toxin has grown out of studies that suggest an association between vinyl chloride–manufacturing plants and (1) increased rates of congenital malformations in the community (36) and

(2) increased rates of spontaneous abortions among wives of exposed workers (38). The first topic is beyond the scope of the current discussion and the interested reader is referred to several publications where this issue is examined (18,31,89,93). Here we consider the studies that suggest rates of spontaneous abortions are increased in wives of exposed workers.

Selikoff (cited in ref. 36) was apparently the first to observe an excess of stillbirths and miscarriages among wives of vinyl chloride monomer workers. Selikoff found a rates for miscarriages and stillbirths of 140/1,000 pregnancies in one plant in Georgia and 72/1,000 pregnancies in another. These rates were 2–4 times the rates for stillbirths and miscarriages registered in the state as a whole (36). As Barlow and Sullivan (4) noted, however, the ascertainment reliability for cases and for Georgia vital statistics data is unknown. Fetal deaths at all stages, particularly spontaneous abortions, are widely recognized to be underreported in vital statistics (32,86), and the rates reported by Selikoff are within the range of "normal" rates (87).

The most widely discussed evidence for an association between male reproductive performance and vinyl chloride exposure comes from a study by Infante et al. (38). Reproductive histories of 95 males exposed to vinyl chloride monomer during polymerization were compared with those of a 158-member control group. The control group included polyvinyl chloride fabrication workers with little vinyl chloride monomer exposure and rubber workers with no vinyl chloride monomer exposure. Rates of fetal deaths were compared between the study and control groups prior to and following exposure, and rates within the study group were compared before and after exposure. Following exposure, the rates in the study group were higher than those in the controls, whereas the reported rates prior to exposure were similar. There was a 2.5-fold increase in the age-adjusted fetal death rate in the study group following exposure. Mean paternal age at conception was similar for the study and control groups, but the majority of fetal deaths in the study group was from husbands younger than 30 years of age. It is possible that younger employees had higher vinyl chloride exposure, with the older employees being in more senior positions with less exposure (4).

A number of methodological issues have been raised regarding the study of Infante et al. (38), which reported an association between exposure of male workers to vinyl chloride and subsequent spontaneous abortions in their wives. It is beyond the scope of this discussion to evaluate these issues here, and the interested reader is referred to papers by Infante et al. (40), Buffler (7), Monson (64), Hatch et al. (31), and Clemmesen (11). It is our opinion that the data of Infante et al. are suggestive of an effect, but additional studies are required. It would be particularly useful if studies were to include sperm analyses and hormonal evaluations in an attempt to elucidate the possible mechanisms for male reproductive toxicity.

Perchloroethylene

Eskenazi et al. studied the effects of perchloroethylene (PCE) exposure on semen quality in dry-cleaning workers (22) and on reproductive outcomes of their wives (21). Exposure was based on PCE levels in expired air and an index of exposure based on job tasks in the 3 months preceding the semen analysis. Reproductive outcomes were also compared between dry-cleaning workers and laundry workers who did not have PCE exposure.

The sperm counts and proportions of motile sperm were not significantly related to exposure (22). While the average percentage of abnormally shaped sperm was similar for the two groups, the dry cleaners had a significantly higher proportion of round sperm than did the laundry workers. The laundry workers had significantly more narrow sperm. Dry cleaners did not have fewer motile sperm than laundry workers, but dose-related differences were observed in the patterns of their swimming paths, based on computer-assisted sperm analysis of videomicrographs. Infertility has been reported in men with mostly round-headed sperm, as such sperm lack an acrosome and are therefore unable to penetrate an ovum. It is not known what the potential implications may be for alterations in swimming patterns, but the findings do suggest some impact of PCE on sperm function (22).

Fertility among the wives of dry cleaners and laundry workers was also compared (21). The numbers of pregnancies, the rates of spontaneous abortion, and the standardized fertility ratios were similar between the two groups. Wives of dry cleaners were more than twice as likely to have a history of attempting to become pregnant for more than 12 months or to have sought care for infertility. A lower percentage of wives of dry cleaners became pregnant in their first and second cycles of unprotected intercourse than did the wives of laundry workers. The wives of dry cleaners had about half the per-cycle pregnancy rate of wives of laundry workers, but this difference was not statistically significant. The wives of the men with higher exposure scores also had somewhat lower fertility. It should be noted that the sample sizes were small in this study, and thus the statistical power to observe an effect(s) was low.

A unique aspect of the study by Eskenazi et al. (21) is that they examined the associations between length of time to conception and 17 semen parameters described in their other report (22). Only the number of ghost sperm and the number of double-headed sperm were related to time to conception. The issue of the effects of sperm parameters, other than motility and count, on fertility has not been studied well, and it is unclear what the impact of some of these on reproductive function may be.

Chloroprene

Chloroprene (2-chlorobuta-1,3-diene) is used as a monomer for the production of synthetic rubber and latexes. One of the major products is polychloroprene (Neoprene) (41). There are close structural similarities between chloroprene and vinyl chloride.

Evidence for an effect of chloroprene on male reproductive function comes from a review by Sanotskii (81). Adverse reproductive effects were observed in female workers, and women were removed from chloroprene production. A questionnaire was developed to study reproductive function in male workers and was administered to 143 exposed workers and 118 unexposed controls. No exposure levels were given, except to note that the concentration levels in air were "several times higher than the former maximum permissible concentration" (2 mg/m^3).

Sanotskii (81) revealed functional disturbances in spermatogenesis, referred to by Barlow and Sullivan (4) as decreased sperm motility, after 6–10 years working in chloroprene production. Morphologic disturbances were reported to be increased after 11 years of exposure. Infante et al. (41) refer to these data as showing "a reduction in the numbers and motility of sperm following occupational exposure to chloroprene." In addition, cases of spontaneous abortion occurred more than three times as frequently in the wives of chloroprene workers as in those of controls.

To our knowledge, the study reported by Sanotskii (81) is the only reproductive outcome study involving male workers. The NIOSH criteria document on chloroprene (68) refers to a study of French workers who manifested symptoms from overexposure. In this group were some individuals with sexual impotency, including reduced libido, and problems of sexual dynamics.

In summary, the available data suggest an effect of chloroprene on the male reproductive system. The animal studies, while equivocal, indicate that a direct toxic effect on the testes is a likely mechanism. It is clear that additional research is needed, and studies of reproductive outcome in rubber workers (64) may shed light on this issue. Infante (37) has also reviewed the available data on chloroprene and points out the need for additional studies.

Ethylene Glycol Ethers

The effects of exposure to ethylene glycol ethers on male reproduction were studied by Welch and colleagues (102,103). The first study (103) was based on semen analysis of shipyard painters and controls who were exposed to these substances, and the second study (102) calculated standardized fertility ratios for the two groups, based on reproductive history questionnaires.

Welch et al. (103) examine several indicators of reproductive toxicity among a group of 73 painters and 40 controls. Semen analyses were carried out, and FSH, LH, and testosterone levels in serum were evaluated. Workers' exposure to glycol ethers was verified by measuring urinary metabolites of 2-ethoxyethanol and 2-methoxyethanol. No quantitative exposure data were provided. While the exposed workers more frequently had low sperm densities ($\leq$20 million/mL) and oligospermia (per-ejaculate count $\leq$100 million/mL), neither of these differences were statistically significant. When workers were stratified on the basis of smoking status, the exposed nonsmokers had a marginally statistically significantly higher rate of oligospermia. In the exposed group, 5% of the workers were azoospermic, compared with an expected 1% based on population data. No differences were observed in hormonal values.

Examining reproductive history questionnaires, Welch and co-workers (102) did not observe any differences in standardized fertility rates for painters exposed to ethylene glycol ethers, when the expected numbers of births were based on either United States fertility tables or data from unexposed workers. Both painters and controls had a standardized fertility ratio >1, and there was no significant difference in the fertility of the two groups during the exposure period. Neither were there significant differences between the two groups when the subjects were married but not yet employed at the shipyard. This finding contrasts with the semen analyses discussed above that identified a significant difference in the rate of oligospermia between the nonsmoking control and exposed groups and a marginally significant difference in the sperm count between all painters and all controls.

Ratcliffe et al. (75) examined semen quality in foundry workers with specific exposures to 2-ethoxyethanol, compared with a group of men without glycol ether exposure. While no effect of exposure duration on semen quality was observed, there were some differences in semen parameters between the exposed and unexposed groups in this cross-sectional study. The average sperm count per ejaculate among the exposed workers was significantly lower than that of the unexposed workers (113 versus 154 million sperm/ejaculate). The mean sperm concentrations did not different significantly between the two groups, but the concentration was lower in the exposed group and the proportion of men with oligospermia (count ≤ 20 million/mL) was greater. The exposed workers had a significantly lower proportion of double-headed sperm and a significantly higher proportion of immature forms. Other semen parameters did not vary between the two groups. The authors note the limitation of the statistical power of their study to observe effects because of the small sample size. They interpret their findings as suggesting a potential effect of exposure to 2-ethoxyethanol on sperm counts (75).

Veulemans et al. (98) used a case-control design to study the possible associations between ethylene glycol ethers and sperm disorders. The approach they used was innovative in that they selected their cases and controls from first-time patients at a clinic for reproductive disorders and determined exposure on the basis of urinary metabolites of ethylene glycol ethers. Cases were men diagnosed as infertile or subfertile on the basis of semen analyses, and the controls were men who were considered to be of normal fertility based on the same assessment. The main metabolites of 2-methoxyethanol and 2-ethoxyethanol and their acetates were analyzed in urine specimens taken at the time of examination. While the metabolite methoxyacetic acid (MAA) was identified in the urine of only three subjects, urinary ethoxyacetic acid (EAA) was detected in 45 subjects. Importantly, 39 of these were cases and only six were controls, giving a highly significant odds ratio for exposure in the cases. In addition, a highly significant clustering of EAA cases was observed in the subcategories of azoospermia and severe oligospermia. Information was also collected on occupational histories, and, importantly, 42 of the EAA-positive subjects were in the same employment for at least 1 year prior to the examination, indicating the potential for long-term exposure and effects on spermatogenesis.

The authors (98) discuss a number of advantages to using a case-control design as opposed to a cross-sectional study. The availability of specific tests for metabolites of the common ethylene glycol ethers clearly offers an advantage over the methods used to determine exposures in most epidemiologic studies of occupational reproductive hazards. The only parallel approach with which we are familiar is the assessment of blood lead levels.

In summary, the studies reviewed are consistent in showing effects of glycol ethers, particularly 2-ethoxyethanol, on sperm counts. Since 2-ethoxyethanol is used in a wide variety of products and a large number of workers are potentially exposed (75), additional studies with quantitative exposure data are indicated. Veulemans et al. (98) make a strong argument for the effectiveness of case-control studies; we suggest that there appears to be a need for a large-scale prospective cohort study.

Anesthetic Gases

The first epidemiologic study to report an adverse effect of anesthetic gases on male reproduction was done by Askrog and Harvald in 1970 (see ref. 16). These authors reported a higher frequency of spontaneous abortions among women whose husbands worked as anesthesiologists. However, the authors compared obstetric histories before and after starting employment in anesthesia and did not control for maternal age as a possible confounder.

In 1974, the American Society of Anesthesiologists (ASA) conducted a national survey by mailing questionnaires to 49,585 exposed operating room personnel and 23,911 unexposed individuals as a comparison group (12). Of the 54.5% that responded to the survey, there was no increased risk of spontaneous abortion for the wives of exposed respondents, compared with the wives of unexposed respondents, but there was a significant increase (25%) in the incidence of congenital abnormalities for the wives of exposed male physician anesthetists, when compared with unexposed male physicians.

Shortly after the ASA survey, another epidemiologic survey was conducted of anesthetic health hazards among dentists (13). A mail questionnaire was sent to 4797 general dental practitioners and 2642 oral surgeons. The responses indicated that 20.2% of the general practitioners (377 of 1866 respondents) and 74.8% of the oral surgeons (1291 of 1727 respondents) had anesthetic exposures exceeding 3 hours per week. In a comparison of the health of individuals exposed and unexposed to inhalation anesthetics, there was a significant increase (78%) of spontaneous abortion in the spouses of exposed dentists.

A mail survey of 7949 male doctors in the United Kingdom was undertaken to determine whether there was a relation between operating room exposure and abnormalities in reproductive history (46). The results of this study showed that paternal exposure did not appear to influence the overall abortion rate, the frequency of major congenital abnormalities, or involuntary infertility. The frequency of minor congenital abnormalities in the children of exposed fathers was higher, 3.09% compared with 2.35% among the nonexposed. The authors conclude, however, that there may be reporting bias toward overreporting of minor birth defects; major problems are less susceptible to this bias.

In a prospective study of 46 male anesthesiologists (each with a minimum of 1 year of work in hospital operating rooms ventilated with modern gas-scavenging devices) and 26 control anesthesiology residents, semen samples were evaluated for differences between the anesthesiologists and residents at the beginning of their residency and then again 1 year later (114). Concentrations of sperm and percentages of sperm having abnormal head shapes were determined for each sample. No significant differences were found between anesthesiologists and beginning residents. Limiting the analyses to men with no confounding factors (eg, varicocele, recent illness, medications, heavy smoking, and frequent sauna use) did not change the results. Sperm concentration and morphology in the 13 residents without any confounding factors did not change significantly after 1 year of exposure to anesthetic gases. However, the group of men who had one or more confounding factors (excluding anesthetic gas exposure) showed significantly higher percentages of sperm abnormalities than did the group of men without such factors. These results suggest that limited exposure to anesthetic gases does not significantly affect sperm production, as indicated by changes in sperm concentration and morphology.

In summary, the effects of anesthetic gases on reproductive outcomes in exposed males are equivocal. The suggestions of increased rates of congenital malformations and spontaneous abortions should not be ignored; the absence of an observable effect on spermatogenesis leaves unresolved the question of the mechanisms of such an effect. The most logical assumption would be that anesthetic gases act as mutagens rather than reproductive toxicants, but this must be considered as conjecture.

CONCLUSION

The substances and studies reviewed clearly show the effects of some occupational and environmental chemicals on the testes and on male reproduction. Although the number of substances with such effects is limited, there is a need for additional studies of suspect chemicals.

Because of the growing concerns regarding the possible reproductive effects of occupational exposure to hazardous substances, particular attention should be paid to noninvasive methods of health surveillance. The collection of reproductive histories from workers can play an important role in identifying potential reproductive toxicants. Methods such as those developed by Levine and associates (56), which involve the routine collection of reproductive history in employee populations, need to be further developed and evaluated. There are a number of epidemiologic methods that can be used to examine suspected reproductive toxicants (89), and additional methodological approaches are being developed. The importance of sperm analyses in studies of male reproductive toxicity should be stressed.

In conclusion, additional attention needs to be paid to the possible adverse reproductive effects of exposure of males to occupational and environmental chemicals. It would be unfortunate if a situation similar to that surrounding DBCP was again first discovered by the affected workers discussing their inability to have the children they desire, rather than by astute clinicians, surveillance programs, or evidence from animal studies.

ACKNOWLEDGMENT

The author thanks Ms. Lila Hurwitz for aid in preparation of the manuscript.

REFERENCES

1. Alexander NJ. Male evaluation and semen analysis. *Clin Obstet Gynecol.* 1982;25:463–482.
2. Assennato G, Paci C, Baser ME, et al. Sperm count suppression without endocrine dysfunction in lead-exposed men. *Arch Environ Health.* 1987;42:124–127.
3. Babich H, Davis DL, Stotzky G. Dibromochloropropane (DBCP): a review. *Sci Total Environ.* 1981;17:207–221.
4. Barlow SM, Sullivan FM. *Reproductive Hazards of Industrial Chemicals.* New York, NY: Academic Press; 1982.
5. Biava CG, Smuckler EA, Whorton D. The testicular morphology of individuals exposed to dibromochloropropane. *Exp Mol Pathol.* 1987;29:448–458.
6. Braunstein GD, Cahlgren J, Loriaux DL. Hypogonadism in chronically lead-poisoned men. *Infertility.* 1987;1:33–51.
7. Buffler PA. Some problems involved in recognizing teratogens used in industry. *Contr Epidemiol Biostat.* 1979;1:118–137.
8. Cannon SB, Veazey Jr JM, Jackson RS, et al. Epidemic Kepone poisoning in chemical workers. *Am J Epidemiol.* 1978;107:529–537.
9. Chyzzer A. Des intoxications par le plomb se presentant dans le ceramique en Hungrie. *Chir Press (Budapest).* 1908;44:906–909.
10. Cirla AM, Bertazzi PA, Tomasini M, et al. Study of endocrinological functions and sexual behavior in carbon disulfide workers. *Med Lav.* 1978;69:118–129.
11. Clemmesen J. Mutagenicity and teratogenicity of vinyl chloride monomer (VCM): epidemiological evidence. *Mutat Res.* 1982;98:97–100.
12. Cohen EN, Brown BW, Bruce DL, et al. Occupational disease among operating room personnel: a national study. *Anesthesiology.* 1974;41:321–340.
13. Cohen EN, Brown Jr BW, Bruce DL, et al. A survey of anesthetic health hazards among dentists. *J Am Dent Assoc.* 1975;90:1291–1296.
14. Cohn WJ, Boylan JJ, Blanke RV, Fariss MW, Howell JR, Guzelian PS. Treatment of chlordecone (Kepone) toxicity with cholestyramine. *N Engl J Med.* 1978;298:243–248.
15. Coste J, Mandereau L, Pessione F, et al. Lead-exposed workmen and fertility: a cohort study on 354 subjects. *Eur J Epidemiol.* 1991;7:154–158.
16. Council on Environmental Quality. *Chemical Hazards to Reproduction.* Washington, DC: U.S. Government Printing Office; 1981.
17. Eaton M, Schenker M, Whorton MD, et al. Seven-year follow-up of workers exposed to 1,2-dibromo-3-chloropropane. *J Occup Med.* 1986;28:1145–1150.

18. Edmonds LD, Anderson CE, Flynt Jr JW, James LM. Congenital central nervous system malformations and vinyl chloride monomer exposure: a community study. *Teratology*. 1978;17:137–142.

19. Egnatz DG, Ott MG, Townsend JC, Olson RD, Johns DB. DBCP and testicular effects in chemical workers: an epidemiological survey in Midland, Michigan. *J Occup Med*. 1980;22:727–732.

20. Epstein SS. Kepone-hazard evaluation. *Sci Total Environ*. 1978;9:1–62.

21. Eskenazi B, Fenster L, Hudes M, et al. A study of the effect of perchloroethylene exposure on the reproductive outcomes of wives of dry-cleaning workers. *Am J Ind Med*. 1991;20:593–600.

22. Eskenazi B, Wyrobek AJ, Fenster L, et al. A study of the effect of perchloroethylene exposure on semen quality in dry cleaning workers. *Am J Ind Med*. 1991;20:575–591.

23. Gennart J-P, Bernard A, Lauwerys R. Assessment of thyroid, testes, kidney and autonomic nervous system function in lead-exposed workers. *Int Arch Occup Environ Health*. 1992;64:49–57.

24. Gennart J-P, Buchet J-P, Roels H, et al. Fertility of male workers exposed to cadmium, lead, or manganese. *Am J Epidemiol*. 1992;135:1208–1219.

25. Gilfillan SC. Lead poisoning and the fall of Rome. *J Occup Med*. 1965;7:53–60.

26. Girgis SM, Hafez ESE. Basic concepts in andrology. In: Hafez ESE, ed. *Human Reproduction: Conception and Contraception*. 2nd ed. Hagerstown, Md: Harper and Row; 1980:123–144.

27. Glass RL. RE: Sperm count depression in pesticide applicators exposed to dibromochloropropane. *Am J Epidemiol*. 1980;112:164–165.

28. Glass RI, Lyness RN, Mengle DC, Powell KE, Kahn E. Sperm count depression in pesticide applicators exposed to dibromochloropropane. *Am J Epidemiol*. 1979;109:346–351.

29. Goldsmith JR, Potashnik G, Israeli R. Reproductive outcomes in families of DBCP-exposed men. *Arch Environ Health*. 1984;39:85–89.

30. Hamilton A, Hardy HL, eds. Hereditary lead poisoning. In: *Industrial Toxicology*, third edition. Acton, Ma: Publishing Sciences Group; 1974.

31. Hatch M, Kline J, Stein Z. Power considerations in studies of reproductive effects of vinyl chloride and some structural analogs. *Environ Health Perspect*. 1981;41:195–201.

32. Hook EB. Incidence and prevalence as measures of the frequency of birth defects. *Am J Epidemiol*. 1982;116:743–747.

33. Henderson J, Baker HWG, Hanna PJ. Occupation-related male infertility: a review. *Clin Reprod Fertil*. 1986;4:87–106.

34. Huff JE, Gerstner HB. Kepone: a literature summary. *J Environ Pathol*. 1978;1:377–395.

35. IARC. *Monographs on the Evaluation of Carcinogenic Risks of Chemicals to Humans. Vol 19: Some Monomers, Plastics, and Synthetic Elastomers and Acrolein*. Lyon, France: International Association for Research on Cancer; 1979.

36. Infante PF. Oncogenic and mutagenic risks in communities with polyvinyl chloride production facilities. *Ann N Y Acad Sci*. 197;271:49–57.

37. Infante PF. Chloroprene: adverse effects on reproduction. In: Infante PF, Legator MS, eds. *Proceedings of a Workshop on Methodology for Assessing Reproductive Hazards in the Workplace*. Cincinnati, Ohio: NIOSH; 1980:87–101.

38. Infante PF, McMichael AJ, Wagoner, JK, Waxweiler RJ, Falk H. Genetic risks of vinyl chloride. *Lancet*. 1976;1:734–735.

39. Infante PF, Tsongas TA. Occupational reproductive hazards: necessary steps to prevention. *Am J Ind Med*. 1983;4:383–390.

40. Infante PF, Wagoner JK, Waxweiler RJ. Carcinogenic, mutagenic and teratogenic risks associated with vinyl chloride. *Mutat Res*. 1976;41:131–141.

41. Infante PF, Wagoner JK, Young RJ. Chloroprene: observations of carcinogenesis and mutagenesis. In: Hiatt HH, Watson JD, Winsten JA, eds. *Origins of Human Cancer. Book A: Incidence of Cancer in Humans*. Cold Spring Harbor, NY: Cold Spring Harbor Laboratory; 1977:205–217.

42. Kahn E, Whorton D. RE: Sperm count depression in pesticide applicators exposed to dibromochloropropane. *Am J Epidemiol*. 1980;112:161–164.

43. Kapp Jr RW, Picciano DJ, Jacobson CB. Y-Chromosomal nondisjunction in dibromochloropropane exposed workmen. *Mutat Res*. 1979;64:47–51.

44. Katz DF. Human sperm as biomarkers of toxic risk and reproductive health. *J NIH Res*. 1991;3:5:63–67.

45. Kharrazi M, Potashnik G, Goldsmith JR. Reproductive effects of dibromochloropropane. *Isr J Med Sci*. 1980;16:403–406.

46. Knill-Jones RP, Newnan BJ, Spence AA. Controlled survey of male anesthetists in the United Kingdom. *Lancet*. 1975;2:807–809.

47. Lancranjan I. Alterations of spermatic liquid in patients chronically poisoned by carbon disulfide. *Med Lav*. 1972;63:29–33.

48. Lancranjan I, Popescu HI, Gavanescu O, Klepsch I, Serbanescu M. Reproductive ability of workmen occupationally exposed to lead. *Arch Environ Health.* 1975;30:396–401.

49. Lancranjan I, Popescu HI, Klepsch I. Changes of the gonadic function in chronic carbon disulfide poisoning. *Med Lav.* 1969;60:566–571.

50. Landrigan PJ, Melius JM, Rosenberg MJ, Coye MJ, Binkin NJ. Reproductive hazards in the workplace: development of epidemiologic research. *Scand J Work Environ Health.* 1983;9-83–88.

51. Lanham JM. Nine-year follow-up of workers exposed to 1,2-dibromo-3-chloropropane. *J Occup Med.* 1987;488–489.

52. Lantz GD, Cunningham GR, Huckins C, Lipshultz LI. Recovery from severe oligospermia after exposure to dibromochloropropane. *Fertil Steril.* 1981:35:46–53.

53. Lerda D. Study of sperm characteristics in persons occupational exposed to lead. *Am J Ind Med.* 1992;22:567–571.

54. Lee IP. Effects of drugs and chemicals on male reproduction.In: Spira A, Jouannet P, eds. Facteurs de la fertilité humaine/Human Fertility Factors. *INSERM.* 1981;103:311–334.

55. Legator MS. Chronology of studies regarding toxicity of 1-2-dibromo-3-chloropropane. *Ann N Y Acad Sci.* 1979;329:331–338.

56. Levine RJ, Symons MJ, Balogh SA, Arndt DM, Kaswandik NT, Gentile JW. A method for monitoring the fertility of workers, 1: methods and pilot studies. *J Occup Med.* 1980;22:781–791.

57. Levine RJ, Symons MJ, Balogh SA, Milby TH, Whorton MD. A method for monitoring the fertility of workers, 2: validation of the method among workers exposed to dibromochloropropane. *J Occup Med.* 1981;23:183–188.

58. Lindbohm M-L, Sallmén M, Anttila A, Taskinen H, Hemminki K. Paternal occupational lead exposure and spontaneous abortion. *Scand J Work Environ Health.* 1991;17:95–103.

59. Lipshultz LI, Ross CE, Whorton D, Milby T, Smith R, Joyner RE. Dibromochloropropane and its effect on testicular function in man. *J Urol.* 1980;124:464–468.

60. Mattison DR. The mechanisms of action of reproductive toxins. *Am J Ind Med.* 1983;4:65–79.

61. McGregor AJ, Mason HJ. Chronic occupational lead exposure and testicular endodrine function. *Hum Exp Toxicol.* 1990;9:371–376.

62. Meyer CR. Semen quality in workers exposed to carbon disulfide compared to a control group from the same plant. *J Occup Med.* 1981;23:435–439.

63. Milby TH, Whorton D. Epidemiological assessment of occupationally related, chemically induced sperm count suppression. *J Occup Med.* 1980;22:77–82.

64. Monson RR. Occupational hazards and fetal deaths. In: Porter IH, Hook EB, eds. *Human Embryonic and Fetal Death.* New York, NY: Academic Press; 1980:159–174.

65. National Research Council. *Biologic Markers in Reproductive Toxicology.* Washington, DC: National Academy Press; 1989.

66. Neshkov NC. The influence of chronic intoxication of ethylated benzene on the spermatogenesis and sexual function of man. *Gig Tr Prof Zabol.* 1971;13:45–46.

67. Ng TP, Goh HH, Ng YL, et al. Male endocrine functions in workers with moderate exposure to lead. *Br J Ind Med.* 1991;48:485–491.

68. NIOSH. *Criteria for a Recommended Standard–Occupational Exposure to Chloroprene.* Rockville, Md: NIOSH; 1977.

69. Olsen GW, Lanham JM, Bodner KM, et al. Determinants of spermatogenesis recovery among workers exposed to 1,2-dibromo-3-chloropropane. *J Occup Med.* 1990;32:979–984.

70. Potashnik G, Ben-Aderet N, Israeli R, Yanai-Inbar I, Sober I. Suppressive effect of 1,2-dibromo-3-chloropropane on human spermatogenesis. *Fertil Steril.* 1978;30:444–447.

71. Potashnik G, Goldsmith J, Insler V. Dibromochloropropane-induced reduction of the sex-ratio in man. *Andrologia.* 1984;16:213–218.

72. Potashnik G, Phillip M. Lack of birth defects among offspring conceived during or after paternal exposure to dibromochloropropane (DBCP). *Andrologia.* 1988;20:90–94.

73. Potashnik G, Yanai-Inbar I. Dibromochloropropane (DBCP): an 8-year reevaluation of testicular function and reproductive performance. *Fertil Steril.* 1987;47:317–323.

74. Potashnik G, Yanai-Inbar I, Sacks MI, Israeli R. Effect of dibromochloropropane on human testicular function. *Isr J Med Sci.* 1979;15:438–442.

75. Ratcliffe JM, Schrader SM, Clapp DE, Halperin WE, Turner TW, Hornung RW. Semen quality in workers exposed to 2-ethoxyethanol. *Br J Ind Med.* 1989;46:399–406.

76. Ratcliffe JM, Schrader SM, Steenland K, et al. Semen quality in papaya workers with long term exposure to ethylene dibromide. *Br J Ind Med.* 1987;44:317–326.

77. Rodamilans M, Osaba MJM, To-Figueras J, et al. Lead toxicity on endocrine testicular function in an occupationally exposed population. *Hum Toxicol.* 1988;7:125–128.
78. Rom WH. Effects of lead on reproduction. In: Infante PF, Legator MS, eds. *Proceedings of a Workshop on Methodology for Assessing Reproductive Hazards in the Workplace.* Cincinnati, Ohio: NIOSH; 1980:33–43.
79. Sallmén M, Lindbohm M-L, Anttila A, et al. Paternal occupational lead exposure and congenital malformations. *J Epidemiol Community Health.* 1992;46:519–522.
80. Sandifer, SH, Wilkins RT, Loadholt CB, Lane LG, Eldridge JC. Spermatogenesis in agricultural workers exposed to dibromochloropropane. *Bull Environ Contam Toxicol.* 1979;23:2703–2710.
81. Sanotskii IV. Aspects of the toxicology of chloroprene: immediate and long-term effects. *Environ Health Perspect.* 1976;17:85–93.
82. Schenker MB, Samuels S, Eaton M. Nine-year follow-up of workers exposed to 1,2-dibromo-3-chloropropane: the authors reply. *J Occup Med.* 1987;29:488–489.
83. Schrader SM, Ratcliffe JM, Turner TW, Hornung RW. The use of new field methods of semen analysis in the study of occupational hazards to reproduction: the example of ethylene dibromide. *J Occup Med.* 1987;29:963–966.
84. Schrader SM, Turner TW, Ratcliffe JM. The effects of ethylene dibromide on semen quality: a comparison of short-term and chronic exposure. *Reprod Toxicol.* 1988;2:191–198.
85. Schrag SD, Dixon RL. Occupational exposures associated with male reproductive dysfunction. *Annu Rev Pharmacol Toxicol.* 1985;25:567–592.
86. Sever LE. RE: Incidence and prevalence as measures of the frequency of birth defects. *Am J Epidemiol.* 1983;118:608–609.
87. Sever LE. The state of the art and current issues regarding reproductive outcomes potentially associated with environment exposures: reduced fertility, reproductive wasteage, congenital malformations, and birth weight. Presented at the U.S. EPA Workshop on Reproductive and Developmental Epidemiology: Issues and Recommendations. Cincinnati, Ohio; 1989. US EPA 600/8-89/103.
88. Sever LE. Congenital malformations related to occupational reproductive hazards. *Occup Med.* 1994;9:471–494.
89. Sever LE, Hessol NA. Overall design consideration in male and female occupational reproductive studies. In: Lockey JE, Lemasters GK, Keye Jr WR, eds. *Reproduction: The New Frontier in Occupational and Environmental Health Research.* New York, NY: Alan R. Liss; 1984:15–47.
90. Sever LE, Hessol NA. Toxic effects of occupational and environmental chemicals on the testes. In: Thomas JA, Korach KS, McLachlan JH, eds. *Endocrine Toxicology.* New York, NY: Raven Press; 1985:211–248.
91. Steinberger E. Current status of studies concerned with evaluation of toxic effects of chemicals on the testes. *Environ Health Perspect.* 1981;38:29–33.
92. Taylor JR, Selhorst JB, Houff SA, Martinez AJ. Chlordecone intoxication in man, I: clinical observations. *Neurology.* 1978;28:626–630.
93. Theriault G, Iturra H, Gingras S. Evaluation of the association between birth defects and ambient vinyl chloride. *Teratology.* 1983;27:359–370.
94. Thrupp LA. Sterilization of workers from pesticide exposure: the causes and consequences of DBCP-induced damage in Costa Rica and beyond. *Int J Health Serv.* 1991;21:731–757.
95. Uzych L. Teratogenesis and mutanagenesis associated with the exposure of human males to lead: a review. *Yale J Biol Med.* 1985;58:9–17.
96. Vanhoorne M, Comhaire F, De Bacquer D. Epidemiological study of the effects of carbon disulfide on male sexuality and reproduction. *Arch Environ Health.* 1994;49:273–275.
97. Vanhoorne M, Vermeulen A, De Bacquer D. Epidemiological study of endocrinological effects of carbon disulfide. *Arch Environ Health.* 1993;48:370–375.
98. Veulemans H, Stenno O, Masschelein R, et al. Exposure to ethylene glycol ethers and spermatogenic disorders in man: a case-control study. *Br J Ind Med.* 1993;50:71–78.
99. Vudelja N, Farago F, Nikolic V, Vuckovic S. Clinical experience with intoxications of fuel containing lead-tetraethyl. *Folia Facult Med Universitas Comenianae.* 1967;5:133–138. (cited in reference 4)
100. Walker AE. A preliminary report of a vascular abnormality occurring in men engaged in the manufacture of vinyl chloride. *Br J Dermatol.* 1975;93:22–23.
101. Walker AE. Clinical aspects of vinyl chloride disease: skin. *Proc R Soc Med.* 1976;69:286–289.
102. Welch LS, Plotkin E, Schrader S. Indirect fertility analysis in painters exposed to ethylene glycol ethers: sensitivity and specificity. *Am J Ind Med.* 1991;20:229–240.

103. Welch LS, Schrader SM, Turner TW, Culler MR. Effects of exposure to ethylene glycol ethers on shipyard painters, II: male reproduction. *Am J Ind Med*. 1988;14:509–526.
104. Whorton D. Dibromochloropropane (DBCP). In: Infante PF, Legator MS, eds. *Proceedings of a Workshop on Methodology for Assessing Reproductive Hazards in the Workplace*. Cincinnati, Ohio: NIOSH; 1980:103–115.
105. Whorton D, Krauss RM, Marshall S, Milby TH. Infertility in male pesticide workers. *Lancet*. 1977;2:1259–1261.
106. Whorton D, Milby TH, Krauss RM, Stubbs HA. Testicular function in DBCP exposed pesticide workers. *J Occup Med*. 1979;21:161–166.
107. Whorton MD. The effects of the occupation on male reproductive function. In: Spira A, Jouannet P, eds. Facteurs de la fertilité humaine/Human Fertility Factors. *INSERM*. 1981;103:339–350.
108. Whorton MD. Male occupational reproductive hazards. *West J Med*. 1982;137:521–524.
109. Whorton D, Foliart D. DBCP: eleven years later. *Reprod Toxicol*. 1988;2:155–161.
110. Whorton MD, Milby TH. Recovery of testicular function among DBCP workers. *J Occup Med*. 1980;22:177–179.
111. Winder C. Reproductive and chromosomal effects of occupational exposure to lead in the male. *Reprod Toxicol*. 1989;3:221–233.
112. Winder C. Lead, reproduction and development. *Neurotoxicology*. 1993;14:303–318.
113. Wong O, Utidjian HMD, Karten VS. Retrospective evaluation of reproductive performance of workers exposed to ethylene dibromide (EDB). *J Occup Med*. 1979;21:98–102.
114. Wyrobek AJ, Brodsky J, Gordon L, Moore DH, Watchmaker G, Cohen EN. Sperm studies in anesthesiologists. *Anesthesiology*. 1981;55:527–532.
115. Wyrobek AJ, Gordon LA, Burkhart JG, et al. An evaluation of human sperm as indicators of chemically induced alterations of spermatogenic function. *Mutat Res*. 1983;115:73–148.
116. Yonay E. The nematode chronicles. *New West*. 1981; May:66-74, 144–153.

Subject Index